Mayo Clinic's Complete Guide for Family Physicians and Residents in Training

Mayo Clinic's Complete Guide for Family Physicians and Residents in Training

EDITOR

ROBERT L. BRATTON, M.D., WITH CONTRIBUTORS

Consultant, Department of Family Medicine
Mayo Clinic Jacksonville
Jacksonville, Florida

Assistant Professor of Family Medicine
Mayo Medical School
Rochester, Minnesota

McGraw-Hill
Health Professions Division

New York St. Louis San Francisco Auckland Bogotá Caracas Lisbon London Madrid Mexico City Milan Montreal New Delhi San Juan Singapore Sydney Tokyo Toronto

McGraw-Hill

A Division of The ***McGraw-Hill*** *Companies*

Mayo Clinic's Complete Guide for Family Physicians and Residents in Training

1234567890DOCDOC99

ISBN 0-07-134683-X

This book was set in Times New Roman by The PRD Group, Inc.
The editors were Martin Wonsiewicz and Steve Melvin.
The production supervisor was Richard Ruzycka.
The cover and text were designed by Joan O'Connor.
The index was prepared by Edwin Durban.

R.R. Donnelley and Sons, Inc., was printer and binder.

This book is printed on acid-free paper.

Cataloging-in-Production Data is on file for this title at the Library of Congress.

DEDICATED TO THE TENS
OF THOUSANDS OF HARDWORKING
FAMILY PHYSICIANS WHO PROVIDE
THE HIGHEST LEVEL
OF COMPASSIONATE AND
COMPREHENSIVE CARE
TO THEIR PATIENTS.

CONTENTS

CONTRIBUTORS

David C. Agerter, M.D.
Chair, Department of Family Medicine, Mayo Clinic and Mayo Foundation; Assistant Professor of Family Medicine, Mayo Medical School, Rochester, Minnesota

Sandra L. Argenio, M.D.
Residency Director and Consultant, Department of Family Medicine, Board of Governors, Mayo Clinic Jacksonville, Jacksonville, Florida; Assistant Professor of Family Medicine, Mayo Medical School, Rochester, Minnesota

Robert F. Avant, M.D.
Past Chair, Department of Family Medicine, Mayo Clinic and Mayo Foundation; former Professor of Family Medicine, Mayo Medical School, Rochester, Minnesota. Present address: Executive Director, American Board of Family Practice, 2228 Young Drive, Lexington, KY 40505.

John W. Bachman, M.D.
Consultant, Department of Family Medicine, Mayo Clinic and Mayo Foundation; Professor of Family Medicine, Parker D. Sanders and Isabella G. Sanders Professor of Primary Care, Mayo Medical School, Rochester, Minnesota

Gregory A. Bartel, M.D.
Consultant, Department of Family Medicine, Mayo Clinic and Mayo Foundation; Instructor in Family Medicine, Mayo Medical School, Rochester, Minnesota

Matthew E. Bernard, M.D.
Family Medicine Residency Program Director and Consultant, Kasson Mayo Family Practice Clinic, Kasson, Minnesota; Instructor in Family Medicine, Mayo Medical School, Rochester, Minnesota

Robert L. Bratton, M.D.
Consultant, Department of Family Medicine, Mayo Clinic Jacksonville, Jacksonville, Florida; Assistant Professor of Family Medicine, Mayo Medical School, Rochester, Minnesota

Harvey D. Cassidy, M.D.
Chair, Department of Family Medicine, Mayo Clinic Jacksonville, Jacksonville, Florida; Assistant Professor of Family Medicine, Mayo Medical School, Rochester, Minnesota

Benjamin W. Chaska, M.D.
Former Consultant, Department of Family Medicine, Mayo Clinic Jacksonville, Jacksonville, Florida; Former Assistant Professor of Family Medicine, Mayo Medical School, Rochester, Minnesota

Francis X. DeCandis, M.D.
Consultant, Department of Family

Medicine, Mayo Clinic Jacksonville, Jacksonville, Florida; Instructor in Family Medicine, Mayo Medical School, Rochester, Minnesota

Frederick D. Edwards, M.D.
Consultant and past Chair, Department of Family Medicine, Mayo Clinic Scottsdale, Scottsdale, Arizona; Assistant Professor of Family Medicine, Mayo Medical School, Rochester, Minnesota

Ted Epperly, M.D., Col. USA
Immediate Past President, Uniformed Services Academy of Family Physicians; Chief, Department of Family and Community Medicine, Eisenhower Army Medical Center, Fort Gordon, Georgia

Robert G. Fish, M.D.
Consultant, Kasson Mayo Family Practice Clinic, Kasson, Minnesota; Instructor in Family Medicine, Mayo Medical School, Rochester, Minnesota

Walter B. Franz III, M.D.
Consultant, Department of Family Medicine, Mayo Clinic and Mayo Foundation; Assistant Professor of Family Medicine, Mayo Medical School, Rochester, Minnesota

Joseph W. Furst, M.D.
Consultant, Department of Family Medicine, Mayo Clinic and Mayo Foundation; Instructor in Family Medicine, Mayo Medical School, Rochester, Minnesota

Michele A. Hanson, M.D.
Consultant, Department of Family Medicine, Mayo Clinic and Mayo Foundation; Instructor in Family Medicine, Mayo Medical School, Rochester, Minnesota

Lori Heim, M.D., LTC. USAF
President, Uniformed Services Academy of Family Physicians; Assistant Professor of Family Medicine, Uniformed Services University of the Health Sciences, Bethesda, Maryland

James R. Keene, D.O.
Senior Resident, Department of Family Medicine, Mayo Clinic and Mayo Foundation, Rochester, Minnesota

Jan M. Larson, M.D.
Senior Associate Consultant, Department of Family Medicine, Mayo Clinic Jacksonville, Jacksonville, Florida

Rhonda M. Medows, M.D.
Consultant, Department of Family Medicine, Mayo Clinic Jacksonville, Jacksonville, Florida; Instructor in Family Medicine, Mayo Medical School, Rochester, Minnesota

Robert E. Nesse, M.D.
Consultant, Kasson Mayo Family Practice Clinic and Clinical Practice Vice Chair for Managed Care Operations, Mayo Clinic and Mayo Foundation; Vice Chair, Board of Governors, Mayo Clinic Rochester, Associate Professor of Family Medicine, Mayo Medical School, Rochester, Minnesota

William J. O'Brien, M.D.
Consultant, Department of Family Medicine, Mayo Clinic Scottsdale, Scottsdale, Arizona; Instructor in Family Medicine, Mayo Medical School, Rochester, Minnesota

R. John Presutti, D.O.
Associate Residency Director and Senior Associate Consultant, Department of Family Medicine, Mayo Clinic Jacksonville, Jacksonville, Florida; Instructor in Family Medicine, Mayo Medical School, Rochester, Minnesota

Jerry W. Sayre, M.D.
Senior Associate Consultant, Department of Family Medicine, Mayo Clinic Jacksonville, Jacksonville, Florida

Mark S. Schwartz, Ph.D.
Chair, Section of Psychology, Mayo Clinic Jacksonville, Jacksonville,

Florida; Associate Professor of Psychology, Mayo Medical School, Rochester, Minnesota

Ruel W. Scott, M.D.
Chief Resident, Department of Family Medicine, Mayo Clinic Jacksonville, Jacksonville, Florida

Robert D. Sheeler, M.D.
Consultant and Clinical Practice Chair, Department of Family Medicine, Mayo Clinic and Mayo Foundation; Assistant Professor of Family Medicine, Mayo Medical School, Rochester, Minnesota

Walter C. Taylor III, M.D.
Consultant, Department of Family Medicine, Mayo Clinic Jacksonville, Jacksonville, Florida; Assistant Professor of Family Medicine, Mayo Medical School, Rochester, Minnesota

Susan L. Wickes, M.D.
Consultant, Department of Family Medicine, Mayo Clinic Scottsdale, Scottsdale, Arizona; Assistant Professor of Family Medicine, Mayo Medical School, Rochester, Minnesota

Susan S. Wilder, M.D.
Senior Associate Consultant, Department of Family Medicine and Family Practice Residency Program Director, Mayo Clinic Scottsdale, Scottsdale, Arizona; Assistant Professor of Family Medicine, Mayo Medical School, Rochester, Minnesota.

John M. Wilkinson, M.D.
Consultant, Department of Family Medicine, Mayo Clinic and Mayo Foundation; Assistant Professor of Family Medicine, Mayo Medical School, Rochester, Minnesota

Floyd B. Willis, M.D.
Consultant, Department of Family Medicine, Mayo Clinic Jacksonville, Jacksonville, Florida; Instructor in Family Medicine, Mayo Medical School, Rochester, Minnesota

Halina Woroncow, M.D.
Consultant, Kasson Mayo Family Practice Clinic, Kasson, Minnesota; Instructor in Family Medicine, Mayo Medical School, Rochester, Minnesota

MAYO FAMILY MEDICINE ALUMNI, MAYO FAMILY MEDICINE CURRENT RESIDENTS, MAYO CLINICS CURRENT PHYSICIAN STAFFS

Mayo Family Medicine Alumni

Rochester

1981	Richard L. Bartsh, M.D.	Jeffrey K. Polzin, M.D.
	Walter B. Franz III, M.D.	John M. Wilkinson, M.D.
1982	David C. Agerter, M.D.	Gary W. Dausman, M.D.
	Bruce D. Cooper, M.D.	Matthew J. Puffer, M.D.
1983	Bradley C. Eichhorst, M.D.	Teresa B. Jensen, M.D.
	James E. Gaede, M.D.	
1984	John B. De Keyser, M.D.	David F. Hogness, M.D.
	Frederick D. Edwards, M.D.	Susan L. Wickes, M.D.
1985	Gregory L. Angstman, M.D.	Mark S. Mellstrom, M.D.
	Craig W. Clanton, M.D.	Julianne Thompson, M.D.
	Martin A. Kanne, M.D.	
1986	Thomas B. Cariveau, M.D.	Robert G. Fish, M.D.
	Benjamin W. Chaska, M.D.	Jeffrey A. Indrelie, M.D.
1987	Steven C. Adamson, M.D.	Jeffrey A. Luerding, M.D.
	Steven D. Hagedorn, M.D.	Cheri L. Olson, M.D.
	Laurie J. Lindor, M.D.	Joseph F. Rinowski, M.D.
1988	Michele A. Hanson, M.D.	Kenneth J. Liesen, M.D.
	Mark S. Hench, M.D.	Daniel G. Pesch, M.D.
	Timothy J. Johnson, M.D.	Carol Simmons (Mitchell), M.D.

1989	Kurt B. Angstman, M.D. Christian D. Herter, M.D. Mary J. Loken, M.D.	James P. Siepmann, M.D. Floyd B. Willis, M.D.
1990	Janet R. Albers, M.D. Jack V. Carlisle, M.D. Jay D. Myers, M.D.	Deborah A. Sailler, M.D. Julie K. Van Beek, M.D. Wade C. Wernecke, M.D.
1991	Frank A. Bock, D.O. Michael L. Bristow, D.O. Tammy R. Ellingsen, M.D.	Annie M. Kontos, M.D. Scott D. Pauley, M.D. Robert F. Reed, M.D.
1992	Paul M. Altrichter, M.D. Nancy N. Fazekas, M.D. David A. Handley, M.D.	Gail G. Knops, M.D. Juan P. Leyva, M.D. Michael L. Rohrenbach, D.O.
1993	Timothy C. Bachenberg, M.D. Matthew E. Bernard, M.D. Robert L. Bratton, M.D.	Gregory B. Mc Callum, M.D. David P. Weismantel, M.D. Halina Woroncow, M.D.
1994	Wendy S. Bartanen, M.D. Thomas J. Chapa, M.D. Robert T. Flinchbaugh, D.O. Vicki L. Jacobsen, M.D.	Bonnie J. Morrill, M.D. Sandhya Pruthi, M.D. Lynda Christine Sisson, M.D. David Wender, D.O.
1995	Anthony F. Chou, M.D. Carlos A. Frias, M.D. Anne Marie Kramlinger, M.D.	Jennifer Horn-Ommen, M.D. Martin F. Waldron, M.D.
1996	Suzanne Blake (Weinrich), D.O. Marites C. Buenafe, M.D. Jon Bylander, M.D. Margaret C. Gill, M.D. Jennifer C. Kaufman, M.D.	Monica Myklebust, M.D. David Nill, M.D. Angela E. O'Neil, M.D. Lori L. Wischnack, M.D.
1997	Vincent Akimoto, M.D. Lori A. Bates, M.D. Lonnie W. Berger, M.D. Victoria J. Hagstrom, M.D.	Kyle J. Kircher, M.D. Michael C. Liu, M.D. James A. Storlie, M.D. Gregory T. Sweat, M.D.
1998	David J. Heine, M.D. James R. Keene, D.O. Sarah L. Ludington, M.D. Michelle Olson, M.D. Emily Onello, M.D.	Parita Patel, M.D. David Vande Merwe, M.D. Jo T. VanWinter, M.D. Todd Wade, M.D. Richard Wehseler, M.D.
1999	Darryl E. Barnes, M.D. Thomas A. Billings, D.O. David H. Haase, M.D. Laura J. Johnston, M.D. Lynn K. Kelley, M.D.	Yale Y. Liang, M.D. Margret K. Rydell, M.D. Todd K. Sommer, D.O. Alice R. Suchomel, M.D. Bosheng Yang, M.D.

Mayo Family Medicine Current Residents Rochester

2000	Robert P. Bonacci, M.D. Jennifer Hartman, M.D.	Julie A. VanEck, M.D. Richard Wells, D.O.

	Susan E. Romanik, M.D.	Victor P. Yapuncich, M.D.
	Grant W. Tarbox, D.O.	
2001	Gregory E. Baker, M.D.	Paula Knapp-Baker, D.O.
	Jennifer J. Boelter, M.D.	Shannon J. Kowal, D.O.
	Mariana Diangiolo, M.D.	John M. Murphy, M.D.
	Gregory M. Garrison, M.D.	Gregory G. Santoscoy, M.D.
	Sharon M. Hammond, M.D.	Ruth J. Tiffault, D.O.
2002	Philip Aponte, M.D.	James W. Ott, M.D.
	Russell Bergum, D.O.	Laura I. Pelaez, M.D.
	Kevin Coleman, D.O.	Anne M. Rutledge, M.D.
	Nima Desai, M.D.	Rohini Singh, M.D.

Mayo Clinic Rochester Department of Family Medicine Current Physician Staff

Steven C. Adamson, M.D.
David C. Agerter, M.D.
Paul Altrichter, M.D.
Gregory J. Anderson, M.D.
Gregory L. Angstman, M.D.
John W. Bachman, M.D.
Gregory A. Bartel, M.D.
Lori A. Bates, M.D.
Matthew E. Bernard, M.D.
Thomas A. Billings, D.O.
Marites C. Buenafe, M.D.
John B. Collins, M.D.
Robert G. Fish, M.D.
Robert T. Flinchbaugh, D.O.
Walter B. Franz III, M.D.
Joseph W. Furst, M.D.
Margaret C. Gill, M.D.
Steven D. Hagedorn, M.D.
Michele A. Hanson, M.D.
Wade P. Hanson, M.D.
Thomas R. Harman, M.D.
Jennifer Horn-Ommen, M.D.
Margaret S. Houston, M.D.
Vicki Jacobsen, M.D.
Michael W. Justice, M.D.
Kyle J. Kircher, M.D.
Anne Marie Kramlinger, M.D.
Robert E. Nesse, M.D.
Angela E. O'Neil, M.D.
Scott D. Pauley, M.D.
Matthew J. Puffer, M.D.
Norman H. Rasmussen, M.D.
Robert D. Sheeler, M.D.
Gregory T. Sweat, M.D.
Eugenia S. Walsh, M.D.
John M. Wilkinson, M.D.
Halina Woroncow, M.D.

Mayo Family Medicine Alumni
Jacksonville

1997	Patricia Amadio, M.D.	Dalia McCoy, M.D.
	Dario Beltran, M.D.	R. John Presutti, D.O.
	Maria I. Lowney, D.O.	David Scheiner, D.O.
1998	Janet V. Attlesey, M.D.	Izabella Z. Riffe, M.D.
	Elizabeth Bozeman, M.D.	Marc W. Thorpe, M.D.
	John D. Pennington, M.D.	Margarita Vendrell, M.D.
1999	Kim Barbel-Johnson, D.O.	Paul F. Roberts, M.D.
	Reuben H. McBrayer, M.D.	Ruel W. Scott, M.D.
	Eduardo Peña Dolhun, M.D.	Thomas A. Waller, M.D.

Mayo Family Medicine Current Residents
Jacksonville

2000	Todd M. Brinker, M.D.	John E. Monnier, M.D.
	Kimberly A. Goodemote, M.D.	Michael B. Mueller, D.O.
	James N. Johnson, M.D.	Martin M. Pinto, M.D.
2001	Kevin S. Adams, M.D.	Antoinette S. Gonzaga, M.D.
	Charles S. Bibbs, M.D.	Daniel P. Montero, M.D.
	Stephanie B. Garrison, M.D.	Clayton M. Ramsue, M.D.
2002	Courtney C. Badour, D.O.	K. Dawson Jackson, Jr., M.D.
	Mary Ann Borgman, M.D.	Mark A. Novas, M.D.
	Amber C. Isley, M.D.	

Mayo Clinic Jacksonville Department of Family Medicine Current Physician Staff

Sandra L. Argenio, M.D.	John D. Pennington, M.D.
Robert L. Bratton, M.D.	R. John Presutti, D.O.
Harvey D. Cassidy, M.D.	Izabela Z. Riffe, M.D.
Francis X. DeCandis, M.D.	Jerry W. Sayre, M.D.
Brian H. Grimard, M.D.	Walter C. Taylor, M.D.
Jan M. Larson, M.D.	Marc W. Thorpe, M.D.
Reuben H. McBrayer, M.D.	Thomas A. Waller, M.D.
Rhonda M. Medows, M.D.	Floyd B. Willis, M.D.

Mayo Family Medicine Alumni
Scottsdale

1998	James Armstrong, M.D.	Richard Fleming, M.D.
	Katayoun Baniriah, D.O.	Timothy Locknane, M.D.
1999	Hollis A. Burggraf, M.D.	J. Warren Willey, D.O.
	Sarah K. Rieves, M.D.	Michael A. Woo-Ming, M.D.
	Dennis Swearingen, M.D.	Andrew L. Wright, M.D.

Mayo Family Medicine Current Residents
Scottsdale

2000	Jennifer W. Boyden, M.D.	Carolyn C. Moats, M.D.
	Stacy J. Clark, D.O.	John W. Whiteside, M.D.
	Andrea L. Darby-Stewart, M.D.	Alice J. Lively, D.O.
2001	Jon L. Belsher, M.D.	Blair A. Nelson, M.D.
	David Galbreath, M.D.	Charles S. Peterson, M.D.
	Mark A. Kropf, M.D.	Robert D. Segal, M.D.

2002

Ryan Abraham, M.D.
Dean Earp, M.D.
Angel Gomez, M.D.
Molly Kresin, D.O.
Laurie Pozun, D.O.
Iris Sadowsky, D.O.

Mayo Clinic Scottsdale Department of Family Medicine Current Physician Staff

Charles E. Basye, M.D.
Frederick D. Edwards, M.D.
D. Scott Endsley, M.D.
Keith A. Frey, M.D.
Michael J. Hovan, M.D.
Jay D. Meyers, M.D.
William J. O'Brien, M.D.
Cathleen J. Smith, M.D.
Wade C. Wernecke, M.D.
Susan L. Wickes, M.D.
Susan S. Wilder, M.D.

PREFACE

The specialty of Family Practice is as diverse as the physicians who make up its membership. This book is a collaborative effort on the part of Mayo Clinic Jacksonville, Rochester, and Scottsdale to describe the specialty of Family Practice to those who may have interest in the field. The book's purpose is to provide a reference that describes in a comprehensive manner most aspects of the specialty. This information will be helpful to medical students during their family practice rotations or to those deciding on specialty training and considering Family Practice. The book may be used as a resource for family practice residents in training and those who have graduated and are currently in practice. Although no one source can be exhaustive in describing our complex field, this text provides a major reference for those who are interested in the specialty.

As editor of this first edition, I thank all the contributors who helped make this text possible. Their hard work and diligence allowed us to produce this valuable reference.

ACKNOWLEDGMENTS

Special thanks to Ms. Andrea Holcombe, Ms. Shannon Richardson, and Ms. Carol Saville who helped with the preparation of this book. Without their diligent efforts, this text would not have been accomplished.

The editor would also like to thank Dr. Carol Kornblith, Mrs. Roberta Schwartz, Mrs. Dianne Kemp, and Mrs. Dorothy Tienter and the rest of the Mayo Clinic Section of Scientific Publications who played such an important role in the preparation of this book.

Finally the editor would like to thank Mr. Marty Wonsiewicz and the McGraw-Hill staff for their support, commitment, and expertise in developing and publishing this project.

Mayo Clinic's Complete Guide for Family Physicians and Residents in Training

1

INTRODUCTION

Robert L. Bratton, M.D.

The *Mayo Clinic's Complete Guide for Family Physicians and Residents in Training* is a coordinated effort by the Departments of Family Medicine at Mayo Clinic, Rochester, Minnesota; Jacksonville, Florida; and Scottsdale, Arizona. As one of the largest departments of Family Medicine in the United States, the "parent department" located in Rochester served as a model for the development of the other Family Medicine departments at the satellite clinics as the need for primary care became obvious to the Mayo Clinic, one of the most subspecialized clinics in the world. Despite its relatively short existence, the specialty of Family Practice is now the second largest specialty and the leader in the delivery of primary care. The purpose of this guide is to explain the evolving field of family medicine and to give helpful and enlightening information to medical students interested in the field of family medicine, family medicine residents who are currently serving in their respective residency programs, or family physicians in practice.

Unlike any other book of its kind, this guide will provide practical advice for performing well on rotations, what to expect once you have graduated from a residency program, and general information for surviving during one of the most challenging and sometimes grueling 3 years a family physician may have to endure. There are many references that provide clinical and scientific material necessary to graduate from medical school and residency training. This guide takes a different approach aimed at the individual physician or resident physician and focuses on what this person can expect and how to survive the labors of residency training and being in family practice.

Although most of us have survived the 4 years of medical school and have muddled through the myriad of facts and details of patient care, many have not received the basic tools necessary to survive during residency and as a family physician in practice. This book is filled with general information gathered from multiple sources and will provide the resident and physician in practice with the confidence and knowledge to perform to the best of their abilities.

As family physicians, we are all unique and come from many different backgrounds. In the future, many of us will be faced with distinctly different practice settings. But above all, we are part of a family of physicians that believes in the same values and quality of care administered to our patients. As described by the American Academy of Family Physicians,

> the specialty of Family Practice is the medical specialty which provides continuing and comprehensive health care for the individual and the family. It is the specialty in breadth which integrates the biological, clinical, and behavioral sciences. The scope of family practice encompasses all ages, both sexes, each organ system and every disease entity. Family practice is the continuing and current expression of the historical medical practitioner and is uniquely defined within the family context.[1]

These principles form the cornerstones of every family physician's practice.

To fully understand the specialty of Family Practice, one must know how the specialty evolved. Knowledge of the trials and tribulations, scrutiny, resistance, and finally acceptance and now respect the family physician enjoys within the medical profession is imperative and paramount to establishing a well-rounded education within the field of Family Medicine. One quickly

General Internal Medicine	Pediatrics	OB/GYN	Psychiatry	Orthopedics, ENT, Gastroenterology, etc.

FIGURE 1-1 Comparison of the body of knowledge of other specialties with that of family practice (striped area). ENT, ear, nose, and throat; OB/GYN, obstetrics and gynecology.

realizes the roots of family practice run deep and are anchored by the public's demand for a physician who provides comprehensive, cost-effective, continuing, and compassionate care.

Often mislabeled as "the jack of all trades and the master of none," the public and medical community are realizing that the family physician is a precious commodity our medical system cannot do without. In fact, we may be the only specialty that is capable of saving our impersonal, costly, and inadequate current medical system. As family physicians, we have repeatedly shown that there is a body of knowledge that our specialty *has* mastered, and it represents the most important aspect of medical care to our patients.

> *"Medicine can be used only as people are educated to its accomplishments."*
>
> —Charles H. Mayo

Critics often boast that the family physician is incapable of learning all the information that is available to medical care providers. In response to this frequent remark, I point out that the field of Family Medicine contains the same amount of learned information as any other specialty. We, as family physicians, are more focused on the presenting symptoms and signs and initial management of patients' problems, whereas the specialist has a narrower focus of knowledge but more depth with respect to atypical presentations or extended or experimental treatments. The body of knowledge remains equal for all physicians (Fig. 1-1). It is true that family physicians cannot master all aspects of medicine, but we can master the body of information that makes up primary care, just as any other specialists can master their own field.

In addition, the family practice "specialist" is able to adequately treat 90% to 95% of all problems that patients present with in the office. In fact, in support of this statement the U.S. Agency for Health Care Policy and Research reports that fewer than 5% of patients presenting to family physicians are referred to specialists.[2] This is evidence that the well-trained family physician has the knowledge and expertise to manage most medical problems.

In describing the specialty of Family Practice, many terms may come to mind. From thoughts of the television character, Marcus Welby, M.D., to the memory of Norman Rockwell's painting of the family physician (Fig. 1-2), we each have our own vision of the "family doctor." The compassion, the genuine interest, and the never-ending commitment over time to the patient's needs come to mind. In many circles, the care provided by family physicians often is referred to as the 4As:

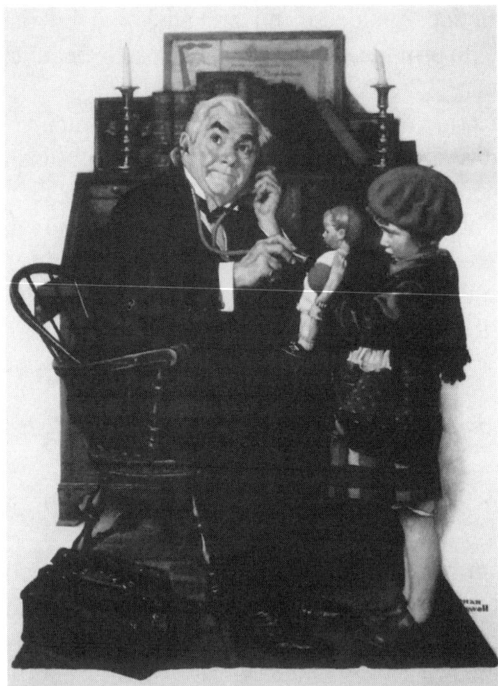

FIGURE 1-2
In describing the family physician, many images come to mind. Norman Rockwell provided this traditional painting in 1929. (By permission of the Norman Rockwell Family Trust. Copyright 1998.)

*A*ffordable

*A*vailable

*A*ffable

*A*ll encompassing

The care provided by family physicians has also been described by the 5 Cs:

*C*ontinuity of care

*C*omprehensive care

*C*oordinated care

*C*are of the patient in the family *c*ontext

Health *c*are in the *c*ommunity *c*ontext[3]

These are hallmark qualities of the practicing family physician and represent the traits the public expects in a primary physician (Box 1-1).

As time has passed, we have witnessed the increased demand for family physicians in our ever-changing medical environment. Salaries have in-

BOX 1-1 ATTRIBUTES OF THE FAMILY PHYSICIAN

The following characteristics are certainly desirable for all physicians, but they are of greatest importance for the physician in family practice:

1. A strong sense of responsibility for the total, ongoing care of the individual and the family during health, illness, and rehabilitation.
2. Compassion and empathy, with a sincere interest in the patient and the family.
3. A curious and constantly inquisitive attitude.
4. Enthusiasm for the undifferentiated medical problem and its resolution.
5. An interest in the broad spectrum of clinical medicine.
6. The ability to deal comfortably with multiple problems occurring simultaneously in one patient.
7. A desire for frequent and varied intellectual and technical challenges.
8. The ability to support children during growth and development and during their adjustment to family and society.
9. The ability to assist patients in coping with everyday problems and in maintaining stability in the family and community.
10. The capacity to act as coordinator of all health resources needed in the care of a patient.
11. A continuing enthusiasm for learning and for the satisfaction that comes from maintaining current medical knowledge through continuing medical education.
12. The ability to maintain composure in times of stress and to respond quickly with logic, effectiveness, and compassion.
13. A desire to identify problems at the earliest possible stage (or to prevent disease entirely).
14. A strong wish to maintain maximum patient satisfaction, recognizing the need for continuing patient rapport.
15. The skills necessary to manage chronic illness and to ensure maximal rehabilitation following acute illness.
16. An appreciation for the complex mix of physical, emotional, and social elements in holistic and personalized patient care.
17. A feeling of personal satisfaction derived from intimate relationships with patients that naturally develop over long periods of continuous care, as opposed to the short-term pleasures gained from treating episodic illnesses.
18. A skill for and commitment to educating patients and families about disease processes and the principles of good health.

The ideal family physician is an explorer, driven by a persistent curiosity and the desire to know more. He is part theologian, as was Paracelsus; part politician, as was Benjamin Rush; and part humorist, as was Oliver Wendell Holmes. At all times, however, the care of the patient—the whole patient—is the primary goal.

From Rakel RE (ed): Textbook of Family Practice, 5th ed. Philadelphia, WB Saunders Company, 1995, p 6. By permission of the publisher.

creased significantly as the government and insurance companies have increased reimbursement for family physicians. Job opportunities have skyrocketed as more and more communities, health plans, and individuals have sought the care and expertise of family physicians. Fortunately for the specialty of Family Practice, this may be just the tip of the iceberg.

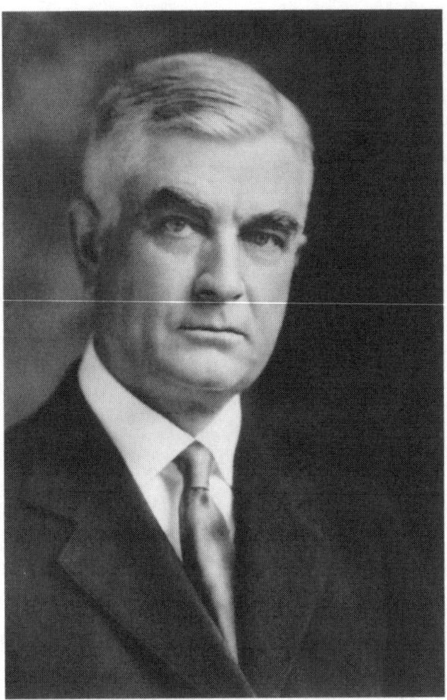

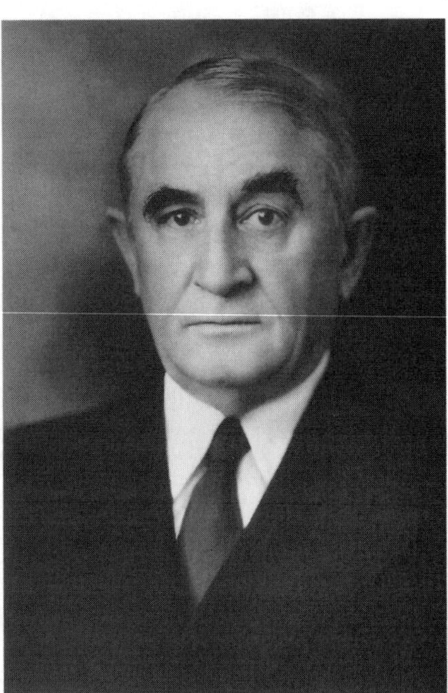

W. J. Mayo C. H. Mayo

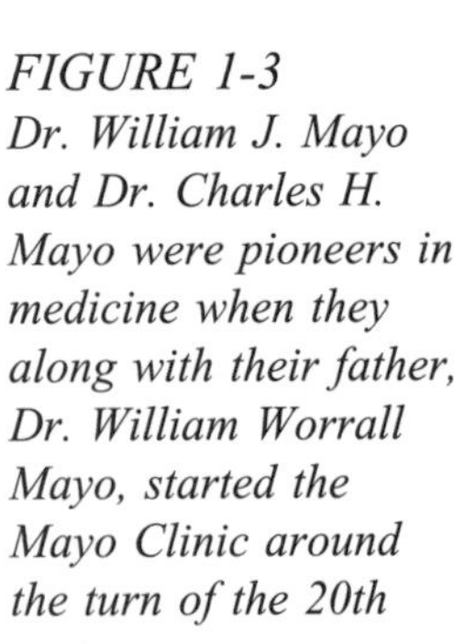

FIGURE 1-3
Dr. William J. Mayo and Dr. Charles H. Mayo were pioneers in medicine when they along with their father, Dr. William Worrall Mayo, started the Mayo Clinic around the turn of the 20th century.

As we approach a new millennium, the field of Family Medicine will be changing constantly to meet the needs of our patients, but the foundation of the specialty is firmly set in the principles that have made the specialty unique. These we must never forget. As these changes do occur we must always look to the future but never forget the past—and in the end always do what is right for our patients. As Dr. William J. Mayo (Fig. 1-3) once stated many years ago, ''I look through a half-opened door into the future, full of interest, intriguing beyond my power to describe, but with a full understanding that it is for each generation to solve its own problems and that no man has the wisdom to guide or control the next generation.''[4] With this statement in mind, the specialty of Family Practice, as a body of dedicated physicians working together for the good of their patients, has been charged with the task of correcting much of what is wrong with our current health care system.

REFERENCES

1. American Academy of Family Physicians: Congress adopts revised definitions concerning family physician. Congress Reporter Oct 5–7:4, 1993

2. Gaus CR, Clancy CM: From the Agency for Health Care Policy and Research: research at the interface of primary and specialty care. JAMA 274:1419, 1995
3. Taylor RB: Family medicine principles: current expressions. In Family Medicine: Principles and Practice. 4th ed. Edited by RB Taylor, AK David, TA Johnson, Jr, DM Phillips, JE Scherger. New York, Springer-Verlag, 1994, p 1
4. Mayo WJ: Seventieth birthday anniversary. Ann Surg 94:799, 1931

2

HISTORY OF THE SPECIALTY OF FAMILY PRACTICE

Robert L. Bratton, M.D.

It is much more important to know what sort of patient has a disease than what sort of disease a patient has.

—Sir William Osler, *Aequanimitas: With Other Addresses to Medical Students, Nurses and Practitioners of Medicine*

The roots of family practice run deep and are anchored in the deepest, most fertile soil of medicine. Perhaps the first reference to family practice was made by Hippocrates (Fig. 2-1) when he wrote, ''It is necessary for the physician to provide not only the needed treatment, but to provide for the patient himself, and those beside him, and for his outside affairs.''[1] It is clear from this statement that Hippocrates realized the importance not only of the disease process but also of viewing the patient as a whole in the setting of the patient's own surroundings, where many factors and influences may affect the patient's well-being. This is a hallmark principle of the specialty of Family Practice.

In more recent times—at the turn of the century—it was not hard to find a general practitioner (Fig. 2-2). In most cases, these physicians were highly respected by those in their communities and fondly referred to as ''family doc.'' However, as medicine advanced and increasingly became based on scientific theory, more and more physicians chose to specialize in different areas of medicine, which were much more narrow in scope and practice.

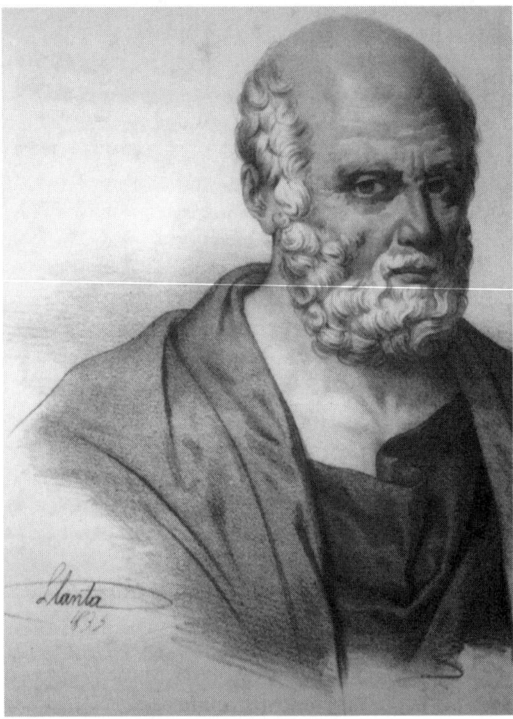

FIGURE 2-1
Hippocrates' beliefs were consistent with the current principles of Family Medicine. (From Yale University, Harvey Cushing/John Hay Whitney Medical Library. By permission.)

"In the study of some apparently new problems we often make progress by reading the work of the great men of the past. . . ."

—Charles H. Mayo

FLEXNER REPORT

In 1910, the status of medical training was poor. A study led by Dr. Abraham Flexner (known as the Flexner Report and funded by the Carnegie Foundation) found medical training was marginal at best. The report cited inadequate faculty training and low standards for medical teaching. Only 5 schools (led by Johns Hopkins University) of the 155 American and Canadian schools examined received approval. After this controversial and enlightening report, a revolution took place in medical education that was funded by more than 600 million dollars donated by wealthy American philanthropists.[1] After the emergence of superior medical schools, most graduates practiced general

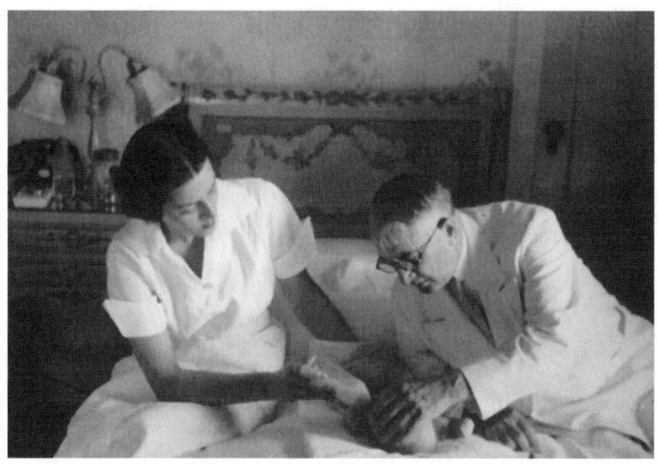

FIGURE 2-2
In many respects the Mayo brothers and their father were family physicians who cared for their patients in a comprehensive, continuous, and compassionate fashion.

medicine, providing various services, including general surgery, obstetrics, pediatrics, and outpatient primary medicine. In fact, in 1930, 80 percent of American physicians were "general practitioners" and only 20 percent considered themselves "specialists."

DECLINE OF GENERAL PRACTICE

In the years that followed the improvement of medical training centers, the specialization of medicine started to emerge. The face of medicine began to change drastically at an alarming pace. With more and more training programs providing additional specialty training, physicians gravitated to more select fields of medicine.

By 1940, experts had commented that the swing of the pendulum toward specialization had reached its peak and that modern medicine had fragmented the health care delivery system to too great a degree. In the years that followed, general practice continued to decline.

In addition, World War II also added to the explosion of specialized care and saw further decline of general practice. Physicians received military exemption if they chose to go into structured residency programs that focused on certain fields of medicine, whereas the field of general practice had no residency training programs to offer medical school graduates. Furthermore, specialists were given higher rank and, therefore, higher salary, leaving the general practitioner dodging bullets on the front lines. At the end of World War II in 1945, the GI bill paid stipends for medical school and up to 4 years of residency training, thus furthering the specialization of medicine.[1]

As the specialty fields grew, the general practitioner almost disappeared. Specialists were more highly respected, earned more money, and worked fewer hours than their colleagues in general practice. In addition, there were no structured residency programs after medical school other than a 1-year internship for those in general practice. Because of this and the rapidly growing field of medicine, most specialists viewed those in general practice as receiving inferior training.

AMERICAN ACADEMY OF GENERAL PRACTICE

In view of these vast changes in medicine and the deterioration of the field of general practice, a few leaders in general practice began advocating for a new specialty for general practitioners. On June 10, 1947, in Atlantic City, New Jersey, a group of about 200 general practitioners formed the American Academy of General Practice, a predecessor to the American Academy of Family Physicians. Although the group floundered in its early years, there remained a core of physicians dedicated to general practice, which grew into the specialty of Family Practice.

> *''Probably the most interesting period of medicine has been that of the last few decades. So rapid has been this advance, as new knowledge developed, that the truth of each year was necessarily modified by new evidence, making the truth an ever-changing factor.''*
>
> —Charles H. Mayo

During the 1950s and the early 1960s, the field of general practice was hidden in obscurity. The general public sought fragmented care from various specialists without calling one physician their family doctor. Despite these changes in public attitudes and demand, there remained a group of general practitioners who envisioned a new specialty that would incorporate the values of the old family doctor who cared for patients ''from the womb to the grave.'' It was this small group, led by such prominent physicians as Dr. Nicholas Pisacano and others (see Table 2-1 and Box 2-1), that continued to fight for a new specialty—the specialty of Family Practice.

REBIRTH OF FAMILY PRACTICE

The year 1966 represented a milestone for the development of family practice. During this year several important declarations emerged supporting the con-

TABLE 2-1
AMERICAN BOARD OF FAMILY PRACTICE
FOUNDING BOARD (1969)

Amos N. Johnson, M.D.	Malcom E. Phelps, M.D.
Herman E. Drill, M.D.	Carroll L. Witten, M.D.
Thomas E. Rardin, M.D.	Vernon L. Wilson, M.D.
Lester D. Bibler, M.D.	Nicholas J. Pisacano, M.D.
Francis L. Land, M.D.	George E. Burket, Jr., M.D.
William J. Shaw, Sr., M.D.	I. Phillips Frohman, M.D.
Arthur D. Nelson, M.D.	John G. Walsh, M.D.

cept of a specialty devoted to ''general'' or, as it became known, ''family practice.''

1 The National Commission on Community Health Services, established by the American Public Health Association and the National Health Council, issued a report (called the Folsom Report, or the Harvard Report) asserting, ''Every individual should have a personal physician who is the central point for integration and continuity of all medical . . . services to his patient. Such a physician will emphasize the practice of preventive medicine. . . . He will be aware of the many and varied social, emotional and environmental factors that influence the health of his patient and his patient's family. . . . His concern will be for the patient as a whole, and his relationship with the patient must be a continuing one.''
2 The Citizens Commission on Graduate Medical Education (the Millis Commission) . . . [established by the American Medical Association issued a report that] called for a physician who ''focuses not upon individual organs and systems but upon the whole man [or woman], who lives in a complex social setting, and . . . knows that diagnosis or treatment of a part often overlooks major causative factors and therapeutic opportunities.''
3 The Ad Hoc Committee on Education for Family Practice ([also known as] the Willard Committee), appointed by the AMA Council on Medical Education, stated that the American public ''does want and need a large number of well-qualified family physicians.'' It further recommended that training should include extensive experiences simulating a family-oriented medical practice—a drastic change from the hospital-based training of other specialties. (From Stanard.[1] By permission of the American Academy of Family Physicians and the author.)

BOX 2-1 Dr. Nicholas J. Pisacano (JUNE 6, 1924–MARCH 11, 1990)

The late Dr. Nicholas J. Pisacano was a Renaissance man (Fig. 2-3). Recognized as one of the founders of the specialty of family practice, Dr. Pisacano believed in the comprehensive, compassionate, and continuing care of the patient, even when the field of medicine was emerging as a subspecialized albatross that focused on a patient's specific organ or physiologic system. Dr. Pisacano realized the public's need for a generalist approach to medical care.

> The time has come when we must act to save medicine as a profession. We not only owe it to ourselves and to the youngsters who follow us, but primarily to the public who needs a revered profession. We . . . [must] *reconsecrate* ourselves to those ancient and cherished values of caring and giving. . . . We must enforce continuing competence and proficiency, but, above all, we must *rededicate* ourselves to public service. We should embrace superspecialism and high technology only as they contribute to the welfare of human beings. . . . We welcome and support scientific inquiry and new technology, but we must maintain a healthy balance of those advances with humanism. . . . Let us not be drawn into mediocrity. . . . Let us show the people we hold high the staff of Aesculapius and that we can, and will, care for all who enter the health system with equal concern and *caritas*. . . . These proposals . . . are not foolish dreams. . . . If we act to *reconsecrate* ourselves as physicians, think of the good that would be accomplished; think of what the public's image of us would be—but most important, think of how you would feel—Doctor!

Relentless in his efforts, Dr. Pisacano and others fought diligently for years against much resistance from the medical community to establish the specialty of family practice. In 1969, Dr. Pisacano realized his dream when the American Board of Family Practice was approved as the 20th medical specialty.

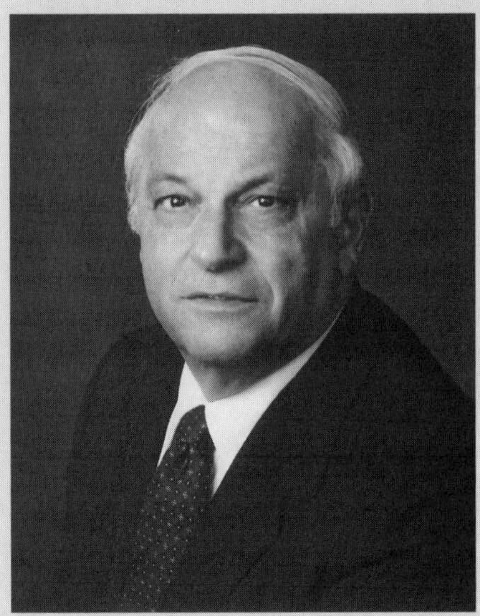

FIGURE 2-3
Dr. Nicholas J. Pisacano was instrumental in the development of the American Board of Family Practice. The Pisacano Memorial Foundation was founded in his honor and awards scholarships to deserving students interested in the field of Family Medicine. (By permission of the American Board of Family Practice.)

BOX 2-1 Continued

Born in Philadelphia, Pennsylvania, Dr. Pisacano was the first executive director for the American Board of Family Practice and led the board in its early years through tumultuous times without compromising the ideals of family practice. For years Dr. Pisacano taught basic biology to undergraduate students at the University of Kentucky—refusing pay and receiving the teacher of the year award in 1965. Dr. Pisacano firmly believed a family physician should have a broad liberal arts education to relate better to patients. In the 1970s and 1980s, he championed the idea of continuing medical education and led the American Board of Family Practice in establishing a certification examination that had to be successfully completed before one received Board certification and a recertification process that had to be successfully completed every 7 years to maintain Board certification.

At the time of his unexpected death in 1990, the specialty of family practice had emerged as the leader in the delivery of primary care. As a tribute to his life of dedicated service to the specialty of family practice, the Nicholas J. Pisacano, M.D., Memorial Foundation was established. This foundation awards scholarships on a yearly basis to outstanding medical students and residents who have shown an interest in family practice. As stated by Eric Crall, M.D., Pisacano scholarship recipient 1993, ''The Pisacano Scholars Award is much more than the distinction that it obviously represents. It is a challenge to shun mediocrity, to hold compassion for all who seek our care, and to strive always for development of our interpersonal skills in addition to our medical knowledge.'' The following is a list of past Pisacano Scholarship recipients.

Pisacano Scholar Alumni

Gaynell S. Anderson, M.D. Univ. Oklahoma (96)/Residency – Wichita, KS, Shawnee, OK

Kirk Bollinger, M.D. Utah (95)/Residency – Casper, WY, Cody, WY

Kara Cadwallader, M.D. UC – San Francisco (95)/Residency – Tacoma, WA, Seattle, WA

Cheng-Chieh Chuang, M.D. Yale (95)/ Residency – Pawtucket, RI, Locum Tenens

Eric Crall, M.D. Emory (94)/Residency – St. Petersburg, FL, St. Petersburg, FL

Dineen Greer, M.D. UC –San Francisco (95)/ Residency – Seattle, WA, Seattle, WA

Kenneth Grimm, M.D. Penn (94)/Residency – Ann Arbor, MI, Dearborn, MI

Jerome Hotchkiss, M.D. Med. Coll. of VA (95)/ Residency – Seattle, WA, Seattle, WA

Penny Jeffery, M.D. Iowa (95)/Residency – Iowa City, IA, Wichita, KS

Seth Koss, M.D. Univ. of Pennsylvania (96)/ Residency – Philadelphia, PA, Valley Center, CA

Kurt Lindberg, M.D. Univ. of Michigan (96)/ Residency – Beverly, MA, Holland, MI

Linda M. C. Lou, M.D. Washington (95)/ Residency – Seattle, WA, Locum Tenens

Thomas McGorey, M.D. Loyola (95)/Residency – Waukesha, WI, Watertown, WI

Trish Palmer, M.D. Rush (95)/Residency – Berwyn, IL, Salt Lake City, UT

Katrina Posta, M.D. UCLA (95)/Residency – Santa Monica, CA, Santa Monica, CA

Jamie Reedy, M.D. UMDNJ-RWJ (95)/ Residency – New Brunswick, NJ, Piscataway, NJ

Sarita Sharma Salzberg, M.D. Ohio State (95)/ Residency – Columbus, OH, Columbus, OH

James Schieberl, M.D. UC – San Diego (95)/ Residency – Sacramento, CA, Woodland, CA

Barbara Troupin, M.D. Penn (95)/Residency – San Diego, CA, Locum Tenens

David Turner, M.D. Dartmouth/Brown (95)/ Residency – Tacoma, WA, Tacoma, WA

BOX 2-1 Continued

Current Pisacano Scholars

Randi Berg, M.D. Wisconsin (96) Resident – Asheville, NC
Erika Bliss. UC – San Diego 4th year
Leslie Brott. Univ. of Texas – San Antonio 4th year
Stephen Cook, M.D. UC – San Francisco (97) Resident – Tacoma, WA
Christine Dehlendorf. Univ. of Washington 3rd year
Jennifer DeVoe, M.D. Harvard (99) Rhodes Scholar – London
Marguerite Duane. SUNY – Stony Brook 4th year
Jill Endres, M.D. Iowa (97) Resident – Winston Salem, NC
Filomeno Gonzalez Univ. of Texas Galveston 3rd year
English [Hairrell]-Gonzalez. Univ. of Alabama – Birmingham (99) Resident – Washington, D.C.
David Hutcheson-Tipton, M.D. Colorado (97) Resident – Denver, CO
Keith Knepp, M.D. Univ. of Illinois – Peoria (97) Resident – Peoria, IL
Nerissa Koehn. Harvard Medical School – WHO Fellowship – Zanzibar, Tanzania
Timothy Leaman, M.D. Temple (98) Resident – Philadelphia, PA
Sarah Lesko, M.D. Penn (98) Resident – San Francisco, CA
James Little, M.D. Colorado (98) Resident – Portland, OR
Jennifer Lochner, M.D. Univ. of Wisconsin (99) Resident – Portland, OR
Steven Lore, M.D. Utah (99) Resident – Pocatello, ID
Alexandra Mazard-Bertini, M.D., M.P.H. Stanford (97) Resident – New York, NY
Sarah Morgan. Stanford Univ. 4th year
Susan Powell, M.D., M.P.H. Washington (97) Resident – Anchorage, AK
Anna Mies Richie, M.D. Southern Illinois Univ. (98) Resident – Springfield, IL
Eowyn Rieke, M.D. Brown (99) Resident – Seattle, WA
Marti Y. Taba, M.D. Hawaii (98) Resident – Columbus, OH
James Toombs. Univ. of Missouri – St. Louis 4th year

For more information concerning the Nicholas J. Pisacano, M.D., Memorial Foundation or the Pisacano Scholarships, contact the NJP Memorial Foundation, 2228 Young Drive, Lexington, Kentucky 40505.

(From Pisacano NJ: Reconsecratio medici [editorial]. J Am Board Fam Pract 2:78, 1989. By permission of the American Board of Family Practice.)

APPROVAL OF FAMILY PRACTICE AS THE 20TH MEDICAL SPECIALTY

The impact of these efforts and declarations was realized on February 8, 1969, when the specialty of Family Practice was approved as the 20th medical specialty board.

The new Family Practice specialty was born out of a need to provide comprehensive and continuing care that viewed the patient as a whole being

BOX 2-2

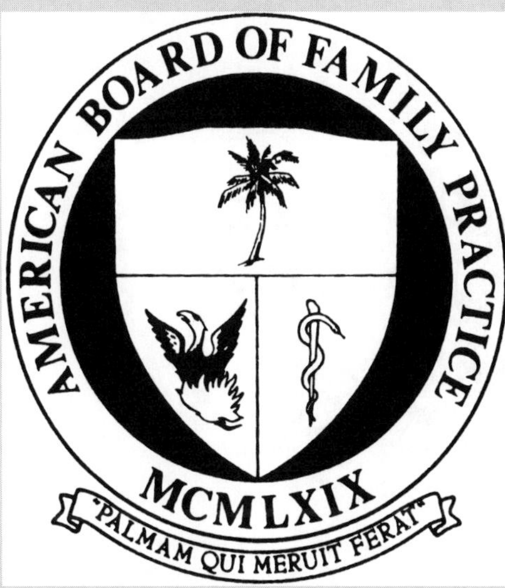

AMERICAN BOARD OF FAMILY PRACTICE

The Emblem of the American Board of Family Practice embodies the story of the specialty of Family Practice.

The upper half of the Emblem pictures a palm tree. The lower half is divided into 2 parts: on the left-hand side is a representation of the mythological bird, the Phoenix, rising out of its nest of fire; on the right-hand side is the standard of medicine, the Staff of Aesculapius.

The palm tree is the Phoenix dactylifera, the Latin name for the date palm, so called because of the ancient idea that if this tree is burned down or if it falls through old age, it will rejuvenate itself and spring up fairer than ever. This symbolizes our specialty arising directly from its general practice heritage.

The Phoenix, the fabulous Arabian mythological bird, lives a certain number of years, at the close of which it makes a nest of spices, sings a melodious dirge, flaps its wings to set fire to the pile and burns itself to ashes and comes forth with new life. This, of course, symbolizes our periodic recertification.

Immediately below the Emblem are the Latin words, ''Palmam Qui Meruit Ferat''—''Let him bear the palm who has earned it.'' This refers to the Roman custom to give the victorious gladiator a branch of the palm tree, the palm leaf being a sign of attainment of victory—symbolizing for us the attainment of Diplomate status by examination.

Nicholas J. Pisacano, M.D.

(From American Board of Family Practice: http//www.abfp.org/abfp.htm. By permission.)

BOX 2-3

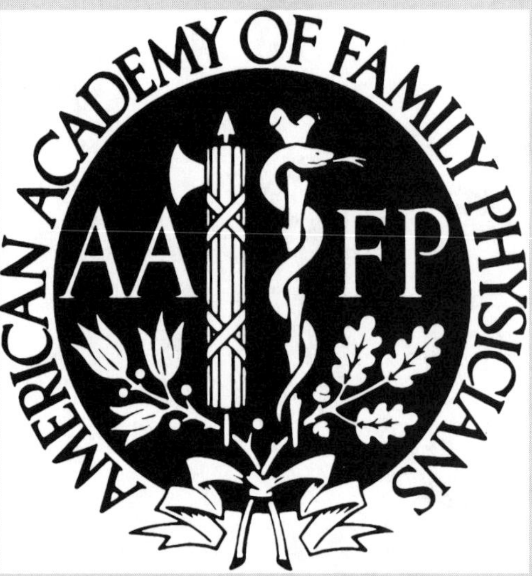

THE AAFP OFFICIAL SEAL

The AAFP seal is rich in symbolism. The circle that forms the basis of the seal stands for ''eternity and unity.'' The laurel branch at left symbolizes ''honor, valor and victory.'' The oak leaves at right signify ''divine knowledge.'' The ax or mace, capable of breaking through the strongest armor, represents ''strength.'' In Greek, it stands for ''the power of light over darkness.'' In Egyptian, the mace signifies ''clever one'' and ''cleaver of the way.'' The staff encircled by the serpent represents ''healing'' and ''the renewing power of life.'' It is the traditional symbol of medicine, not to be confused with the Caduceus (a double-winged staff), which is the insignia of the military medical corps. (From the Archives for Family Practice—American Academy of Family Practice Foundation. By permission.)

instead of as a set of specialized organ systems that the specialists had carved out. The American Board of Family Practice (Box 2-2) was the specialty's governing body that required certification and recertification examinations for its diplomates every 7 years. It was the first specialty board to require this. In 1970, the American Board of Family Practice offered its first certification examination, and in 1971 the American Academy of General Practice changed its name to the American Academy of Family Physicians (Box 2-3). The specialty of Family Practice grew rapidly (Box 2-4). In 1969, there were 15 original residency programs. By 1975, there were 250 programs training 3,720 family practice residents. By 1985, this number had doubled, and in 1998, there were 452 programs with more than 10,000 residents in

BOX 2-4 THE HISTORY OF FAMILY MEDICINE AT THE MAYO CLINIC

Mayo Clinic Rochester
Reflections from Sharon J. Krier, former medical secretary as well as education secretary, 1988-1998, and now supervisor and administrative secretary for the department (Fig. 2-4).

Even though I was born and raised in Rochester, Minnesota, and the Mayo Clinic served as my family's health care provider, I was not aware of the concept of family medicine until I began my employment in the Department of Family Medicine. I must admit I questioned if family medicine could or would be successful among the specialty giants in the Mayo system. My positive experiences in family medicine began in a small rural community 25 miles from Rochester when a satellite clinic was opened in 1976 at Plainview, Minnesota. I recall thinking how mature (polite way of saying old) the attending family physician appeared to me as I began working at the Plainview facility. This mature physician has become a special friend over the years, and at the age of 76 years, he is still actively involved in education at Mayo. Residents are experiencing the unique opportunity of learning from his wealth of wisdom, knowledge, and experience in patient care.

As family medicine at Mayo developed and the department consisting of 3 physicians (one of them being that mature physician from Plainview) moved into the existing Baldwin Building in 1978, I thought we were viewed as a threat in regard to space and care—"is there a need for family medicine at Mayo?" I think physicians as well as paramedical personnel thought we had to prove ourselves—that indeed there was a place for family medicine at Mayo. Twenty-two years later, with a combined staff of 40 providers, family medicine is well respected and valued within the Mayo system.

It was the vision of Dr. Robert Avant that a residency program in family medicine be developed. This became a reality in 1978, with 4 residents/year to the present program consisting of 25 residents. Many changes have occurred in the curriculum of the residency program as well as the depth and breadth of training. During this time the caliber of applicants to the residency program has improved.

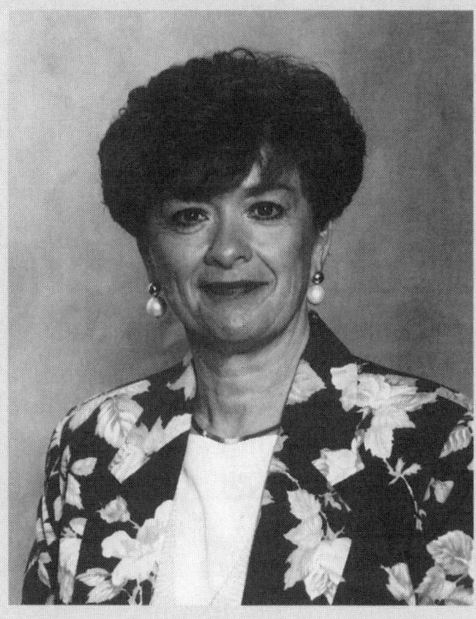

FIGURE 2-4
Sharon J. Krier, a medical and education secretary, was instrumental in founding the Department of Family Medicine in Rochester, Minnesota, in 1978.

BOX 2-4 Continued

Family medicine at Mayo has experienced the finest leadership over the years in the residency program as well as within the department. I consider myself fortunate to have worked with family medicine greats, including Drs. Robert Avant, Robert Nesse, David Agerter, and Matthew Bernard. It is thrilling to watch Mayo-trained family medicine residents grow and become well-respected physicians and staff members at Mayo. What's more, I've even inherited ''grandchildren'' through these former residents—now staff members. These are extra perks that make family medicine at Mayo even more special!

I am often asked ''aren't you burned-out; don't you want to go somewhere else?'' I can honestly say I enjoy family medicine as much today as when I began in 1976. There is no room for burnout as we continue to grow and change at an alarming rate. I must admit the stress level has increased because growth in staff, patient panel sizes, new programs, and Mayo's tremendous appetite for sophisticated technology has not always been accompanied by adequate space and support staff. However, because the feeling of family in family medicine at Mayo prevails, I know I made the right choice 22 years ago as I started working in that little community of Plainview, Minnesota, with my good friend.

Mayo Clinic Jacksonville

Reflections from Shannon Richardson, former medical secretary and now Residency Coordinator for the department.

Life as a secretary in the Department of Family Medicine when it was born was a lot different than it is now. We had to define our roles as part of primary care, a new concept to Mayo Clinic Jacksonville. Not only were we responsible for typing the patient notes for more than 20 patients per physician per day before the patient's next appointment, but we were responsible for answering incoming telephone calls from all of those patients. In addition, we were responsible for scheduling patient appointments and for making sure the physician's schedule was correct in all aspects. Sometimes it felt like we were trying so hard to get the work accomplished that there was not time to make ourselves more efficient. And as time passed, more physicians were hired and the Family Medicine residency program was born, ultimately adding 18 resident physicians to the practice.

With that growth came change. Paramedical staff have been added, and technologic advancements have changed our secretarial role. A transcription department was developed, and the physicians dictate by telephone. An appointment office was created, and patients began to schedule their visits through appointment schedulers. The biggest change was the conversion to an electronic medical record, which eliminated the movement and tracking of paper charts.

Finally, the administrative component of our role surfaced. We have been able to devote ourselves to our physicians and concentrate on what they need from the beginning to the end of the day.

BOX 2-4 Continued

We now have been able to go that extra mile and provide the quality they need. After all, life as a secretary has never been as simple as dotting i's and crossing t's in a manuscript. It is much more. It involves critical-thinking skills and anticipating the physicians' needs. Most people cannot reach the physician without speaking with the secretary first. Our goal as family medicine secretaries is to make sure that the physician is not inundated with the unnecessary and is as efficient as possible. Each secretary can take pride in knowing that everything we do is important and knowing that we are an integral part of making sure each physician's day proceeds as it should.

Mayo Clinic Scottsdale

Reflections from Frederick D. Edwards, M.D., Consultant, Department of Family Medicine, Mayo Clinic Scottsdale, Scottsdale, Arizona; Assistant Professor of Medicine, Mayo Medical School, Rochester, Minnesota.

The Department of Family Medicine at Mayo Clinic Scottsdale had its origin at Mayo Clinic Rochester in 1993 when Dr. Bradley C. Eichhorst was named the founding Chair for the department in Scottsdale and he began recruiting physicians from a nationwide applicant pool to be founding members of the department. Patient care began in January 1994, when the first family physician in Scottsdale started seeing patients at the main clinic building. Over the next 6 months, 4 additional members were added to the department and the Mayo Thunderbird Family Practice Center was constructed in Scottsdale, Arizona. This state-of-the-art facility included on-site laboratory and radiology facilities, a completely electronic medical record, and teleconferencing capabilities that linked the center via satellite to the main Mayo Clinic Scottsdale.

At the same time, the clinical aspects of the department were being founded, and the residency program was begun. Initial work on the residency application was begun in January 1994, with completion of the application during May of that same year. The application was submitted during the summer of 1994 and was finally approved by the Residency Review Committee for Family Medicine during 1995 (with permission to accept the inaugural class of residents in 1996).

The most significant growth within the department occurred in September 1994, when the Mayo Fountain Hills Family Practice Center was acquired with the addition of 2 more family physicians to the department. Since that time, the Fountain Hills practice has been moved to a completely new Family Practice Center. There have been 2 faculty members added to the Thunderbird site as well as a nurse practitioner and a third physician at the Fountain Hills site (bringing the department up to 10 family physicians and a nurse practitioner).

The Family Medicine Department continues to thrive, with the growth of its patient population and the maturation of the residency program to include 6 residents for each of the 3 years of the program. The department is proud to uphold the 3 shields of the Mayo Clinic, with active involvement in areas of clinical practice, education, and research.

training. As of 1997, close to 50,000 physicians had graduated from accredited family practice residencies and there was now (unlike any other specialty) a family practice residency program in every state.[1]

At the present rate of growth, the field of Family Medicine will continue to prosper and remain the leader in the delivery of primary care. The public has demanded a physician who specializes in comprehensive, cost-effective, and continuing care of the individual. Family practice has successfully and honorably fulfilled this important role in our advanced medical system.

REFERENCE

1. Stanard JR: Caring for America: The Story of Family Practice. Virginia Beach, Virginia, Donning Company Publishers, 1997

SUGGESTED READING

Rakel RE: Textbook of Family Practice, 5th ed. Philadelphia, WB Saunders, 1995, pp 3-19

THE SPECIALTY OF FAMILY PRACTICE

3

Robert G. Fish, M.D.

With the support of the American Medical Association, the American Academy of General Practice, and the United States general practitioners, family practice became the 20th American medical specialty in 1969. The initial definition of the specialty, by agreement of the American Board of Family Practice and the American Academy of Family Physicians stated the following:

> Family Practice is the specialty in breadth which builds upon a core of knowledge derived from other disciplines—drawing most heavily on internal medicine, pediatrics, obstetrics and gynecology, surgery and psychiatry—and which establishes a cohesive unit, combining the behavioral sciences with the traditional biological and clinical sciences.[1]

"Medicine is the best of all professions, the most hopeful."

—William J. Mayo

In a sense, the early family practitioners acknowledged that they were practitioners lacking their own body of knowledge and they applied but did not contribute to the body of medical knowledge. Since that time, the above statement has proved to be a good foundation for the specialty; however, in 1986 the American Board of Family Practice adopted the current definition of family practice:

> Family Practice is the medical specialty which is concerned with the total health care of the individual and the family. It is the specialty in breadth which integrates the biological, clinical, and behavioral sciences. The scope of family practice is not limited by age, sex, organ system, or disease entity.[2]

BOX 3-1 DEFINITIONS

Family Practice

The official definition of Family Practice as adopted by the American Board of Family Practice is as follows:

> Family Practice is the medical specialty which is concerned with the total health care of the individual and the family. It is the specialty in breadth which integrates the biological, clinical, and behavioral sciences. The scope of family practice is not limited by age, sex, organ system, or disease entity.

Family Medicine

There is a fine but distinct difference between Family Practice and Family Medicine. The two terms are often erroneously used synonymously. The specialty is named Family Practice and represents a special method of health care delivery. Family Medicine, on the other hand, is regarded as the unique academic discipline for the specialty. Family Practice is a quintessential specialty consisting of the integration of several disciplines along with the unique discipline—still evolving—called Family Medicine. Family Medicine is emerging as a body of knowledge or system (discipline, if you will) which is being continuously developed, studied (research base), and taught as an integrative entity.

From American Board of Family Practice.[2] By permission of the publisher.

Family practice now had a specific body of medical knowledge that defined its existence (Box 3-1). From this foundation, the specialty could develop into the leading specialty that delivered primary care.

A PERIOD OF CHANGE

The 1990s have seen many changes that favor generalist health care, and several of these changes allow the next major step in developing the scientific discipline of Family Medicine. The first of these changes is to move to evidence-based teaching in medical school, in which educational content and clinical decisions are based on critical review of published research studies.[3,4] The second change is the emergence of managed care and the need for data to show the best ways to provide cost-effective, quality care in a competitive environment.

From humble beginnings in 1969 when there were 15 pilot family practice residency programs, the specialty of family practice has now expanded to 452 family practice residency programs. In 1996, for the first time, there was a family practice residency program located in each of the 50 states and in Puerto Rico.[5–7] The total number of residents in training in 1973 was 1,754, and this number surpassed 7,000 only 8 years later.[8] In 1997 a major milestone was reached when more than 10,000 residents were training in family practice residency programs, with 3,200 to 3,500 residents in each residency class. Two all-time highs were set in July 1996, when there were 3,572 first-year positions and 3,494 (97.8 percent) of them were filled. As of January 1996, 46,800 physicians had completed family practice residency programs.

> *"Perhaps the ability not only to acquire the confidence of the patient, but to deserve it, to see what the patient desires and needs, comes through the sixth sense we call intuition, which in turn comes from wide experience and deep sympathy for and devotion to the patient, giving to the possessor remarkable ability to achieve results."*
>
> —William J. Mayo

Currently, there are 670,000 physicians in the United States. Of this number, 52,000 are family physicians and 20,000 are general practitioners.[8] As mentioned above, there are 452 family practice residency training programs in community hospitals and academic medical centers, and in 1997 in the United States 16 percent of graduating medical students chose careers in family practice.

Family physicians often are the first contact for patients and place a high premium on being the physicians who coordinate care for their patients. The family physician often makes sure that proper referrals are made to specialists in an economical way. Therefore, they are the ideal primary care providers in managed care settings (Box 3-2).

BOX 3-2

Family Physician's Creed

I am a family physician
one of many across this country.

This is what I believe:

You, the patient
are my first professional responsibility
whether man, woman or child
ill or well
seeking care, healing, or knowledge.

You and your family deserve high quality,
affordable health care including treatment,
prevention and health promotion.
I support access to health care for all.

The specialty of family practice
trains me to care for the whole person
physically and emotionally,
throughout life
working with your medical history
and family dynamics
coordinating your care
with other physicians when necessary.

This is my promise to you.

From American Academy of Family Physicians: *F.Y.I.: Information for You on the Latest Academy Services and Products.* American Academy of Family Physicians, Fall 1997. By permission of the publisher.

DEMOGRAPHICS OF FAMILY PRACTICE

The demographic composition of family physicians with respect to sex and minority status has shifted dramatically since 1981. Fewer than 10 percent of the residents in training during each year before 1976 were women.[8] After 1987, more than 30 percent of the residents in training each year were women, and after 1994, more than 40 percent.[8] Since 1973, the American Academy of Family Physicians has collected information with respect to the minority status of residents in training. Minorities include African Americans, Mexican Americans, American Indians, and others. Before 1977, fewer than 10 percent of the residents in training during any particular year belonged to minority groups. This percentage increased to 27.7 percent in July 1995.[8]

The practice patterns of graduates of family practice residencies vary widely. More than 10 percent of graduating family practice residents during each year before 1988 entered solo practice.[9] For each year after 1988, fewer than 10 percent of graduating family practice residents chose to practice alone, with only 5 percent of the 1996 graduates choosing a solo practice. The percentage of graduates choosing a family practice group increased from 20 percent in 1984 to 46 percent in 1996. Without question, the major trend among graduates is to enter group rather than solo practice, unlike the general practitioners of previous years. Of all family physicians practicing in 1995, those who did not complete a family practice residency program were twice as likely to have a solo practice as were graduates of family practice residency programs: 53 percent and 25 percent, respectively.[8]

FAMILY PHYSICIAN ENCOUNTERS

The family physician sees 20 to 30 patients per day on average (Fig. 3-1). Family practitioners perform many procedures, and 36 percent of U.S. family practice residency graduates provide obstetric services for their patients.[8] The family practitioner is likely to perform office surgery, flexible sigmoidoscopy, colposcopy, and casting of simple fractures. Most U.S. family practitioners provide hospital services for their patients and care for their patients in nursing homes. The problems attended to by U.S. family practitioners vary from practice to practice according to the emphasis of the physician. The problems seen most frequently in family practice offices are listed in Table 3-1.

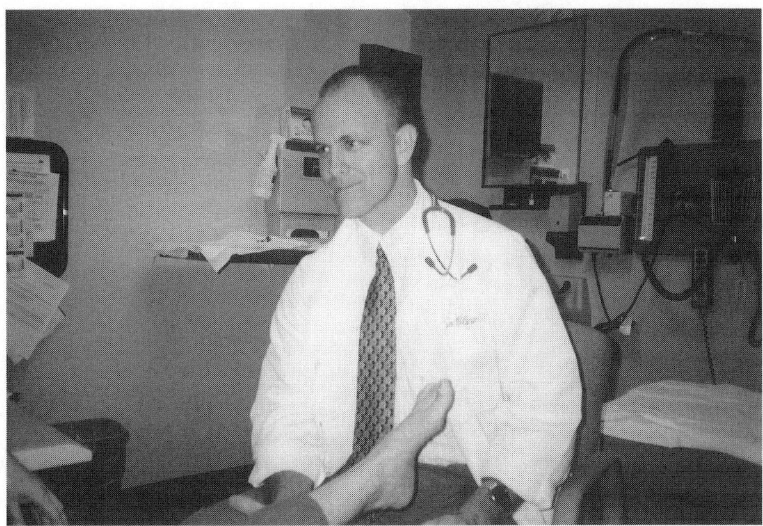

FIGURE 3-1
The family physician typically sees 20 to 30 patients per day in the clinic setting.

TABLE 3-1
PROBLEMS SEEN MOST FREQUENTLY BY FAMILY PHYSICIANS

Essential hypertension
General medical examination
Chronic sinusitis
Acute upper respiratory infection
Bronchitis
Acute pharyngitis
Otitis media
Diabetes mellitus
Sprains and strains of the back
Normal pregnancy
Asthma
Depressive disorder
Health supervision of infant or child
Gastroenteritis or colitis
Contact dermatitis and eczema

Modified from American Academy of Family Physicians.[8] By permission of the publisher.

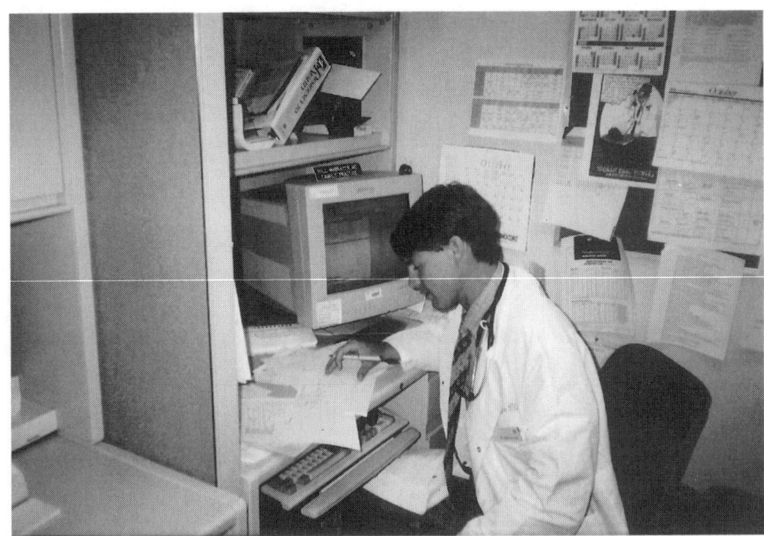

FIGURE 3-2 Family physicians are trained to care for most of the problems that patients present with.

> *"Every part of the body is dependent on the whole and to develop a specialty more fully is to study what constitutes health and disease."*
>
> —Charles H. Mayo

Family physicians manage most of the problems encountered in their practices (Fig. 3-2). The U.S. Agency for Health Care Policy and Research reported that only 4.5 percent of patients seen by primary care physicians are referred to specialists.[10] In addition to full scope office-based practice, many family physicians develop special interests in their practice. Sports medicine and geriatric care are 2 of the more common interests of family physicians, and currently there are certificates of added qualifications available for each of these areas (see Chaps. 24 and 25).

FAMILY PHYSICIAN PRACTICE SITES

Family physicians settle in communities that represent the full spectrum of size and location of communities in the entire United States. Approximately 37 percent of graduates in 1996 located in towns of fewer than 25,000 people

TABLE 3-2
DISTRIBUTION OF 1998 GRADUATING RESIDENTS BY COMMUNITY SIZE

CHARACTER AND POPULATION OF COMMUNITY	REPORTING GRADUATES		
	NO.	%	CUMULATIVE %
Rural area or town (< 2,500)			
Not within 25 miles of large city	115	4.8	4.8
Within 25 miles of large city	61	7.6	7.4
Small town (2,500–10,000)			
Not within 25 miles of large city	234	9.8	17.2
Within 25 miles of large city	144	6.0	23.2
Small city (10,000–25,000)			
Not within 25 miles of large city	181	7.6	30.8
Within 25 miles of large city	203	8.5	39.3
Medium city (25,000–100,000)	423	17.7	57.0
Suburb of small metropolitan area	71	3.0	59.9
Small metropolitan area (100,000–500,000)	287	12.0	72.0
Suburb of large metropolitan area	318	13.3	85.3
Large metropolitan area (500,000 or more)	215	9.0	94.3
Inner city/low income area (500,000 or more)	137	5.7	100.0
Total	2,389	100.0	100.0

From American Academy of Family Physicians: *Report on Survey of 1998 Graduating Family Practice Residents.* Kansas City, Missouri, American Academy of Family Physicians. Reprint 155x. By permission of the publisher.

(Table 3-2). Approximately 6 percent of graduates in 1996 settled in rural towns of fewer than 2,500 people and 15 percent settled in large metropolitan areas of more than 500,000 people. These proportions did not differ substantially from the distribution of all family physicians, regardless of the completion year, as indicated in the American Academy of Family Physicians data collected in May 1995.[8]

Although family physicians in the United States practice primarily in the office setting, approximately 87 percent of active members of the American Academy of Family Physicians had hospital admission privileges in May 1995. Of these physicians, 86 percent indicated that the privileges they were granted were "generally about right." Both the percentage of family physicians with hospital privileges and the satisfaction rates are similar to the results published in previous years.[8,11–13]

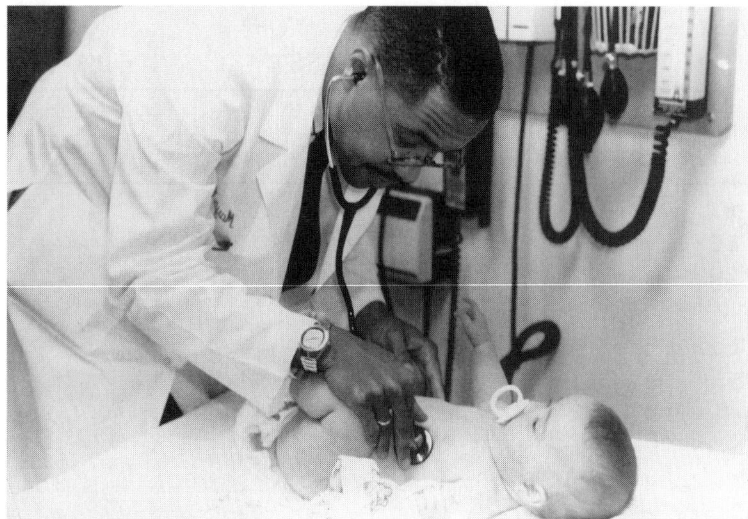

FIGURE 3-3
Family physicians play an important role in the lives of their patients, from the womb to the grave.

CONCLUSIONS

Family physicians are increasingly in high demand in all areas of the U.S. health care system and particularly in areas where there are high percentages of managed care patients. The fact that 9 of 10 graduates of family practice residencies continue to practice as family practice physicians has significant personnel policy implications: family practice residency programs are an effective mechanism for the production of generalist physicians.[14] The demand for family physicians will continue to grow. As the health needs of the United States change, the practice profile of the family physician may change as well, but the family physician's practice will remain broad based, with attention to the patient in the context of the family as a whole (Fig. 3-3).

REFERENCES

1. American Board of Family Practice and American Academy of Family Physicians: Cited by Taylor RB: Family medicine: current issues and future practice. In Family Medicine: Principles and Practice. Fifth edition. Edited by RB Taylor, AK David, TA Johnson Jr, DM Phillips, JE Scherger. New York, Springer, 1998, pp 1–5
2. American Board of Family Practice: 1997 Directory of Diplomates. Lexington, Kentucky, American Board of Family Practice, 1997, p iii
3. Silagy C, Lancaster T: The Cochrane Collaboration in Primary Care: an interna-

tional resource for evidence-based practice of family medicine. Fam Med 27:302, 1995

4. Hayward RS, Wilson MC, Tunis SR, Bass EB, Guyatt G, for the Evidence-Based Medicine Working Group: Users' guides to the medical literature. VIII. How to use clinical practice guidelines. A. Are the recommendations valid? JAMA 274:570, 1995
5. Ostergaard DJ: Career alternatives. In Family Medicine: Principles and Practice. Edited by RB Taylor et al (eds). New York, Springer-Verlag, 1978, pp 1093–1100
6. Ostergaard DJ: Career alternatives. In Family Medicine: Principles and Practice. Second edition. Edited by RB Taylor et al. New York, Springer-Verlag, 1983, pp 1741–1749
7. Ostergaard DJ. Appendix II: Statistical data from the American Academy of Family Physicians. In Family Medicine: Principles and Practice. Third edition. Edited by RB Taylor, JL Buckingham, EP Donatelle, TA Johnson Jr, JE Scherger. New York, Springer-Verlag, 1988, pp 16–18
8. American Academy of Family Physicians: Facts About: Family Practice. Kansas City, Missouri, American Academy of Family Physicians, 1996
9. American Academy of Family Physicians: Report on Survey of Graduating Family Practice Residents. Kansas City, Missouri, American Academy of Family Physicians
10. Gaus CR, Clancy CM: From the Agency for Health Care Policy and Research: research at the interface of primary and specialty care. JAMA 274:1419, 1995
11. Survey shows private practice dominant among AAGP members. Group Practice 1:N-7, 1970
12. Clinton C, Schmittling G, Stern TL, Black RR: Hospital privileges for family physicians: a national study of office based members of the American Academy of Family Physicians. J Fam Pract 13:361, 1981
13. Schmittling G, Tsou C: Obstetric privileges for family physicians: a national study. J Fam Pract 29:179, 1989
14. Kahn NB Jr, Schmittling G, Ostergaard D, Graham R: Specialty practice of family practice residency graduates, 1969 through 1993. A national study. JAMA 275:713, 1996

4 FAMILY PHYSICIAN RELATIONSHIPS

Francis X. DeCandis, M.D.

The family physician wears many hats during the course of the day. From conducting rounds in the hospital to interacting with specialists, providing care in the clinic, and finally providing physician coverage at the local high school football game, the job of a family physician is varied and often never ending. In most cases, the work of the family physician has a great impact on the residents of a community as well as the community itself. The family physician is respected as a patient advocate and a community advocate. With this respect comes the responsibility to do what is right for the welfare of the patients, often at the expense of the physician's own free time and privacy. No one knows this better than the small town family doctor. Family physicians, no matter where they practice, are often deeply involved with their patients, both in and out of the office. The field of Family Medicine is often thought of in terms of 2 components, clinical medicine and the art of medicine. Much of what is discussed in this chapter constitutes the art of family practice.

PATIENT-FAMILY PHYSICIAN RELATIONSHIPS

The cornerstone of family practice is the patient-physician relationship. No specialty provides this level of comprehensive, continuous care as does family practice. Family physicians provide medical care throughout their patients' lifetimes, from birth to death. They may provide prenatal care, delivery of newborns, well-child care, school physicals, general examinations for adults, management of chronic medical problems, nursing home care, and finally hospice care. No other physician is trained to provide so many levels of care.

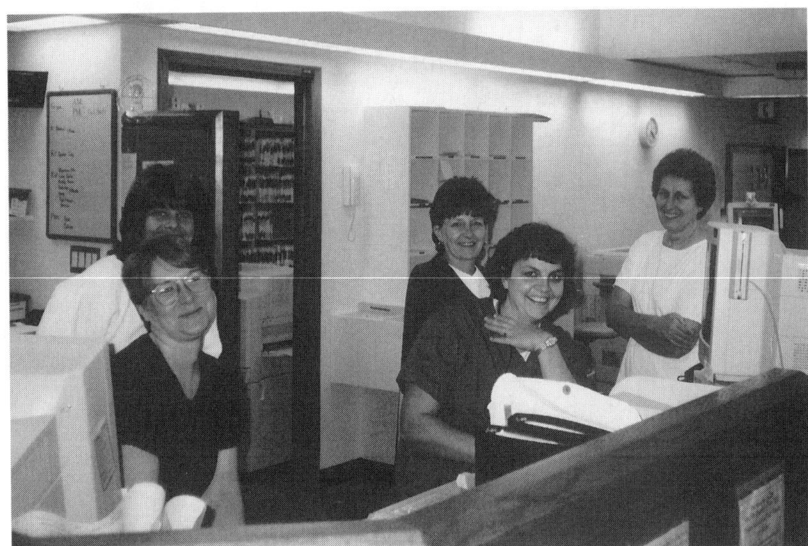

FIGURE 4-1
A warm, congenial staff can help to make a good first impression for new patients in a family physician's office.

Ideally, family physicians are caring, compassionate individuals who are concerned about the overall well-being of the patient (Fig. 4-1). They often become acquainted with the entire family and gain a deep understanding of that family's dynamics. It has been said that a great number of patients present to the family physician's office with complaints that are related to underlying psychosocial problems. Understanding the patient as a whole within the context of complex interpersonal relationships allows the family physician to give better treatment. Many patients feel so close to their family physicians that they invite them to important events such as high school graduations, weddings, christenings, and various other life-changing events.

Professionalism

When patients feel close to their family physicians, they may think of them as family friends. Despite this level of comfort, the family physician must maintain a professional relationship. To help ensure this relationship, the use of the physician's first name should be discouraged in the office. This will help maintain the professional relationship. Every family physician has been in a situation in which a patient appears friendly, calling the physician by the first name and then expecting the physician to honor an inappropriate request (eg, treating over the telephone). Beware of these patients and try to remain professional when faced with requests.

On the other hand, the family physician should always keep the patient's best interest in mind. In some cases, this may require that the physician make an exception to the regular delivery of care to better serve the patient. Each patient is unique and may require a different approach to care. An excellent example is the use of a home visit (house call) for a patient who is unable to travel to the clinic. These types of accommodations may build trust and respect with the patient and reflect a deep sense of caring.

Emotions

Many emotions are involved in the care of patients, and family physicians must be careful not to allow their own emotions to impair the decision-making processes. Whether the physician is experiencing anger, fear, anxiety, sadness, joy, sympathy, or empathy, the physician should remain objective. When experiencing strong emotion, it is only natural to express these feelings and in some situations it may be beneficial. Patients may be comforted by knowing that they matter to their physician. However, the expression of emotion by the physician must always be for the benefit of the patient. In view of this family physicians should understand their own feelings and be able to modify their expression: to understand others one must know oneself.

Addressing the Patient

Proper introduction is important in establishing good rapport with patients. In most cases, a patient who is younger or about the same age as the physician may be addressed by the first name. On the other hand, older patients may be offended by the use of their first names. To avoid these situations, it is best to address older patients by Mr. or Mrs. ___________ and at a later time ask for permission to use the first name, if you feel comfortable with that. Remember, whenever in doubt, use the patient's surname.

Chaperones

When examining the private areas of a patient of the opposite sex, it is necessary to have a chaperone present to avoid misinterpretation of the examination.

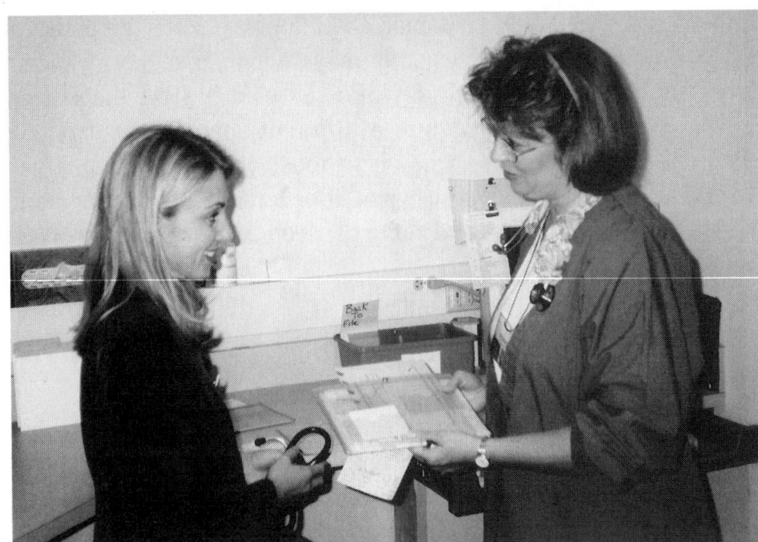

FIGURE 4-2
Throughout the day, family physicians have many important interactions with office staff, nurses, and patients.

Supervision

Resident physicians should always inquire about the department's policy on supervision of patient care. In most cases, the resident physician will need to discuss the patient's case with the staff preceptor and, if appropriate, should have the physician examine the patient. Medicare reimbursement policy often requires that the patient be examined by the staff physician whose name is used for billing purposes. In addition, this reexamination can enhance education by exposing the resident to different approaches and treatment modalities (Fig. 4-2).

FAMILY PHYSICIAN—PHYSICIAN RELATIONSHIPS

During the course of the day, family physicians may have multiple interactions with other physicians involved in their patients' care (Fig. 4-3). With this in mind, the family physician should remain in control of the overall care of the patient unless other specific arrangements are made. Interactions with specialists should always be documented if they affect patient care. The ordering of additional tests by specialists should be discussed beforehand with the family physician. Nothing is more frustrating to a primary care provider than to have a specialist see a patient and order an abundance of tests and further consults with other specialists without first discussing the recommendations with the family physician. This should not be tolerated

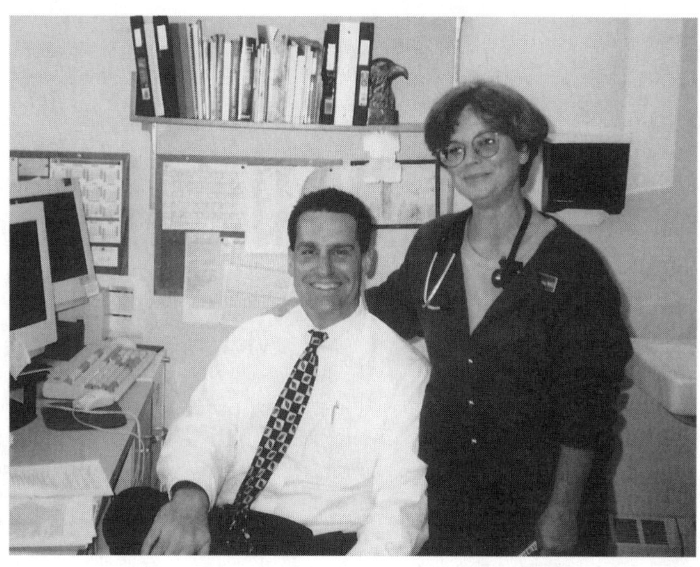

FIGURE 4-3
A good working relationship with colleagues is paramount to a successful practice.

because it destroys the underlying relationship between the family physician and patient, and the control of the patient is lost to the specialist who, in many cases, provides no follow-up care.

Keep in mind, the criticism of fellow physicians should be discouraged. In many cases, all the details of a specific situation are not known, and as a result premature and incorrect conclusions may be drawn. In view of this, it is important to avoid critical remarks directed at other physicians. After all, at some point, you may be the target of such inaccurate and unfair comments.

Family physicians must also work together to promote the specialty. Others may be quick to criticize family physicians, but most of these critics are not knowledgeable about the specialty of family practice. We must, therefore, work together as a specialty to educate our patients and the medical community about the role of the family physician in the delivery of medical care.

Family physicians should seek out and serve in leadership positions in medical or community organizations. By participating in a leadership role, the individual physician promotes the specialty of family practice and helps bring respect and understanding to our profession.

FAMILY PHYSICIAN AND THE COMMUNITY

Family physicians serve patients not only with an individual approach but also from a community-based approach. In urban areas family physicians

BOX 4-1 LaVILLA INDIGENT CARE CLINIC

Marc W. Thorpe, M.D. *Senior Associate Consultant, Department of Family Medicine, Mayo Clinic Jacksonville, Jacksonville, Florida*

The LaVilla Indigent Care Clinic began operating on September 11, 1997, as part of the *We Care Jacksonville* network, a program designed to provide care to Jacksonville's less-fortunate population.

The idea of LaVilla began with Dr. Floyd B. Willis. Dr. Willis is a physician in the Mayo Clinic Jacksonville Department of Family Medicine and a member of the board of directors for The Help Center, a local service-oriented program for the poor. The Help Center is a residence for men and women in downtown Jacksonville that helps with drug rehabilitation and assists in finding employment. Dr. Willis had been working at another downtown free clinic and felt that working at such a clinic would provide a unique opportunity for our residents. The Help Center was an ideal location for such a clinic. I approached Dr. Willis around this time and asked about working at a free clinic. He suggested we start our own.

We Care Jacksonville is part of the Duval County Medical Society. It helps to provide medical care and organize referrals for those without means or access to medical care. Legislation was passed in Florida that provides sovereign immunity to those giving free care. Several clinics have opened in the Jacksonville area as part of *We Care Jacksonville.* Our clinic became the 11th such free clinic (Fig. 4-4).

We started the clinic with old furniture from the Mayo warehouse. We also received a generous donation of office supplies from the family of the late Dr. John R. Nelson of Jacksonville. We filled a modest pharmacy with multiple contributions from drug companies. Mayo Clinic provided those essential supplies we could not find elsewhere and helped design and install a sink, divider curtains, and electrical outlets at The Help Center. When not in use, the curtains can be pulled back and examination tables pushed against the wall to allow the room to be used for other activities.

The clinic operates every other Thursday morning from 8:00 AM to noon and will soon be open every Thursday. Two residents, one staff physician, and a volunteer are present to help with check-in and referrals.

may donate time and resources to care for indigent patients (Box 4-1). In rural communities, family physicians may care for uninsured migrant workers. They are also asked to serve in volunteer charitable organizations, which provide valuable services to the community. Some may serve on school boards or as city council members and decide on important issues that affect our children and families. Others may take a less formal approach in helping the community: a school team physician or perhaps a coach of a soccer team. No matter what their contributions, family physicians shape and impact the world in which they live (Box 4-2). Physicians have a responsibility to give back to the community which has given so much to their careers. It is this spirit of giving that may make our careers even more satisfying.

BOX 4-1 Continued

Initially, many of the patients seen were residents of The Help Center. However, word is slowly getting out about our clinic, and our patient numbers are growing.

The clinic is run by the family practice residents in our program. It provides an opportunity for residents to be intimately involved in what it takes to run a clinic. The clinic also allows the residents to be exposed to a different patient population.

FREE
DOCTOR'S
VISIT
Where: LaVilla Clinic at
The Help Center
When: Today
8:00 am - Noon

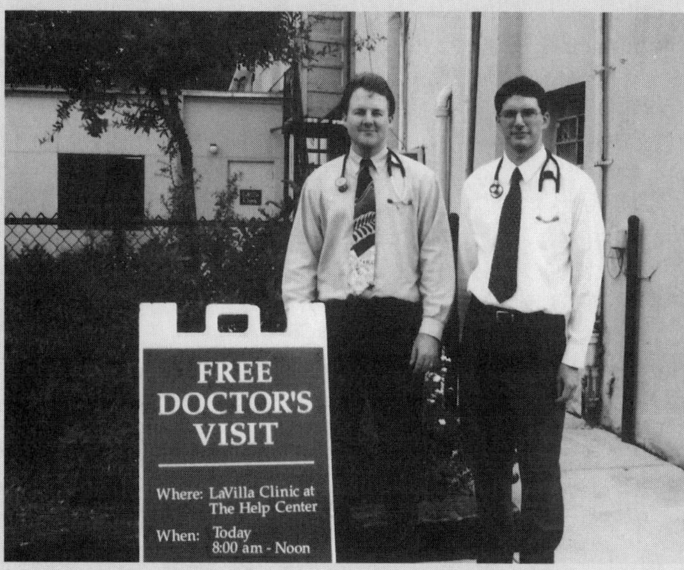

FIGURE 4-4 Family physicians as well as family medicine residents often donate their time to serve at free clinics for the medically underserved.

As Dr. Will wrote on February 15, 1934:

> Our father recognized certain definite social obligations. He believed that any person who had better opportunity than others, greater strength of mind, body or character, owed something to those who had not been so provided; that is, that the important thing in life is not to accomplish for one's self alone, but for each to carry his share of collective responsibility.
>
> In 1894, having paid for our homes and started a modest life insurance program, my brother and I decided upon a plan whereby we could eventually do something worthwhile for the sick. The plan was to put aside from our earnings any sums in excess of what might be called a reasonable return for the work we accomplished.

(*Continues on page 42*)

BOX 4-2 OUR THANKSGIVING

Antoinette Gonzaga, M.D. *First-year Resident, Department of Family Medicine, Mayo Clinic Jacksonville, Jacksonville, Florida*

In appreciation to a community that has welcomed us with open arms, the family medicine residents at Mayo Clinic Jacksonville decided to host a community health fair (Fig. 4-5), and what better time to do so than in October—Family Health Month. Our goal was a celebration of personal wellness by providing a cornucopia of helpful and healthful information.

The residents have been active proponents of health in the community. They are involved with the local school system and provide free physician advice on local nightly television newscasts. However, although the idea of a health fair was not new, it had not been attempted in the 6 years since the start of the Mayo Jacksonville Family Medicine residency program.

Motivation was key to this resident-driven activity. Liaisons and contact persons were approached, telephoned, faxed, and interrogated about the most efficient and effective way to approach this low-budget but well-supported endeavor. As with any of the best-laid plans, changes and compromises were common. Financial problems and personnel issues could not stop the spirit of the Health Fair Committee. Details were dissected, plans projected, and order organized. We rallied the troop of residents for a fun-filled event. Eventually even more people were telephoned, faxed, and interrogated. Added support from staff and faculty and independent health and drug company sponsors arrived in timely fashion.

We managed to send public announcements to the radio and television news programs, and our event was advertised in local newspapers. After months of planning, the fair was ready. If we build it, will they come?

That Saturday morning was clear and bright, with more wind than was needed, but the preparations went smoothly. The site of our event was the parking lot of the Beaches Primary Care Center. Tables were set up, the tent was assembled, and boxes were unloaded. Banners were displayed and balloons drifted in the wind to signal our presence. Residents took their stations.

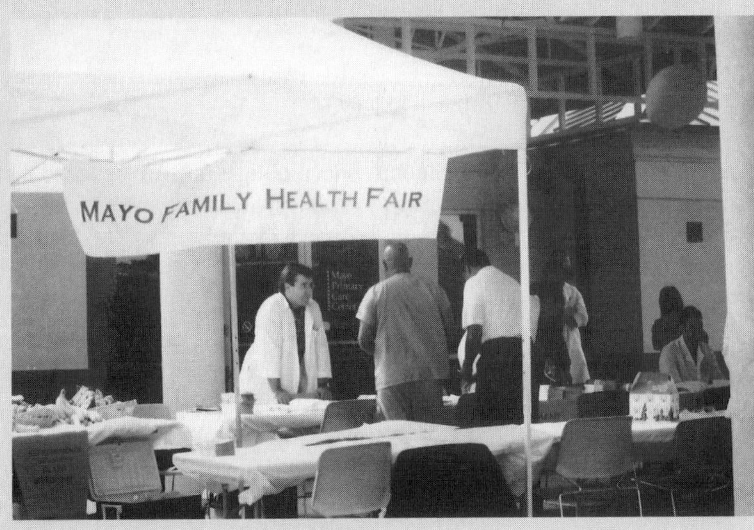

FIGURE 4-5 Residents at Mayo Clinic Jacksonville provided a health fair as a service to the community.

BOX 4-2 Continued

There was urgency mixed with excitement as the residents raced to have everything in place by the designated start time. Ten resident physicians in crisp white coats lined up behind the expertly decorated tables. Representatives from various groups were also positioned and prepared to educate the attendees. The following participants were present: the American Cancer Society, whose focus was to discuss and teach breast self-examination; the Florida/Georgia Blood Alliance, collecting pints of blood; Genesis Rehab Center, which displayed and demonstrated gadgets to increase function; and St. Luke's Home Health, which emphasized environmental safety.

Everyone was ready on time. All that was left to do was to wait. The people came: motorists who had seen our sign from Route A1A, patients at the Clinic who were scheduled for a weekend appointment, and shoppers from the nearby shopping mall. Individuals, couples, and sometimes whole families visited until the final tally reached more than 100 visitors.

Ample information was available to address issues such as children's health and immunizations, pregnancy, nutrition and weight control, cholesterol and blood pressure, and mental health. We distributed brochures, handouts, stickers, magnets, booklets, and other gizmos. Not only did we provide items to quench the intellect, we had a generous array of fruits, juices, and snacks to satisfy the appetite. There was plenty to attract the attention of every member of the community.

People perused the displays, accepted our information, and chatted with the residents. Many people related health care stories. One woman talked about her sister who cannot stop smoking. Another spoke of her uncle who had suffered from a stroke and is slowly starting to recover. Others talked about their own experiences as patients under the care of Mayo physicians. Most everyone was grateful for the care that they had received. Thanks and praise were welcome. Residents saw the impact of medical care on a community (Fig. 4-6). And although it was not the goal of the fair, the compliments and positive feedback from the community were added perks.

The day was a success. And it was a starting ground for a tradition of future fairs.

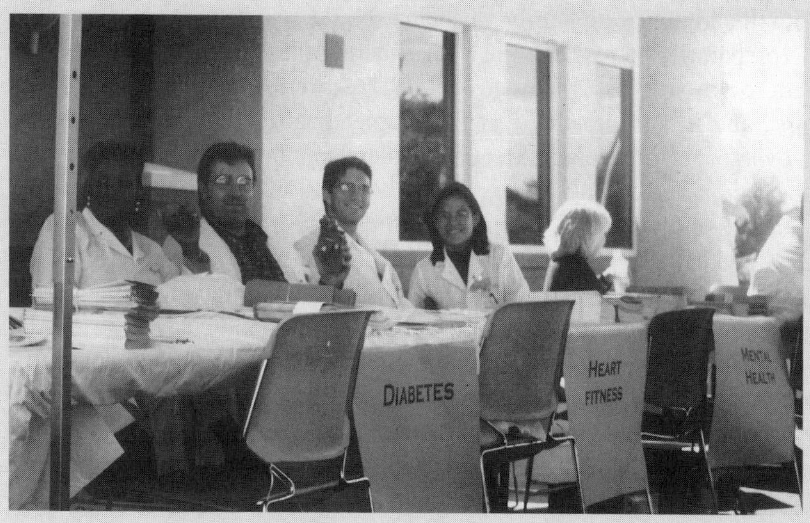

FIGURE 4-6 Residents fortunate to have bright futures ahead give back to the community through service projects such as a health fair.

> The fund which we had built up had come from the (people) and we believed that it ought to return to (them) in the form of advanced medical education, which would develop better-trained physicians, and to research to reduce the amount of sickness. The people's money, of which we have been the moral custodians, is being irrevocably returned to the people from whom it came. (From *Mayo Magazine*, Fall/Winter 1998, p. 23.)

FAMILY PHYSICIAN—NURSE RELATIONSHIPS

In family practice, the physician-nurse relationship is important in the delivery of primary care (Box 4-3). The nurse interacts with the patients on a regular basis and serves as an extension of the physician. The ideal nurse should be congenial, knowledgeable, trustworthy, efficient, and accurate (a scout). An effective nurse can make a physician's life much easier (Fig. 4-8). However, a poor physician-nurse relationship can be extremely detrimental to patient care and one's sense of well-being.

> *"The trained nurse has given nursing the human, or shall we say, the divine touch, and made the hospital desirable for patients with serious ailments regardless of their home advantages."*
>
> —Charles H. Mayo

In today's changing medical care environment, physician extenders (physician assistants and nurse practitioners) are becoming increasingly popular. With this in mind, the family physician should always give adequate thought and preparation to research the laws affecting these individuals before hiring them to provide care. Many government restrictions apply to these relationships, and it is imperative that family physicians involved with employing or overseeing physician extenders understand the regulations involved in supervision and billing of services.

Nurses and physician extenders also play an important role in answering telephone calls in a busy family practice. Family physicians must review a clear triage system with their staff to handle requests and problems generated by patient telephone calls. Some problems may be handled over the telephone, whereas some patients may need to come in for an appointment, and still others may even need to go to the Emergency Department immediately. Poor care may be delivered to patients who are not adequately assessed and triaged over the telephone, and lawsuits may result. When in doubt, it is always better to err on the conservative side and have the patient come to the office for further evaluation.

Box 4-3 A NURSING PERSPECTIVE OF FAMILY PRACTICE

Randi E. McCullough, LPN *Department of Family Medicine, Mayo Clinic Rochester, Rochester, Minnesota*

So, you are going to enter family practice. Personally, I think you are making an excellent choice. In what other field of medicine can you watch the face of a couple who have just received the news that they are going to have their first child? And you can see their faces when you tell them they are going to have twins! Then, years later, you deliver their fourth child. What a joy it is to witness their children grow. Think of the times you sent them home with a diagnosis of croup and times you told their parents that they are supposed to be taking two of the green pills and four of the small, pink ones. Someday you watch the health of their grandparents (whom you also care for) decline and eventually they pass on. Not everything is rosy, as you must already know, but there are some great times to be had. This is what family practice is about.

The nursing staff of the Department of Family Medicine at the Mayo Clinic consists mostly of Licensed Practical Nurses with supervision by a Registered Nurse. We have many different duties, the main purpose of which is to make the patient feel at ease and comfortable while at the same time we assist the physician. As a family physician, having a caring, trustworthy relationship with your nurse will be the basis of your practice. If you develop trust in your nurse, then I believe you will have a satisfying working environment. Your relationship with your nurse is probably one of the most important aspects of your practice. If you have the chance to be part of the hiring process, I encourage you to take an active role. If you are assigned a nurse, hopefully you will be compatible. You may laugh, but it is really no laughing matter when I tell you that how you treat your nurse will come back to haunt you or benefit you in the long run.

The ''warm fuzzies,'' as I call them, are an important part of your relationship with your nursing staff. ''Thank you'' and ''please'' as well as many other pleasantries go a long way. A kind comment, constructive criticism, or positive feedback is always welcomed, whereas sharp accusatory criticism or complaints often do not help the situation and may make it worse. As a resident physician or a physician in practice, I am sure you have had experiences with a nurse who was positive and beneficial. On the other hand, you have probably encountered a nurse who was worse than a rattlesnake to work with (those are the nurses who have come across too many grumpy physicians). Really, with all jokes aside, the relationship with your nurse will be an extremely important factor in providing the best care to your patients and enjoying your practice of medicine. If you choose to be happy, then so can we. Unfortunately, some situations work the other way around. Always sit down with your nurses and let them know of any changes you would like; ask their opinions to make them feel included and an active part of your practice. Suggesting change tactfully is far better than telling your nurses what they have to do.

Talking to patients on the telephone is probably the most time-consuming and important job that nurses have. This may not be true in some practices, because some physicians may want to make their own telephone calls, but this is not a common practice and in most cases is inefficient. I cannot imagine how you could see 20 to 30 patients in a day and find time to make multiple telephone calls. Again, the secret to effectively and efficiently handling telephone calls is based on the trust you have in your nurses, their advice, their ease of handling the patients, their accurate documentation, and the way they come across on the telephone. This may not be evident right away, but this will come across

BOX 4-3 Continued

later in the office when your patients come in to see you. In most cases, patients will tell you if they were comfortable with how their care was handled over the telephone. Telephone calls can range from a new, inexperienced mother calling daily to make sure that a newborn's stools are normal to elderly people calling because they are lonely and need to hear a caring voice. The spectrum of telephone calls varies from seemingly benign to life-threatening situations. The family practice nurse must be trained in appropriate triage to counsel patients properly.

It is not difficult to see that a well-trained nurse can save you time. Most physicians want to spend more time with their patients. In view of this, if your nurse spends more time obtaining necessary information, it eventually allows physicians to spend more time with their patients. The nurse-physician relationship is a working relationship that improves the delivery of care. Working closely is necessary and trust is important. Supporting each other should not be a thought but rather an automatic reaction. The more honest and open you are with your nurses, the more open and honest we can be with you. A successful working relationship is often a "two-way street." I think trusting and enjoying the person you work with reflects on your satisfaction in practice and as a person.

All practices run differently from the time patients check in to the time they leave. This can go smoothly or patients can be dissatisfied with their care. Long waiting time in a physician's office is one of the more common complaints. Allowing your nurse to visit with the patients and explain that your appointments are running late may help defuse the situation. Often a simple comment with a brief explanation to patients is all that is necessary. As a nurse, I feel that these tasks are also our responsibility and represent another way we help patients (Fig. 4-7).

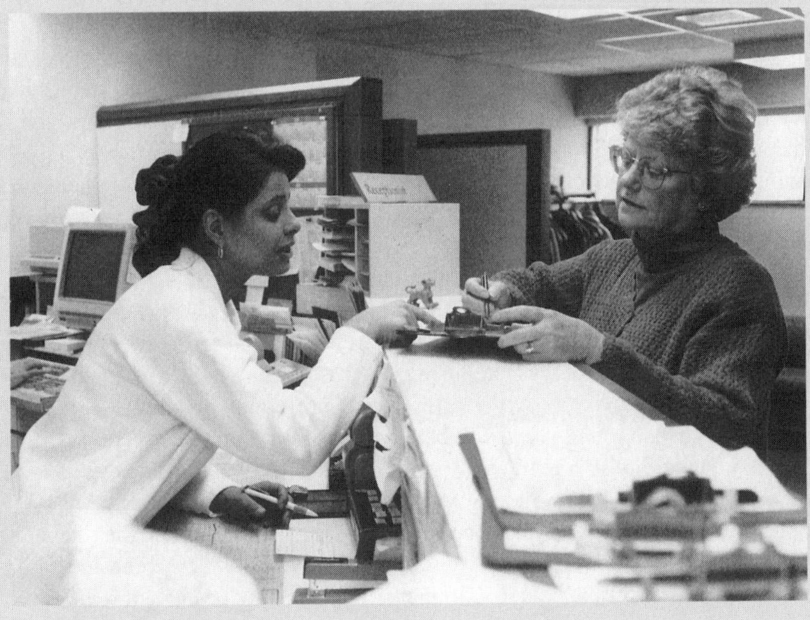

FIGURE 4-7
A helpful staff can make a family physician's practice successful.

BOX 4-3 Continued

From my own experience, I feel that house calls are often beneficial. Some are extremely helpful to ensure good care and a compassionate relationship with your patient. Recently, I received a telephone call from a patient requesting results of a test that had been done earlier that morning. Biopsy specimens were taken, and the patient was worried. Unfortunately, the results showed cancer. Although the physician I worked with was on vacation, I called him at home to report the results. He made a house call to visit and share the unfortunate diagnosis with the anxious patient. Even though the news was bad, the patient's fears were somewhat relieved, and the patient-physician bond was strengthened. Fortunately, the patient did well, and this act of compassion by the patient's physician will never be forgotten. It is this type of care that makes family practice special.

The family physician-nurse relationship is a special relationship. Often the success of a family physician's practice hinges on the help of a hard-working, efficient nurse. Through a cooperative and trusting relationship, the care delivered to your patients can be greatly enhanced. With this in mind, do not underestimate the physician-nurse relationship—it can make your practice as family physician much more enjoyable.

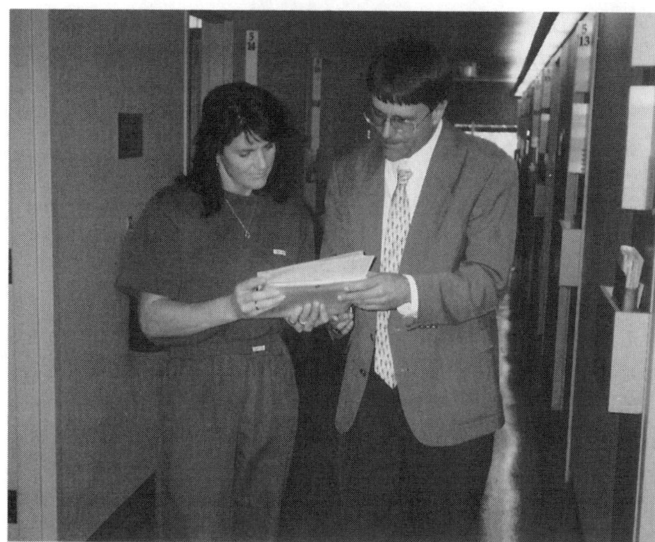

FIGURE 4-8
One of the most important relationships for family physicians is their relationship with their nurse.

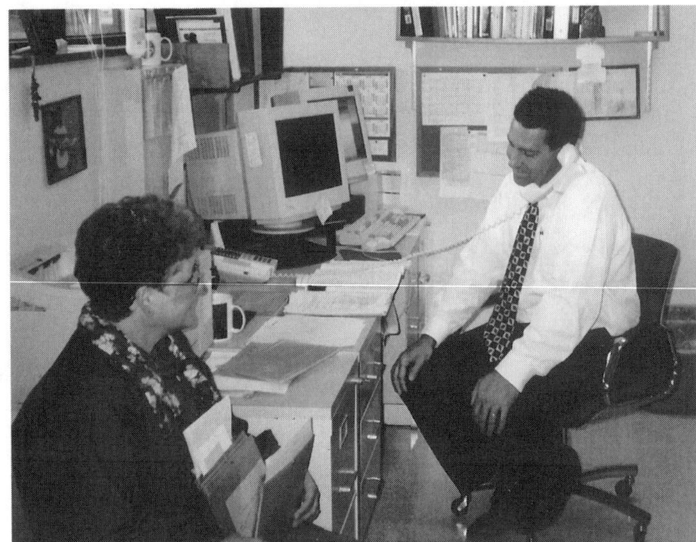

FIGURE 4-9
Interactions with insurance providers can often translate to multiple telephone calls to obtain approval for further tests or consultations.

FAMILY PHYSICIAN—INSURANCE COMPANY RELATIONSHIPS

In the years to come, family physicians and their staffs will have to interact more and more with insurance carriers. Unfortunately, this is often a time-consuming and unpleasant task, but one that must be undertaken for patients to receive appropriate care (Fig. 4-9). Primary care physicians, including family physicians, have assumed this thankless task. Despite the obvious time requirements, staff resources, and hassles of dealing with carriers that may not be agreeable to a plan of care, the family physician must remain dedicated to provide the best care to each individual patient. Through government and specialty influence, unnecessary hassles will, hopefully, be avoidable, and physicians will be justly compensated for their efforts. But this job will not be an easy one. A positive attitude, patience, and understanding from physicians, patients, and insurance providers may help the transition. This is not a trend that is likely to go away in the near future; therefore, we must adapt in the best way we can and in a way that does not jeopardize the care of our patients.

FAMILY PHYSICIAN—FAMILY RELATIONSHIP

In providing good care to your patients, interacting with specialists, dealing with insurance companies and managed care, and working on hospital committees and community organizations, it is easy to have so much demand for time and attention that you may find it difficult to give enough to your own family. Your nuclear and extended family are probably your most important relationship, so save some of yourself for them.

CONCLUSIONS

Family physicians have a complex role in the delivery of medical care. The physicians' service and influence affect not only the patients but the entire community. Family physicians *can* and *do* make a difference.

SELECTING THE RIGHT FAMILY MEDICINE RESIDENCY PROGRAM

5

Sandra L. Argenio, M.D.

The selection of a residency program may be one of the most important career decisions made by a physician. Other aspects of the resident's life often stop for the vigorous demands of residency. The resident's closest friends become colleagues as they search for support in often new surroundings (Fig. 5-1). Many are uprooted from their hometowns and families, and many eventually practice in the general location of their residency program. Without a doubt, the 3 years spent in residency training are among the most formative years in both the medical and professional development of a family physician because they provide the educational foundation on which successful careers are established.

NUMBER OF FAMILY MEDICINE PROGRAMS AND RESIDENTS

Since family medicine became the 20th American medical specialty in 1969, the number of family medicine residency programs has dramatically increased to the present number of 452. In 1996, for the first time, there was a training program in each of the 50 states and in Puerto Rico. Student interest in family medicine has been especially high over the last 5 years. In 1997, more than 10,000 residents were in training in family medicine residency programs. In 1998, more than 2,800 students began family medicine residencies. Despite this influx of bright minds and willing bodies into the specialty, there continues to be a need for well-trained high-quality family physicians. For students who select family medicine residencies, the future offers a wide variety of exciting opportunities.

This chapter reviews many of the important factors that students consider

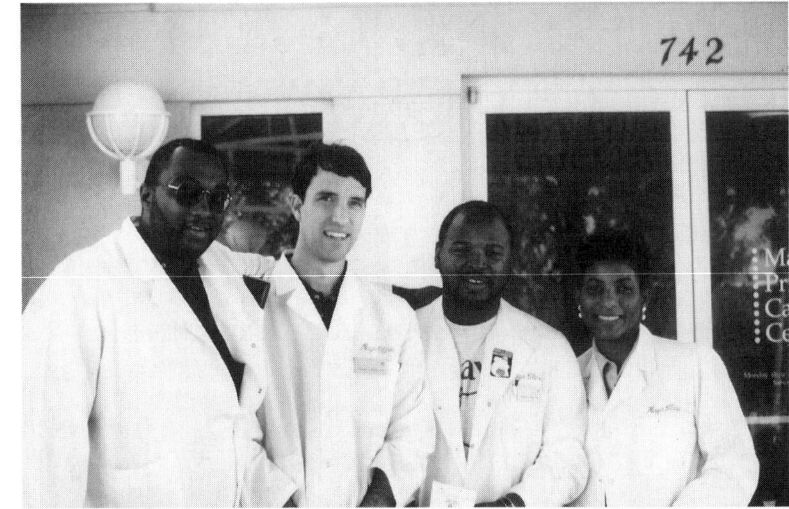

FIGURE 5-1 Lasting relationships often develop among family medicine residents during their training. Therefore, it is important to meet residents during the interview process.

when selecting a residency program. However, it is often a feeling of "the right fit" that leads many students to their final decisions about their future residency programs. Impossible to quantify or describe, this feeling is often a premonition that the student is right for the program and the program is right for the student. After all, the resident will spend the next 3 years in the selected program, and to make life bearable the student must feel comfortable and confident with the decision.

Selecting a family medicine residency is a process that can start early in a student's medical school career. Important factors when selecting a program should include familiarity with a residency program (many students spend a medical school rotation at a residency program); location of the residency program; factors about the program such as practice setting (urban or suburban), educational setting (university or community), and size and number of residency programs at the training site. Other aspects include demographics of the patient population, resources available to the resident, number of residents in training, and the applicant's interactions with residents in a prospective program.

> *"The glory of medicine is that it is constantly moving forward, that there is always more to learn."*
>
> —William J. Mayo

RESOURCES FOR MEDICAL STUDENTS

Students can gather needed information about family medicine residency programs from many resources. A visit to the office of the dean of the medical school can often supply a student with basic information about medical specialties and residencies (Fig. 5-2). The American Academy of Family Practice publishes *The Directory of Family Practice Residency Programs* each year as a service to medical students seeking careers in family practice. The directory supplies significant information about each residency program, including location, size, curriculum and call schedules, salaries, and benefits. The directory is available from the American Academy of Family Practice (telephone: 1-800-944-0000). An online version is available

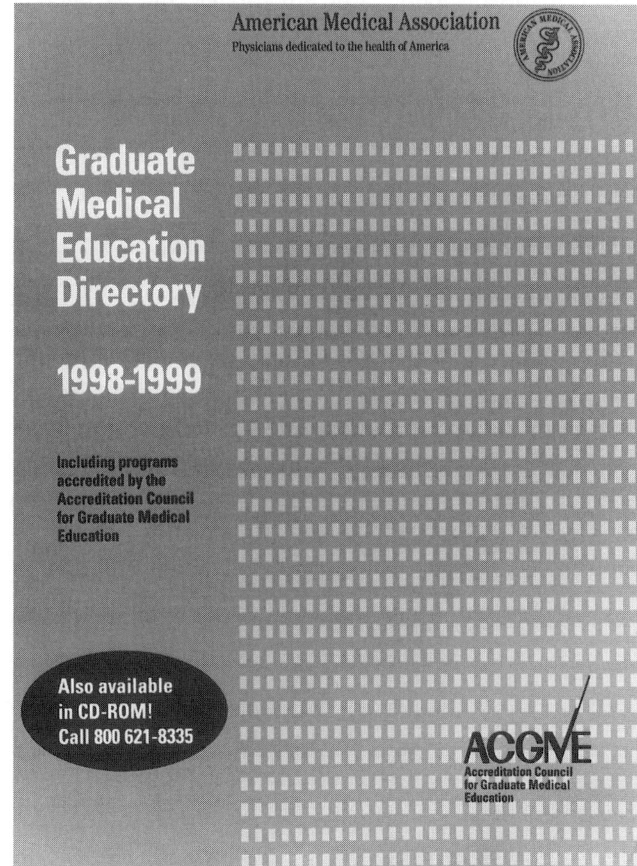

FIGURE 5-2
The Graduate Medical Education Directory is published by the American Medical Association. This resource describes in detail various aspects of each accredited residency program. Students are encouraged to use this resource when selecting a residency program. (From American Medical Association: Graduate Medical Education Directory. Chicago, American Medical Association, 1998. By permission of the publisher.)

on the American Academy of Family Practice's World Wide Web site: http://www.aafp.org/residencies/website.html. Students also can obtain information about family practice training from the Society of Teachers of Family Medicine.

Most medical schools now have their own Department of Family Medicine. The Chair and faculty members in these departments are excellent sources of information about residency programs. They often have personal knowledge and contacts in many family medicine residency programs. In addition, over the last several years, medical students themselves have become one of the best sources of information for those interested in family practice. Many medical schools have active Student Family Medicine interest organizations. These student organizations often sponsor recruitment fairs or dinners to which they invite residents and faculty from many of the family medicine residency programs in their state or region. These activities provide excellent opportunities for students to learn about family medicine and to interact with representatives of residency programs at which they may later interview.

MEETINGS THAT INVOLVE FAMILY PRACTICE PROGRAMS

National meetings also offer information concerning residency programs. The American Academy of Family Practice sponsors the National Conference of Family Practice Residents and Medical Students in Kansas City each summer. This meeting offers a great opportunity for students to interact with residents and faculty from all over the country. This meeting also provides many opportunities for students to become involved in family medicine projects and activities. Many state chapters of the American Academy of Family Practice also sponsor similar activities. In addition, the American Academy of Family Practice hosts a national scientific assembly and convention every fall. Each year the convention is held at a different location and offers the medical student the opportunity to review various residency programs that are represented there.

"The mere possession of a diploma does not endow one with extraordinary knowledge on all possible medical subjects."

—William J. Mayo

FACTORS THAT SHOULD BE CONSIDERED

Once the student has begun to narrow down the choice of residency programs to a few sites, the best way to evaluate a program is to do a rotation at that

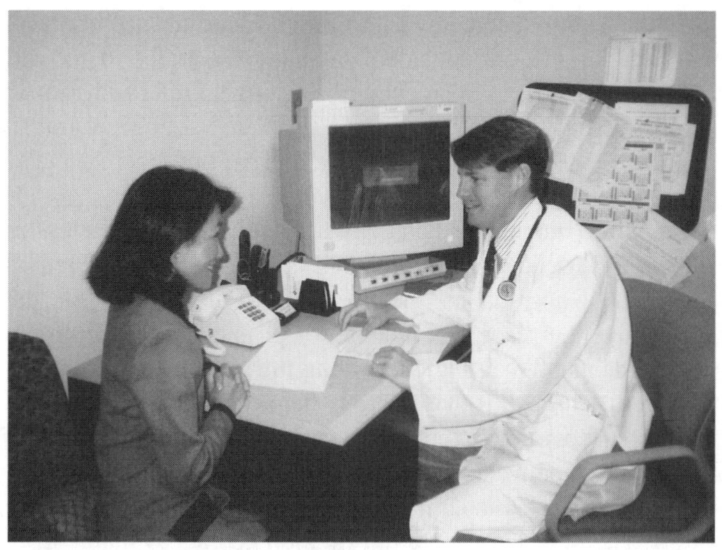

FIGURE 5-3
Resident applicants are interviewed by staff and resident physicians. Applicants and programs are then ranked, and a computer process determines where the applicant will be a resident.

site. Most family medicine residency programs are eager to accept students on required and elective rotations and consider a rotation to be the best way for them to evaluate a student's potential as a future resident in their program. This approach may help solidify a student's choice by allowing the experience of the actual "day in and day out" routine of the residency training program.

In the fall of the fourth year of medical school, students begin their interview process. After completing the application process, if invited, the student travels to the site of the residency program. Costs of travel are usually the responsibility of the student, but many programs will pay for lodging. Careful planning must be followed to receive permission for absence while interviewing. Most students interview at 5 to 10 programs (Fig. 5-3). The first consideration is often location of the program. Students may choose a specific area of the country or an area where they think they may eventually wish to practice. Family medicine residency programs are located in all areas of the country: in inner-city, urban, suburban, or rural locations. An individual residency program may offer experiences in several different environments. The prospective family medicine resident has a wide variety of choices when it comes to selecting a residency program.

Family medicine residency programs are located in various medical structures or settings. Some programs are based in community hospitals and may be the only residency program in the hospital. Other programs are located in large universities where there may be a wide variety of other residency and fellowship programs. Many programs are located at community hospitals and are affiliated with or administered by a university. There are also military-based programs. Students should consider whether they prefer to be in a setting where the family medicine residency is the only training program or whether they prefer to interact with residents in other training programs. The various advantages and disadvantages to the presence of other specialty residents should be explored at the interviews.

Programs differ in the number of hospitals or family practice centers in which the residents experience their training. For instance, the obstetrics rotation may occur at a hospital on the west side of town whereas the pediatrics rotation may take place at a hospital or physician's office on the east side of town. Students often ask about driving time involved in traveling between training sites. Although it may seem to be more convenient to have all activity at one site, most practicing physicians and residents in training actually do have to travel between their offices and hospitals.

Information about rotations and call schedules should be reviewed at the student's interview. The most up-to-date information is often available from the residents currently enrolled in the residency program. As mentioned previously, this information is summarized for all programs in the American Academy of Family Practice's *Directory of Family Practice Residency Programs* and should be reviewed before selecting a residency site. Other factors that may relate to the educational experience include lecture schedules, ratio of faculty to residents, size of the training program, resident research, and medical student rotations at the residency. Students should review salaries and benefits provided by the programs they are considering.

> *''Let there be education in medicine commensurate to instruction; let the young physician be sound in the fundamentals, so that he may see his problem as it is, and his duty to himself, his patients and the science of medicine.''*
>
> —Charles H. Mayo

Actual selection of a first-year position in a residency program almost always proceeds through the National Residency Matching Program (Fig. 5-4), also known as ''the Match.'' At the end of the third year of medical school, students should start to gather information about residency programs as well as schedule dean's letter appointments and request letters of recommendation from medical school faculty members with whom they have worked. Important dates for the Match process can be obtained from the National Residency Matching Program. Applications and letters of recommendation should be sent between July and November of the fourth year

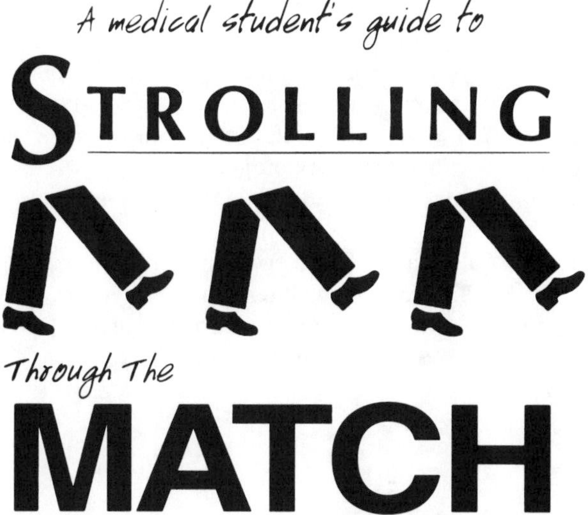

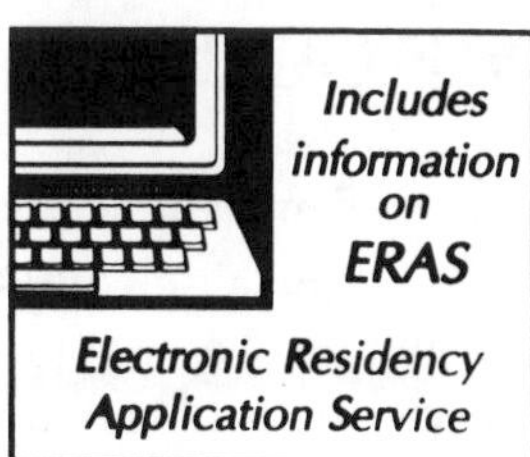

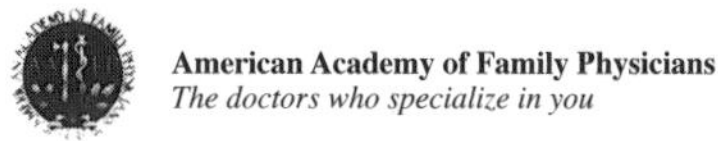

FIGURE 5-4
The American Academy of Family Physicians publishes this guide to assist medical students in their task of applying to family medicine residency programs. (From American Academy of Family Physicians: A Medical Student's Guide to Strolling Through the Match: the What, Where, When, Why, and How of Residency Selection. Kansas City, Missouri, American Academy of Family Physicians, 1997. By permission of the publisher.)

of medical school. Dean's letters are sent to the selected residency programs by November 1. Interviews at residency programs usually occur between November and January of the student's fourth year. Most programs require only 1 day of interviews, during which the student will meet the Program Director and many of the faculty and residents. The student will receive a tour of the Family Medicine Center, the hospital, and often the community. Although most programs do not require a second interview, some students may wish to return to their top choices to gather more information about the residency or the community. Following the interview process, students submit ranked lists to the National Residency Matching Program in February. Students (and programs) must wait patiently until mid-March when the Match results are announced. Students are committed to the program with which they match for at least 1 year, so it is important for students to list only programs where they think they would want to train.

BOX 5-1 TIPS ON SELECTING A RESIDENCY PROGRAM

1. Review important details concerning the program (e.g., salary, call schedule, ratio of staff to residents, facilities).
2. Discuss strengths and weaknesses of the program with residents who are currently enrolled in that program.
3. Contact the residency director and inquire about the program well in advance of your interview.
4. Arrange a rotation at or a visit to the program in which you are most interested.
5. Review the community and location of the residency program.
6. Involve family, spouse, or significant other in making your choice.
7. Try to meet all staff and residents associated with a residency program.
8. Make sure residency is accredited by the Residency Review Committee.
9. Research if residency program has had problems matching all residency slots—if so, why?
10. Make sure you feel comfortable and welcomed by residents and staff.

ELECTRONIC RESIDENCY APPLICATION SERVICE

In 1997, for the first time students applied for residency programs by using the Electronic Residency Application Service. This is a computer-based program designed to transmit residency applications, letters of recommendations, dean's letters, transcripts, personal statements, photographs, and National Board of Medical Examiners or U.S. Medical Licensure Examination scores to each residency program via the internet (http://www.aamc.org/about/progemph/eras).

BOX 5-2 INTERVIEW TIPS

1. Dress professionally
2. Research program before interview
3. Ask intelligent questions, avoid controversy
4. Maintain eye contact
5. Maintain good posture
6. Make sure shoes are polished
7. Smile
8. Focus on positive aspects of the program and positive aspects of your curriculum vitae
9. Be personable
10. Remain relaxed
11. Be honest
12. Address staff and residents by name
13. Allow interviewer to conduct interview and ask you questions. Ask your questions at appropriate times
14. Share a personal experience if appropriate
15. Be courteous to other candidates
16. Make follow-up calls to residency director and write thank-you letters to those with whom you interviewed

Students complete their applications on student workstation data disks, specify the residencies to which they are applying, and deliver the disks to the medical school dean's office. Because the application process is centralized, most students find the Electronic Residency Application Service program more convenient and less cumbersome to use.

CONCLUSIONS

For many students, the road to the family medicine residency starts early in their medical school careers. Many students bring a desire to be a family physician from their early childhood years. Other students may not make their decisions until early in their fourth year of medical school. For all students, however, the selection of a residency program will have a major impact on their personal and professional futures. The factors discussed in this chapter will help students narrow the choice of programs. For most students, the final decision is made by a general feeling about where they will be able to get the best educational preparation for their future careers and where they will be the happiest.

SUGGESTED READINGS

American Academy of Family Physicians: *Facts About: Family Practice.* Kansas City, Missouri, American Academy of Family Physicians, 1997

American Academy of Family Physicians: Directors' Newsletter. Mar. 19, 1998

American Academy of Family Physicians: *The Directory of Family Practice Residency Programs.* Kansas City, Missouri, American Academy of Family Physicians, 1998

Career Insights M.D.: *The Medical Student's Guide to Residencies,* vol 5. New York, Career Publications, pp 137–139, 146–148, 1996

Mandel LP et al: One residency's experience with the Electronic Residency Application Service. Fam Med 29:209, 1997

6

FAMILY MEDICINE RESIDENCY ROTATIONS

Matthew E. Bernard, M.D.

This chapter concentrates on the curriculum components of family medicine residency programs. The 3-year curriculum is arranged into various rotations making up the basic foundation of knowledge and includes general medicine, pediatrics, obstetrics and gynecology, psychiatry, general surgery, and various other fields of medicine to accomplish the requirements set forth by the American Medical Association's Accreditation Council for Graduate Medical Education (ACGME) Residency Review Committee. Over 3 years, family medicine residents are required to rotate through various specialty rotations. Family medicine residency programs take advantage of staff members from various departments and the unique training experience each department offers. At the end of the rotation, the resident should possess a basic knowledge of how to diagnose and treat common illnesses that are likely to be seen in a family physician's office.

BLOCK VERSUS LONGITUDINAL ROTATIONS

In general terms, there are 2 ways to accomplish the family practice curriculum components: block rotation and longitudinal experience. A block rotation (eg, internal medicine, pediatrics, obstetrics, critical care unit) consists of a rotation that ranges from 2 weeks to 3 months and is done at specific times during the 3 years (Box 6-1). Longitudinal experiences are done in small increments throughout the 3 years of the residency. Both block rotations and longitudinal rotations are typically used throughout the family medicine residency training program.

BOX 6-1 PROGRAM DESCRIPTION

You will gain invaluable experience with outpatient continuity of care at the Family Medicine center by caring for your own group of patients throughout the 3-year program. As a first-year resident, you must attend the family practice clinic a minimum of 1 half-day per week. As a second-year resident, the minimum increases to 2 half-days per week. During your third year, the minimum is 3 half-days per week. You will receive on-site supervision and teaching from the Family Medicine faculty.

ROTATION SCHEDULE	MONTHS
First Year	
Family Medicine Inpatient	2
Internal Medicine Inpatient	2
Intensive Care Unit or Cardiac Care Unit	1
Emergency Department	1
Pediatrics Inpatient	2
Obstetrics and Gynecology	2
General Surgery	2
Second Year	
Family Medicine Inpatient	2
Neurology	1
Cardiology	1
Gastroenterology	1
Newborn Nursery and General Pediatrics	1
Pediatrics Emergency Department	1
Gynecology Outpatient	1
Orthopedics Outpatient	1
Psychiatry and Psychology Outpatient	2
Third Year	
Family Medicine Inpatient	2
Community Medicine	1
Pediatrics Outpatient	2
Dermatology	1
Ophthalmology	0.5 to 1
Otorhinolaryngology	0.5 to 1
Urology	0.5 to 1
Electives	3.5 to 4.5

ROTATIONS

To accomplish the required curricular components set forth by the Residency Review Committee, it is necessary to have both inpatient and outpatient rotations. The following describes each required curricular component and the amount of time required in each area. Whether each of the curricular areas is done in the outpatient or inpatient setting or in longitudinal or block rotation depends on each program's unique approach to the family medicine curriculum. The following areas are required to successfully complete an accredited family residency program.

Adult Medicine

Training in this area during residency must allow the resident to acquire the knowledge and skills necessary for the diagnosis, nonsurgical treatment, and management of diseases affecting female and male adults. The Residency Review Committee sets a minimum of 8 months of experience in adult medicine. Of this 8 months, 6 months must be in the inpatient hospital setting. The inpatient experience is accomplished on either a family medicine or internal medicine service and in some cases, both. In addition, there must be a 1-month experience or its equivalent in both the critical care arena and cardiology. The curriculum must also incorporate subspecialties of adult medicine (eg, rheumatology, gastroenterology, oncology, endocrinology) in the training experience. This is one of the major areas in the education of family physicians. The resident is expected to gain an understanding of the diagnosis and treatment of medical conditions that affect adult patients.

> *"While medicine is a science, in many particulars it cannot be exact, so baffling are the varying results of varying conditions of human life."*
>
> —Charles H. Mayo

Pediatrics

Training in pediatric principles is completed in both ambulatory pediatric clinics and inpatient experiences. There must be at least 4 months of pediatric experience (Fig. 6-1). Principles to be covered include common illnesses as well as surgical problems in pediatrics. In addition, the family medicine resident also has a longitudinal pediatric experience as pediatric patients are followed in the family practice outpatient clinic. In some programs, pediatric

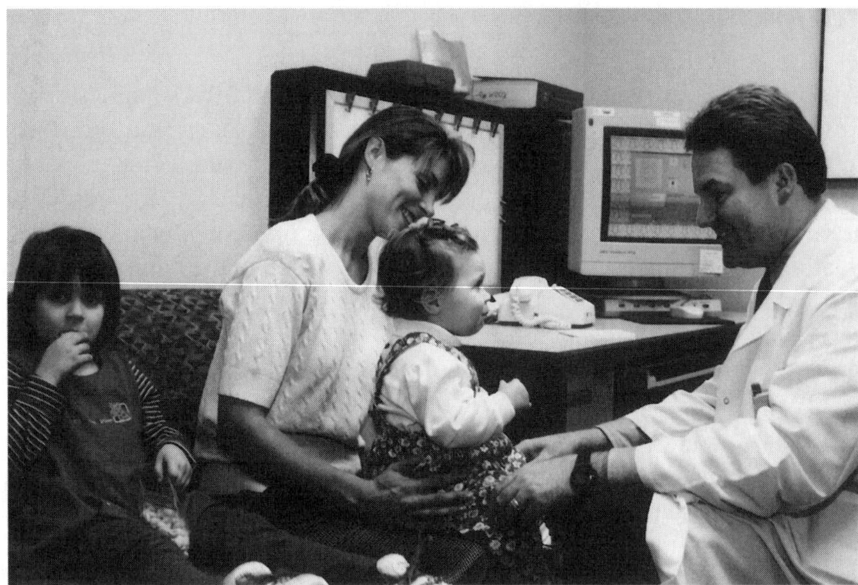

FIGURE 6-1
Comprehensive care, which may involve multiple fields of medicine, is a hallmark of residency training in family medicine.

patients are also cared for by the family practice inpatient hospital service. Newborn care is also an important aspect of the pediatric experience.

Obstetrics and Gynecology

To fulfill the requirements involving obstetrical care, the residency experience must include teaching in the areas of pregnancy, delivery, and care of the newborn. The minimum requirement is 2 months of experience in these areas. Residents are expected to care for pregnant patients through delivery, which provides for a longitudinal experience over the course of 3 years of residency. There also must be training in genetic counseling. In addition, each residency program is required to make available additional training in maternity care during the 3-year curriculum to any resident who may have a special interest in obstetrics.

In the area of gynecologic care, a total of 140 hours that focus on women's health issues must be incorporated into the curriculum during the 3 years of residency. This area of the curriculum covers the areas of normal growth and development, menopause, sexually transmitted diseases, fertility, and human sexuality.

Human Behavior and Mental Health

Training in this area is done by integrating behavioral science and psychiatric knowledge and skills throughout the residency period. There must be instruction in all ages in the areas of sexual orientation and cultural differences. In addition, psychopharmacology, alcohol abuse, and substance abuse must be incorporated into the family medicine curriculum. Other areas of this curriculum that must be addressed are domestic violence and medical ethics. In many programs, this training is accomplished through block and longitudinal experiences. Residents may rotate through psychiatry and in addition treat patients on an ongoing basis as outpatients in the Family Practice Clinic.

Care of the Surgical Patient

The family medicine curriculum must teach residents principles in the perioperative care of the surgical patient. This instruction includes diagnosis of surgical emergencies, appropriate and timely referrals of surgical cases for specialized care, principles of presurgical assessment of patients, and postoperative care of the patient. The following are requirements in each of the surgical areas.

General Surgery There is a 2-month requirement in general surgery, including ambulatory and operating room experience. The resident should gain competency in performing simple office surgery (eg, removal of cysts and lesions) and assisting in major surgery.

Orthopedic Disorders A minimum of 140 hours experience in the care of orthopedic disorders must be covered during the 3 years. It is expected that this curriculum will be accomplished through the use of didactic conferences and clinical experiences that focus on common orthopedic problems (eg, reduction of simple fractures, casting, aspiration of joints) encountered by family physicians.

Surgical Subspecialties In addition, there must be experiences incorporated into the curriculum for disorders of the genitourinary tract (urology); eye (ophthalmology); and ear, nose, and throat (otorhinolaryngology). The resident will be expected to learn the diagnosis and management of problems commonly encountered by family physicians.

"It is unfortunate that so few appreciate from what small causes diseases come."

—Charles H. Mayo

Care of the Elderly Patient

Care of the geriatric patient is accomplished in the family medicine center, long-term nursing care facility, home, and hospital. All areas of care, including physical and psychological issues of the geriatric patient, must be included. Residents may participate in home visits during their geriatric rotation.

Community Medicine

Residents are taught during the 3 years to assess and understand the important health needs of the community in which they work. Areas to be covered include occupational medicine, employee health, public health, community service agencies available for patient help, disease prevention, and healthy lifestyles. Many programs offer a clinical experience with indigent patients, which allows the resident to treat patients who have limited access to health care.

"The examining physician often hesitates to make the necessary examination because it involves soiling the finger."

—William J. Mayo

Emergency Care

Requirements for emergency care include a 1-month block rotation in the delivery of emergency care. There must be adequate patient volume and supervision to ensure adequate exposure to common emergencies. In addition, it is recommended that all standard life-support skills (cardiopulmonary resuscitation, advanced cardiac life support, advanced trauma life support) and procedures for both trauma and medical emergencies be incorporated into this curriculum.

Dermatology

It is expected that the bulk of the dermatology education occurs in the outpatient setting. Residents are taught to properly diagnose and treat skin conditions and skin cancer as well as office procedures. There must be at least 60 hours spent in this area.

Sports Medicine

Sports medicine principles must be incorporated into the 3-year curriculum. The curriculum components are accomplished through didactic conferences, seminars, and clinical experiences. In many residency programs, the resident will have the opportunity to work with a local high school or college athletic team.

Radiology

Residency programs must give residents in training an opportunity to learn the principles and correct cost-effective use of diagnostic imaging and nuclear medicine therapy. Residents will learn the basics of reading chest radiographs, plain films, computed tomographic scans, and magnetic resonance images.

Practice Management

Family medicine residents are taught the importance of finances in medicine in didactic lectures and in the family practice clinic. Such areas as personal finance, office and personnel management, managed care, and professional liability should be covered during the 3 years.

Electives

A minimum of 3 months and maximum of 6 months may be allocated for residents to do elective rotations. The variety of electives will be affected by the available resources of the program. Some programs allow residents to travel to rural areas or abroad to participate in their desired rotation.

Evaluations

The content of a family medicine residency program's curriculum is evaluated continually to determine that the educational experience is beneficial for the resident and that the goals and objectives are being met. Evaluations of residents in training by supervising faculty are generally done after completion of each block rotation. In the case of longitudinal experiences, evaluations are done on a regular basis, which is generally quarterly to biannually. A sample evaluation form for residents in training covers specific areas of performance (Fig. 6-2).

FAMILY MEDICINE RESIDENT EVALUATION FORM

_____ **Check if you did not work with this Resident.**

	Unsatisfactory			**Satisfactory**			**Superior**		
	F	**D**	**C**	**B-**	**B**	**B+**	**A-**	**A**	**A+**
History & Exam Skills	1	2	3	4	5	6	7	8	9
Procedural Competence	1	2	3	4	5	6	7	8	9
Fund of Knowledge	1	2	3	4	5	6	7	8	9
Case Presentation	1	2	3	4	5	6	7	8	9
Organization & Synthesis: Ability to formulate differential diagnosis	1	2	3	4	5	6	7	8	9
Patient Management/Attention to Detail	1	2	3	4	5	6	7	8	9
Clinical Judgment; Ability to choose diagnostic studies	1	2	3	4	5	6	7	8	9
Reading/Self-directed Learning	1	2	3	4	5	6	7	8	9
Professional Relationships with Colleagues (Attitude)	1	2	3	4	5	6	7	8	9
Professional Relationships with Patients and Families (Compassion, empathy, communication skills)	1	2	3	4	5	6	7	8	9
OVERALL CLINICAL COMPETENCE	**1**	**2**	**3**	**4**	**5**	**6**	**7**	**8**	**9**

Length of Exposure ____________________ Resident's Workload: Heavy _____ Average _____ Light _____

Your evaluation should be discussed with the resident. Was this done? Yes _____ No _____
Please take a moment to fill in your comments. They are EXTREMELY valuable to our grading system.

Resident's Strengths:

Areas for Improvement:

____
Signature of Physician Completing Evaluation

____
Signature of Family Medicine Advisor

____
Signature of Resident

A

FIGURE 6-2
Family Medicine Resident Evaluation Form.

Unsatisfactory	**Satisfactory**	**Superior**
1 2 3	**4 5 6**	**7 8 9**
Low Descriptors		**High Descriptors**

History and Exam Skills

Low	High
Needs work on acquiring, recording, analyzing database. Unable to demonstrate basic skills of interviewing and of physical examination appropriate for level of training.	Database and assessment skills outstanding. Extremely thorough but highly efficient. Demonstrates mastery of exam skills; performs far in advance of training level.

Procedural Competence

Low	High
Unable to demonstrate basic skills appropriate for level of training. Disregard for risk to patient and patient's anxiety and comfort.	Demonstrates mastery of procedural skills. Minimizes risk and discomfort to patients. Provides proper explanation of the purpose of the procedure.

Fund of Knowledge

Low	High
Limited, fragmented, poorly organized and applied. Inadequate knowledge of medical principles and pathophysiology related to patient's problems.	Shows superior knowledge of the basic medical principles related to patient's problems. Consistently up to date.

Verbal Case Presentation

Low	High
Inaccurate, disorganized, incomplete and/or verbose.	Accurate, organized, and succinct.

Organization and Synthesis

Low	High
Has difficulty identifying key problems. Poor ability to formulate differential diagnosis. Demonstrates little independence.	Identifies major and minor problems in perspective. Superior grasp of information.

Patient Management

Low	High
Overreliance on tests and procedures. Incomplete therapeutic plans. Misses major problems. Fails to monitor case appropriately.	Appropriately monitors and modifies management. Attention to detail. Very efficient use of lab and other services.

Clinical Judgment

Low	High
Often fails to consider risks and benefits. Is unaware of limitations of knowledge and skills. Frequently uses diagnostic procedures or therapies inappropriately. Indecisive in difficult management situations.	Weighs alternatives, understands limitations of knowledge, and incorporates consideration of costs, risks, and benefits. Wise use of diagnostic and therapeutic procedures. Reasons well in ambiguous situations.

Initiative/Self-Directed Learning

Low	High
Not well motivated. Avoids "doing" when possible. Appears disinterested. Never volunteers. Little evidence of independent reading.	Works exceptionally hard. Active leader/participant. Seeks new learning experiences. Reads and discusses literature.

Professional Relationships with Physicians

Low	High
Behavior interferes with satisfactory performance. Discourteous to nurses and other support staff. Hostile or uncooperative. Poorly receptive to constructive criticism.	Works very well with others. Consistently courteous. Has admiration and respect for coworkers. Gives clear and appropriate information. Accepts constructive criticism.

Relationships with Patients and Families

Low	High
Often discourteous and/or nonempathic with patients. Puts personal convenience above patient's needs.	Consistently courteous and empathic. Gives patient's needs priority even with unpleasant or hostile patients. Educates patients and families; keeps them regularly informed.

B

Advisors

In most residency programs, each resident is assigned an advisor at the start of residency training. The advisor is available for the resident to seek input regarding the electives chosen and serves as a confidant if problems or questions arise. In addition, the advisor may serve as an important mentor who may set an example for the resident to follow during the 3 years of residency training.

Conclusions

The 3-year family medicine residency is a structured program that draws information and teaching from many specialty areas. The goal of the family practice resident should be to master the diagnosis and treatment of medical problems with which patients present to the family physician's office. Family physicians are often the first medical resource the patient encounters. It is important to be competent in managing common medical illnesses and making proper referral when necessary.

7

WEEKLY OUTPATIENT CLINICS

Halina Woroncow, M.D.

The focal point of the family practice residency is the weekly outpatient clinic. This is the "primary setting for training in the knowledge, skills, and attitudes of family practice . . ."[1] Here we develop a panel of patient families whom we come to know over the 3 years of residency. What helps make family practice so intellectually stimulating is that we see these patients for such a broad array of health care needs. These patients could be seen for routine health maintenance, prenatal care, childhood immunizations, tobacco cessation counseling, psychiatric issues, orthopedic procedures, lesion excision, flexible sigmoidoscopy, or geriatric assessment—to name just a few possibilities! Over 3 years, the resident physician acts as an educator, counselor, and confidant as well as the occasional broker of bad news. The outpatient clinics allow us not only to grow in skills and technical expertise but also to mature as interpreters of human behavior. We deal with the psychosocial aspects of the human experience in the clinic on a daily basis. Our skills are honed with each patient interaction.

> *"There are lots of people who think they are sick and who are not sick."*
>
> —Charles H. Mayo

LOGISTICS

The clinic is a full-service practice setting and thus includes diagnostic laboratory and imaging services (a wonderful source of review in microscopy and radiology), an office library, adequate examining rooms to ensure efficient patient flow, resident work space, and office space that can be used for counseling, conferences, or other educational experiences (Box 7-1). The clinic will be reasonably close to the hospital to minimize travel time to and from inpatient rotations. The American Medical Association's Accreditation Council for Graduate Medical Education (ACGME) Residency Review Committee requires that the outpatient clinic be ''appropriately staffed with nurses, technicians, clerks, and administrative . . . personnel to ensure efficiency and adequate support for patient care and educational needs.''[1] The patient population should represent a broad spectrum of problems for the resident to manage. Naturally, the physical location of the clinic (ie, urban, suburban, or rural) with its surrounding community provides a different set of patient experiences for physicians in different clinical sites (Fig. 7-2). You will need to consider this as you commit yourself to a practice site. The ''flavor'' of each clinic varies with its demographics; however, the challenges of patient care in any setting provide rich educational opportunities for the resident and experienced family physician.

PATIENT CONTACT

In the first year, the family practice resident spends 1 half-day a week in the clinic; in the second year, 2 half-days a week; and in the third year, 3 to 5 half-days a week. Outpatient elective months throughout the residency may allow additional time in the clinic. Although initial patients may present with acute concerns (upper respiratory infections, ear pain, urinary tract infections), these visits serve as an opportunity to review health maintenance needs and ''acquire'' patients who do not have an identified primary physician. I'll never forget a patient who presented for evaluation of a sore throat, but who, on review, was overdue for a mammogram. The mammogram was arranged as a result of that acute visit, and her early-stage breast cancer was diagnosed and treated. She's a 3-year survivor of breast cancer at the time of this writing.

> *''It must be remembered that physicians of today are trained to treat the sick, and they must learn how to examine so-called well persons to prevent them from getting sick.''*
>
> —Charles H. Mayo

Often, one goes on to ''adopt'' family members as well—from siblings to grandparents—to provide true cross-generational care. Meeting family members, of course, deepens the physician's understanding of the psychosocial structure from which any patient presents with physical complaints.

BOX 7-1 JOURNAL CLUB

Every month most family practice residency programs hold a journal club at a staff member's home or a local restaurant. The meetings are usually held at night, and in some cases a pharmaceutical company may provide food or snacks. The purpose of journal club is to review recent journal articles or topics of interest (Fig. 7-1). In most cases residents will present an article taken from a major medical journal (*New England Journal of Medicine, Journal of the American Medical Association,* or the *American Family Physician*). Residents often select articles of interest or perhaps related to a recent patient. The meetings allow for a relaxed environment to discuss relevant medical topics that add to the residents' and staff members' knowledge base. A good tip to remember is to present an article relevant to the family practice. Don't select in-depth articles taken from subspecialty journals unless there is a specific topic or point you would like to cover. In most cases, these types of articles may be boring or overembellished with facts that family physicians are not interested in. Always make sure your presentations are clinically relevant. Topics may be selected from *Journal Watch,* a publication that reviews specific articles that are deemed important by a board to the medical community as a whole. Always remember when presenting an article to focus on 2 to 3 important points made by the article—any more will be easily forgotten. Handouts summarizing the important points are often helpful. If you have questions regarding a specific presentation, it may be helpful to discuss your plans with your residency director. Always approach journal club as a means to broaden your educational base in a relaxed environment.

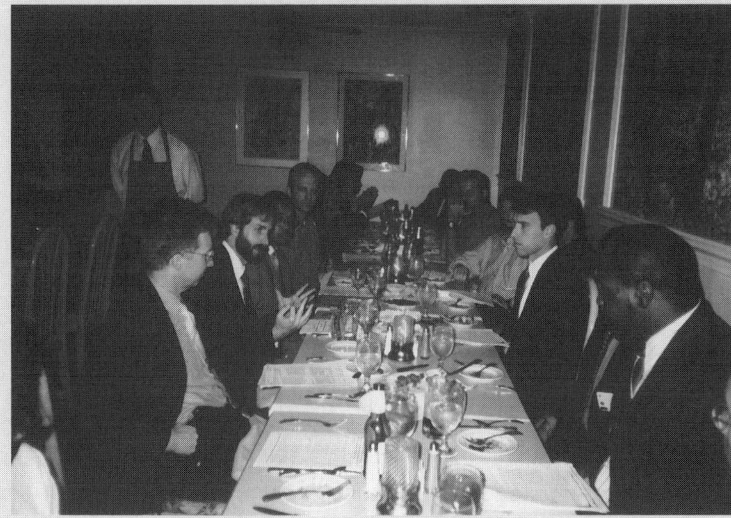

FIGURE 7-1 Journal club allows staff and residents to gather outside of the clinic or hospital to discuss journal articles of interest.

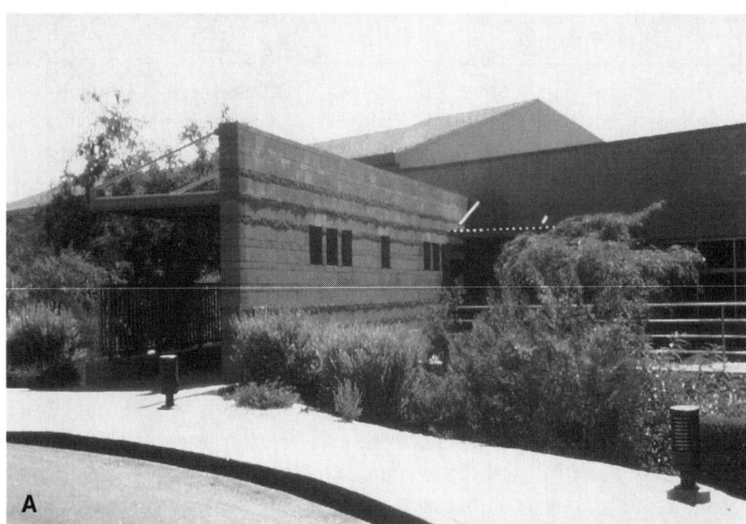

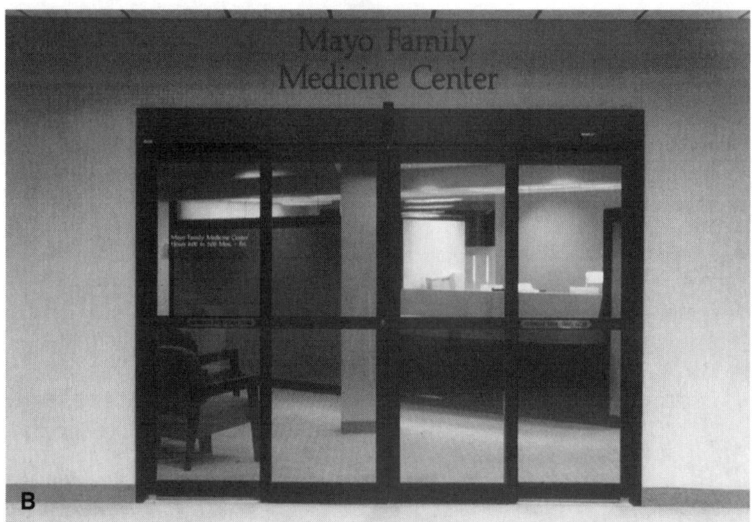

FIGURE 7-2
A. *The Thunderbird Primary Care Clinic at Mayo Clinic Scottsdale is the site where the majority of outpatient teaching takes place for family medicine residents.* B. *Family Practice Outpatient Clinic, Mayo Clinic Jacksonville, where the bulk of training takes place for family medicine residents.*

Family practice is the business of providing continuing, comprehensive medical care. I have several patients whom I cared for as a resident and whom I continue to see today. Once you are identified as an individual's primary care provider, your patient might contact you by phone or at the office for anything from advice for a cold, to questions regarding press coverage of medical issues, to health maintenance needs and medication refills. You might be asked to help facilitate visiting nurse home care for an elderly patient or to do actual house calls yourself. You could be asked

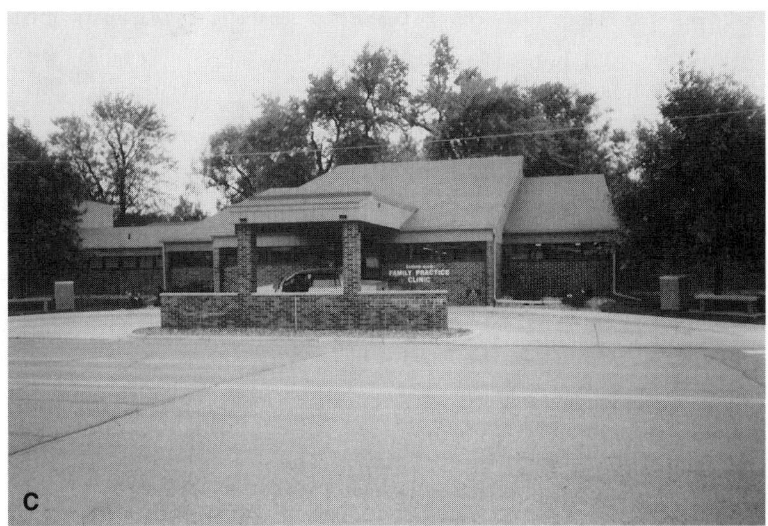

FIGURE 7-2 continued
C. *The Kasson Clinic, located 20 miles west of Rochester, has a small-town, community-based setting that allows family medicine residents to care for their patients with a multitude of services available.*

to certify a child to be fit for school sports or to confirm that a debilitated patient meets criteria for a handicapped sticker for a car. The family physician becomes the primary contact for the family's ongoing medical needs. This requires that the patient have continuing access to medical advice, even when the outpatient clinic is not open. Your residency program will have a plan for handling patient calls after hours.

THE CLINICAL RECORD

All office visits are recorded in a patient chart. This enhances patient care because the physician has readily available the patient's medical history, current list of medications, drug allergies, and reports of recent visits, phone calls, and medication refills. An up-to-date record is particularly important for elderly patients, who are often on complicated, multidrug regimens for their multiple health problems and may not recall the names and doses of their medications. With incomplete information, one could easily stumble into an unwanted drug interaction that could be deleterious to the patient. Clear documentation of prescribed controlled substances (eg, narcotic analgesics) is likewise imperative to help identify any inappropriate, drug-seeking behavior among the patient population.

Some physicians also use flow sheets in their charts to keep track of recommended health maintenance schedules: in diabetes management (Fig.

Diabetes Diabetes Diabetes Diabetes Diabetes Diabetes Diabetes Diabetes Diabetes

No. ____________________

Diabetes Flow Sheet
Kasson Mayo Family Practice Clinic

mayo Sheet Number ______

Name ____________________

Suggested Interval	Initial	3 Month	6 Month	9 Month	Annual	3 Month	6 Month	9 Month	Annual	3 Month	6 Month	9 Month
Date												
Complete Hx & Phys												
Weight												
Blood Press												
Oph Exam												
Foot Exam												
Interim Hx & Phys												
Laboratory												
Hb A1c												
Fasting Glucose												
Chol/HDL												
Trig/LDL												
Urinary Microalbumin												
Creatinine												
ECG												
Other												
Dietician												
Diet/Ex												
Insulin												
Oral Agents												

FIGURE 7-3
Diabetes flow sheet.

7-3), to track blood pressure or cholesterol trends, or to easily compare laboratory test values requiring frequent rechecks (eg, the prothrombin time or INR for a patient who is receiving anticoagulant drugs). Childhood preventive services are often recorded on a flow sheet that identifies the currently recommended frequency of well-child visits, heights and weights, immunization schedule, and some prompts regarding age-appropriate safety and guidance issues (Fig. 7-4). Prenatal care can be organized effectively with a flow sheet (Fig. 7-5). Flow sheets can facilitate the physician's ability to efficiently glean specific information about a patient and ensure health care services delivered are consistent with the standard of care. Get to know the forms available in your clinic.

The patient record is a medicolegal document. Discussions regarding treatment options; informed consent for procedures, including review of risks and benefits; or a patient's choice to decline such treatment all need

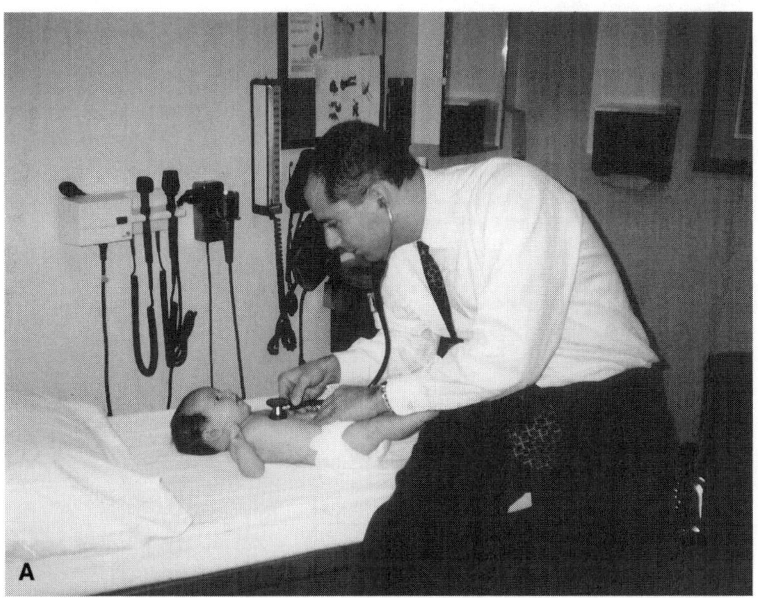

FIGURE 7-4
A. *Well-child visits are an important part of a family physician's practice.*

to be documented. There may be specific work restriction forms that need to be completed and on record in the event of a workers' compensation case. A motor vehicle accident that might be pending litigation obviously requires documentation of a thorough examination and review of appropriate ancillary testing. Alleged physical or sexual abuse cases are among the most emotionally charged visits; however, the examination demands meticulous execution in securing specific physical evidence and providing detailed documentation in the chart for possible use in court. Poor documentation and a sloppy examination can damage a case that might otherwise have deserved legal consideration.

Despite our best efforts to the contrary, any one of us can make a mistake in patient care. We all experience negative patient outcomes at one time or another. The best defense in the case of a poor outcome is a good relationship with the patient, forthright discussion of the outcome, and thorough notes in the chart outlining the physician's clinical thought process throughout. Because court cases may not occur for months to years after an office visit—during which time the details of the patient interaction and physical examination might become understandably blurred in the physician's memory—thorough, timely documentation is key.

(*Continues on page 82*)

Well-Child Record

Primary Medical Care Provider ____________

Mother's Name ____________ Home Phone ____________

Work Place ____________ Work Phone ____________

Father's Name ____________ Home Phone ____________

Work Place ____________ Work Phone ____________

Birthdate: ______ Weight: ______ Height: ______ Head Circumference: ______

Pregnancy and Birth History: ____________

Previous Medical History: ____________

Maternal HBsAg: ☐ Neg ☐ Pos

HBIG ☐ HBV #1 ________ (date)

MN Newborn Screen: ☐ Neg ☐Pos

Water: ☐ City ☐ Well (tested fluoride ________)

Family History: ____________

Single parent: ☐ Adopted: ☐

Siblings: Name / Year of Birth

1. ______ / ____ 2. ______ / ____ 3. ______ / ____

PREVENTIVE HEALTH CARE SCHEDULE

	2 wk	2 mo	4 mo	6 mo	9 mo	15 mo	18 mo	2 yr	3 yr	4 yr	5 yr
Date											
Age											
Measurements											
Weight	%	%	%	%	%	%	%	%	%	%	%
Height	%	%	%	%	%	%	%	%	%	%	%
Head Circumference	%	%	%	%	%	%	%	%	%	%	%
Blood Pressure											
Physical Exam (√ normal, * abn)											
HEENT											
Lungs											
CVS											
Abdomen											
GU											
Skin											
Neuro											
Musculoskeletal											

Development (√ if approp. age or indicate age attained)

90%ile	Personal-Social	Fine Motor	Language	Gross Motor
2 wks	__ Regards face	__ Hands fisted	__ Alert to sound	__ Prone chin up
2 mos	__ Smiles responsively	__ Follows to midline	__ Coos	__ Lifts head 45° (prone)
4 mos	__ Regards own hand	__ Hands together	__ Squeals	__ Pushes up
6 mos	__ Work for toy	__ Reaches for object	__ Turns to voice	__ Pull to sit - no head lag
9 mos	__ Feeds self cracker	__ Assisted pincer grasp	__ Da/da ma/ma nonspecific	__ Stand holding on
15 mos	__ Waves bye-bye	__ Neat pincer grasp	__ 1-2 words	__ Walks well
18 mos	__ Uses cup well	__ Scribbles	__ 3 words	__ Runs
2 yrs	__ Removes garment	__ 2-cube tower	__ Combines 2 words	__ Kicks ball forward
3 yrs	__ Wash and dry hands	__ 6-cube tower	__ Speech ½ understandable	__ Throw ball overhand
5 yrs	__ Dresses without supervision	__ Draws person	__ Defines ⅝-ball, lake, desk, house, banana, curtain, fence, ceiling. (use shape, material, category)	__ Balance each foot-4 seconds

Anticipatory Guidance

	2 wk	2 mo	4 mo	6 mo	9 mo	15 mo	18 mo	2 yr	3 yr	4 yr	5 yr
Immunizations (circle if given)		DPT OPV HbOC HBV #2	DPT OPV HbOC	DPT HbOC	HBV #3	HbOC MMR	DPT OPV				DPT OPV
Tests					Hearing Hgb ______ PPD ______ Ipecac				Hearing Vision	Hearing Vision	Hearing Vision
Safety/Guidance (circle items discussed)	2 wk	2 mo	4 mo	6 mo	9 mo	15 mo	18 mo	2 yr	3 yr	4 yr	5 yr
	Pets Car Seats Falls Water Heater <120° Smoke Alarms	Car Seats Falls Small toys Burns No Walkers	Falls Small toys Burns No walker Fluoride/Teeth Plastic	Small objects Gates/steps Car Seats Burns Cords/plants Water safety	Shoes Poisoning/Ipecac Foods/choking Toddler Car Seat Biking Separation/strangers	Choking Gates Water Burns Falls Behavior/Tantrum	Streets Falls Water Burns Toileting Behavior/Tantrum	Burns Streets Water Car Seat Crib/bed Toileting	Streets Pets Water Stranger TV Dental	Bikes Helmet Streets Water TV	Matches Seatbelts Swim Water Streets TV

B

FIGURE 7-4
B. *Well-child record.*

DATE	AGE	SUBJECTIVE (concerns, nutrition, social, etc.)	OBJECTIVE	ASSESSMENT	PLAN

FIGURE 7-4 continued

MATERNAL RECORD

Corrected EDD ______ MONTH DAY YEAR

Menstrual EDD ______ MONTH DAY YEAR

MARITAL STATUS:
☐ Married ☐ Single
☐ Divorced ☐ Widowed

RELIGION ☐ PRO ______
☐ CAT ☐ JRF ☐ JRO ☐ MOS
☐ OTHER ______

PHYSICIAN SERVICE: ☐ OBSTETRICS ☐ FAMILY MEDICINE ROCHESTER ☐ FAMILY MEDICINE KASSON

MAIDEN NAME ______ LAST FIRST MIDDLE FATHER'S NAME ______ LAST FIRST MIDDLE

ADDRESS ______ PHONE ______

	AGE	BIRTHDATE	BIRTHPLACE CITY	BIRTHPLACE STATE	EDUCATION YRS COMPLETED	OCCUPATION	RACE/ETHNICITY
PATIENT							
FATHER							

Patient Referred: ☐ Yes ☐ No Referring Physician: Name ______ Phone ______
Address ______

OBSTETRICAL HISTORY

LMP ______ Frequency ______ Note if: ☐ Irregular ☐ Abnormal Amount/Duration

On BCP at Conception: ☐ Yes ☐ No HCG+ __/__/__ DATE __/__/__ DATE ☐ Home ☐ MC ☐ Other

On Fertility Medication: ☐ Yes ☐ No Medication ______ NAME Procedure ______ Date ______

PAST PREGNANCIES:

DATE MO / YR	GA WEEKS	LENGTH OF LABOR	BIRTH WEIGHT (GMS)	SEX M/F	TYPE DELIVERY	ANES.	PLACE OF DELIVERY (Hospital, City, State)	PRETERM LABOR YES / NO	COMMENTS/ COMPLICATIONS

TOTAL PREGNANCIES	FULL TERM	PREMATURE (20-37 WKS)	AB. INDUCED	AB SPONTANEOUS	ECTOPICS	MULTIPLE BIRTHS	LIVING

Date, Signature, Pager, Service ______

Reviewed:
☐ CVI dated ______
☐ PFH dated ______

PAST MEDICAL HISTORY

MEDICAL DISEASE
☐ Allergy; specify ______
CARDIOVASCULAR
☐ Hypertension
☐ Murmur
☐ Rheumatic heart disease
Valve involvement ______
☐ Congenital
☐ Cardiac surgery
☐ Mitral valve prolapse
☐ Arrhythmia
☐ Needs SBE prophylaxis
☐ Thrombophlebitis
☐ Superficial, year ______
☐ Deep, year ______
☐ Embolism, year ______

RESPIRATORY
☐ Asthma
☐ Bronchitis
☐ Pneumonia
☐ Viral
☐ Bacterial
☐ Other
METABOLIC
☐ Diabetes
☐ Thyroid
☐ Other
GASTROINTESTINAL
☐ Cholecystitis
☐ Cholelithiasis
☐ Ulcer
☐ Inflam BD
☐ Appendicitis
☐ Hepatitis
☐ Other

NEUROLOGIC
☐ Epilepsy ☐ Other
PSYCHIATRIC
☐ Eating Disorder
☐ Other ______ Year ______
☐ MALIGNANCY
Specify ______
☐ AUTOIMMUNE
Specify ______
RENAL
☐ Cystitis, year ______
☐ Pyelonephritis, year ______
☐ Polycystic kidney
☐ Other
HEMATOLOGIC
☐ Anemia, year ______
☐ Blood disorder
☐ Transfusion, year ______
☐ Other
☐ RH Sensitized

SOCIAL HISTORY
☐ Alcohol
drinks/week ______
☐ Smoking
PPD ______
☐ Cats ☐ Street Drugs
☐ Caffeine ☐ Other Teratogens
☐ Domestic Abuse/Trauma
GYNECOLOGIC DISEASE
Infertility
☐ Primary
☐ Secondary
☐ Pelvic inflammatory disease
☐ Abnormal PAP
☐ CA in situ
☐ Clomiphene
☐ HMG
☐ In vitro fertilization
☐ DES Exposure
☐ Uterine Anomalies
☐ Breast Disease

SURGICAL PROCEDURE
(List with Date)
______
______
______
______
______

Anesthesia Complications
☐ Yes ☐ No

MEDICATIONS
Dosage
______ ______
______ ______
______ ______
______ ______
______ ______
______ ______
______ ______

INFECTION HISTORY

☐ HIGH RISK FOR HIV
☐ HIGH RISK FOR HEPATITIS B
☐ IMMUNIZED
☐ LIVE WITH SOMEONE WITH TB OR EXPOSED TO TB
☐ PATIENT OR PARTNER HAS HISTORY OF GENITAL HERPES
☐ HISTORY OF STD, GC, CHLAMYDIA, HPV, SYPHILIS
☐ HISTORY OF POSITIVE PPD
☐ OTHER (List) ______

Date, Signature, Pager and Service

Comments on Positive Findings ______

FIGURE 7-5
Maternal record.

GENETICS SCREENING/TERATOLOGY COUNSELING

INCLUDES PATIENT, BABY'S FATHER, OR ANYONE IN EITHER FAMILY WITH:

Corrected EDD ______ MONTH DAY YEAR

	AT RISK YES	AT RISK NO
1. Patient's Age ≥ 35 Years	☐	☐
2. Thalassemia (Italian, Greek, Mediterranean, or Asian Background): MCV < 80	☐	☐
3. Neural Tube Defect (Meningomyelocele, Spina Bifida, or Anencephaly)	☐	☐
4. Down Syndrome (first degree relative)	☐	☐
5. Tay-Sachs (eg, Jewish, Cajun, Fr. Canadian)	☐	☐
6. Sickle Cell Disease or Trait (African)	☐	☐
7. Hemophilia	☐	☐
8. Muscular Dystrophy	☐	☐
9. Cystic Fibrosis	☐	☐
10. Huntington Chorea	☐	☐
11. Mental Retardation If Yes, Fragile X ☐ Positive ☐ Negative	☐	☐
12. Patient or Baby's Father had a Child with Birth Defects Not Listed Above	☐	☐
13. ≥3 First-Trimester Spontaneous Abortions, or a Stillbirth	☐	☐
14. Other Inherited Genetic or Chromosomal Disorder	☐	☐
15. Other ______		

Date, Signature, Pager, Service

Note Number and Add Comments and Counseling: ______

PRENATAL EDUCATION	DATE	INITIALS/COMMENTS
EARLY PREGNANCY APPOINTMENT		
PRENATAL CLASSES (LIST BY NAME):		
1.		
2.		
3.		
4.		
PRETERM LABOR: REVIEW AT 18-20 WKS.		
REVIEW AT 28 WKS.		
BREASTFEEDING		
CIRCUMCISION		
POSTPARTUM CONTRACEPTION		
OTHER:		

INITIAL EXAM

Date, Signature, Pager and Service							Comments on Positive Findings
1. GEN APPEARANCE	☐ NORMAL	☐ OTHER	13. URETHRA	☐ NORMAL	☐ OTHER		
2. SKIN	☐ NORMAL	☐ OTHER	14. PELVIMETRY	☐ NORMAL	☐ OTHER		
3. HEENT	☐ NORMAL	☐ OTHER	15. UTERUS SIZE	____ WEEKS	☐ OTHER		
4. LYMPH NODES (neck, axilla, groin)	☐ NORMAL	☐ OTHER	16. ADNEXA	☐ NORMAL	☐ OTHER		
5. THYROID	☐ NORMAL	☐ OTHER	17. CERVIX	☐ NORMAL	☐ OTHER		
6. BREASTS	☐ NORMAL	☐ OTHER	18. VAGINA	☐ NORMAL	☐ OTHER		
7. PULSES	☐ NORMAL	☐ OTHER	19. VAG. INFECT. SCREEN	☐ NEG	☐ POS		
8. HEART	☐ NORMAL	☐ OTHER	20. VULVA	☐ NORMAL	☐ OTHER		
9. LUNGS	☐ NORMAL	☐ OTHER	21. RECTUM, ANUS, PERINEUM	☐ NORMAL	☐ OTHER		
10. ABDOMEN, LIVER, SPLEEN	☐ NORMAL	☐ OTHER	22. EXTREMITIES	☐ NORMAL	☐ OTHER		
11. HERNIA (Femoral, Inguinal)	☐ ABSENT	☐ PRESENT	23. MENTAL STATUS (mood, orientation)	☐ NORMAL	☐ OTHER		
12. BLADDER	☐ NORMAL	☐ OTHER	24. OTHER ______				

LABORATORY

INITIAL LABS	DATE	RESULT	OPTIONAL INITIAL LABS	DATE	RESULT
BLOOD/Rh TYPE	/ /		HGB ELECTROPHORESIS	/ /	
ANTIBODY SCREEN	/ /		CHLAMYDIA	/ /	
HGB	/ /	______ g/dl	PPD	/ /	
PAP SMEAR	/ /	☐ NORMAL ☐ ABNORMAL ______	GC	/ /	
RUBELLA	/ /		SICKLE CELL SCREEN	/ /	
RPR	/ /		TAY-SACHS	/ /	
URINE CULTURE/SCREEN	/ /			/ /	
HBsAg	/ /			/ /	
HIV	/ /			/ /	

8-18 WEEK LABS (WHEN INDICATED/ELECTED)	DATE	RESULT	24-28 WEEK LABS (WHEN INDICATED)	DATE	RESULT	32-36 WEEK LABS (WHEN INDICATED)	DATE	RESULT
MSAFP/MULTIPLE MARKERS	/ /		HGB	/ /	______ g/dl	RPR	/ /	
			DIABETES SCREEN	/ /	1 HR ______	GC	/ /	
	/ /		GTT (IF SCREEN ABNORMAL)	/ /	___ FBS ___ 1 HR	HGB (RECOMMENDED)	/ /	______ g/dl
	/ /				___ 2 HR ___ 3 HR	CHLAMYDIA	/ /	
	/ /		D (Rh) ANTIBODY SCREEN	/ /		GROUP B STREP	/ /	
	/ /		D IMMUNE GLOBULIN	/ /	GIVEN (28 WKS)		/ /	
	/ /			/ /			/ /	

FIGURE 7-5 continued

PRENATAL VISITS	Corrected EDD ______ MONTH DAY YEAR
Date	
Weeks Gestation	
Fundal Hgt (cm)	
Presentation	
FHR	
Fetal Movement: +Present - Absent ↓Decreased	
Contractions: +Present - Absent	
Blood Pressure 200	
190	
180	
170	
160	
150	
140	
130	
120	
110	
100	
90	
80	
70	
60	
Weight (lbs/kgs)	
Weight Gain or Loss (+/-, lbs/kgs)	
Edema (0, +1, +2, +3, +4)	
Urine Protein (0, +1, +2, +3, +4)	
Return Appointment	
Pager	
Other:	

Height: in/cm /

Normal Weight: lbs./kgs /

ULTRASOUND								
SCAN NO.	DATE	PRESENTA-TION	CRL/ BPD	GESTATIONAL AGE BY: HISTORY	US	PLACENTA	FHT/FM	COMMENT

Date, Signature Pager and Service	PROBLEM LIST/SUMMARY
	☐ VBAC/CS risks and benefits discussed ☐ Not a VBAC candidate.
	☐ VBAC candidate (refer to class) plans: ☐ VBAC ☐ C/S Indication(s) for a repeat C/S are:

FIGURE 7-5 continued

DATE, SIGNATURE PAGER, SERVICE	PRENATAL NOTES	Corrected EDD ____ MONTH DAY YEAR

DATE, SIGNATURE PAGER, SERVICE	POST PARTUM NOTES (Outpatient, prior to 6 week exam)

POST PARTUM PHYSICAL EXAM

BP: ___ / ___	WT (lbs/kgs) ____		VULVA	☐ NORMAL	☐ OTHER____	ADNEXA	☐ NORMAL	☐ OTHER ____
BREASTS	☐ NORMAL	☐ OTHER____	VAGINA	☐ NORMAL	☐ OTHER____	RECTAL-VAGINAL	☐ NORMAL	☐ OTHER ____
ABDOMEN	☐ NORMAL	☐ OTHER____	CERVIX	☐ NORMAL	☐ OTHER____	PAP SMEAR DONE?	☐ YES	☐ NO
			UTERUS	☐ NORMAL	☐ OTHER____			

DATE, SIGNATURE PAGER, SERVICE	Comments

FIGURE 7-5 continued

WRITING NOTES

Documentation in a chart might be done by hand, through dictation and transcription by a secretary, or, increasingly, via an electronic record, accessed through a computer in each examining room. A common method of documenting a problem-oriented office visit is the SOAP note.

SUBJECTIVE: the problem or complaint

OBJECTIVE: findings on physical examination

ASSESSMENT: the physician's evaluation of the problem, differential diagnoses

PLAN: treatment, diagnostic testing

A sample entry might be:

01/02/98 Otitis Media John Smith Clinic #0-000-000

S: 5-year-old with no significant medical history presents with 2-day history of right ear pain. Recent upper respiratory tract infection symptoms. Afebrile. Medications: None. Allergies: Sulfa.

O: HEENT (head, eyes, ears, nose, throat): 1+ anterior cervical adenopathy. Left ear canal and tympanic membrane clear. Right tympanic membrane erythematous and bulging, landmarks obscured. Oropharynx nonerythematous, no tonsillar hypertrophy.
HEART: Regular rate, no murmur, not tachycardic.
LUNGS: Clear to auscultation.

A: Right otitis media.

P: Amoxicillin chewable tablets 250 mg, 1 by mouth 3 times a day for 10 days, #30, no refills. Acetaminophen for pain. Return if persistent complaints.

When seeing a patient for a health maintenance visit (eg, general physical examination, Papanicolaou test, and pelvic examination), it is useful to organize the patient's medical information in the following fashion:

CC (chief complaint): 1, 2, 3, etc.
eg, shortness of breath

HPI (history of present illness): 1, 2, 3, etc.
eg, 59-year-old smoker with 2- to 3-month history of dyspnea on exertion

No chest pain. Recent orthopnea. Symptoms more prominent in cold weather. No weight changes. No lower extremity edema.

PMH (past medical history):
eg, hypertension, asthma, coronary artery disease

PSH (past surgical history):
eg, appendectomy, hysterectomy, coronary artery bypass

MEDS (medications):

ALL (allergies):

FH (family history):
eg, diabetes, heart disease, breast cancer

SH (social history):
eg, divorced, 2 children at home, works as a nurse

ROS (review of systems): systematic review of each organ system from HEENT to Neuro

PHYSICAL EXAM:

ASSESSMENT:

PLAN:

This document serves as a handy reference when the patient returns.

PRECEPTORS

There is no substitute for hands-on patient care to build one's confidence and clinical database in primary care (Fig. 7-6*A*). The family practice residency program ensures that patient interactions are adequately supervised each day through the use of a preceptor. The preceptor is available to help assess patients during their office visits and to assist with any procedures. The preceptor also reviews residents' records from recent patient visits, providing clinical wisdom whenever possible while offering quality control (Fig. 7-6*B*). This system serves both as an educational tool for the resident and as a checkpoint for ensuring appropriate patient care. The preceptor is an experienced family physician either on staff with the residency program or in community-based practice and affiliated with the training program. The Residency Review Committee requires a ratio of at least one preceptor per four residents in the clinic at any given time. First-year residents (G1) are

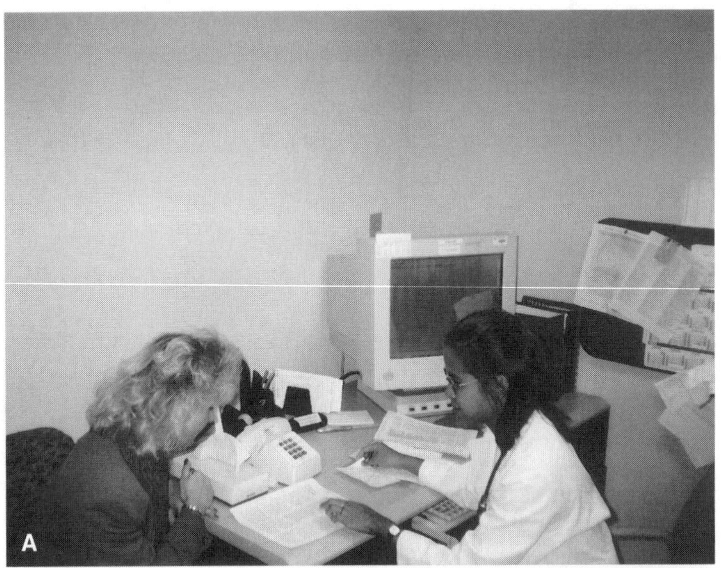

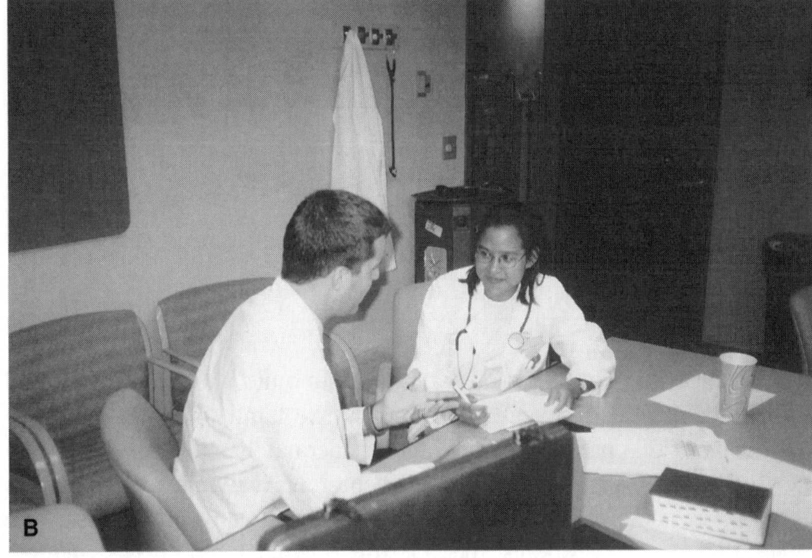

FIGURE 7-6
A. *Resident with patient in clinic.*
B. *After the interview and examination, the resident discusses the patient's case in detail with the supervising staff physician.*

required to review each patient with the preceptor, who confirms findings and helps determine the plan. The preceptor documents knowledge of the case with a note in the patient chart and needs to co-sign any prescriptions given to the patient. This is a medicolegal requirement because G1 residents have not yet obtained their medical licenses. Second- and third-year residents have the same access to the preceptor and can discuss differential diagnoses and treatment options or review physical findings as needed. Such "bedside" teaching can leave the most lasting clinical impressions.

BILLING

Last, but not least, is learning to charge for each office visit. Careful documentation of patient discussion and examination is key here as well to support appropriate charges for the physician's services. As residents, we are allotted extra time to meet and assess patients and discuss them with a preceptor—particularly early in residency training. Thus, the final patient charge is not always based on the amount of time spent during the visit. Commonly, charges are determined by the number of complaints and complexity of the problem presented. The otitis media case presented earlier would be an example of a simple problem-focused visit that would generate one of the lowest charges. A complete physical examination with review of the patient's PMH, PSH, MEDS, ALL, FH, SH, ROS would generate the highest charge for a non-procedure-oriented office visit. In Fig. 7-7, you can see how charges are derived at our clinic. Please note the importance of recording the completeness of your review of systems and physical examination. If one is billing for time spent counseling rather than in examination of a patient, one needs to clarify the issues discussed and log the amount of time involved in face-to-face contact with the patient.

You may have a charge slip that needs to be completed for the billing to be submitted. Procedures usually generate higher charges. Each office will have its own cost structure for everything from the simple, problem-focused visit to cast application to vasectomy. Often with procedures, one must also document suture and tray set-up equipment used to recapture the cost of these supplies. In some offices, these may be built into the cost of the procedure. In obstetric care, it is not uncommon to have a "package cost" to encompass routine prenatal visits, the routine vaginal delivery, and the postpartum visit. Although there is no separate charge then for each prenatal visit, the physician will still likely need to log the office visit on a billing slip or service record for tracking purposes. You will need to learn the particulars of billing in your office.

CONCLUSIONS

Although there is a good bit of nitty-gritty in the outpatient setting with regard to paperwork, billing, and the medical record, all this will become

HISTORY GUIDELINES

Comprehensive

- Chief complaint
- HPI: 4 - 8 elements
- ROS: 10 - 14 systems (or CVI)
- Past, Family, Social History: 1 from each area (or PFH)

Detailed

- Chief complaint
- HPI: 4 - 8 elements
- ROS: 2 - 9 systems
- Past, Family, Social History: 1 from any area

Expanded Problem Focused

- Chief complaint
- HPI: 1 - 3 elements
- ROS: 1 system

Problem Focused

- Chief complaint
- HPI: 1 - 3 HPI elements

History of the Present Illness (HPI elements)

1. Location	5. Timing
2. Quality	6. Context
3. Severity	7. Modifying Factors
4. Duration	8. Associated signs/symptoms

Review of Systems (ROS) (or CVI)

1. Allergic/Immunologic	8. Hematologic/Lymphatic
2. Constitutional Symptoms (fever, weight loss, etc.)	9. GI
	10. GU
3. Psychiatric	11. Musculoskeletal
4. Eyes	12. Integumentary (skin &/or breast)
5. Ears, Nose, Mouth & Throat	
6. CV	13. Neuro
7. Respiratory	14. Endocrine

EXAMINATION GUIDELINES

Comprehensive

General multi-system [8 to 12 organ systems] or complete single organ system

Detailed

An extended examination of the affected body area(s)and other symptomatic or related organ system(s) [Recommend at least 5-7]

Expanded Problem Focused

A limited examination of the affected body area or organ system and other symptomatic or related organ system(s) [Recommend at least 2-4]

Problem Focused

A limited examination of the affected body area or organ system [At least 1]

General Multi-System Examination

Constitutional (VS and General Appearance)
Eyes
Ears, Nose, Mouth, and Throat
Cardiovascular
Respiratory
Gastrointestinal
Genitourinary
Skin
Musculoskeletal
Neurologic
Heme/Lymph/Immun
Psychiatric

Body Areas

Head (including face)	Back
Neck	Genitalia, groin, and buttocks
Chest	Each extremity
Abdomen	

MEDICAL DECISION MAKING GUIDELINES

High Complexity

- Extensive **diagnoses** or management options
- Extensive amount of **data** ordered/reviewed
- High **risk** of complications and/or morbidity or mortality

Moderate Complexity

- Multiple **diagnoses** or management options
- Moderate amount of **data** ordered/reviewed
- Moderate **risk** of complications and/or morbidity or mortality

Low Complexity

- Limited number of **diagnoses** or management options
- Limited amount of **data** ordered/reviewed
- Low **risk** of complications and/or morbidity or mortality

Straightforward

- Minimal number of **diagnoses** or management options
- Minimal **data** reviewed/ordered
- Minimal **risk** of complications and/or morbidity or mortality

DOCUMENTATION SUGGESTIONS:

To support complexity of medical decision making document the following:

- Impression: Diagnosis(es) and co-morbidittes considered
- Plan of care (include tests ordered).
- Review and summarization of outside records
- Personal review of a film, tracing, or specimen
- Discussion of test results with the performing physician
- Decision to obtain/obtaining old records

FIGURE 7-7
Derivation of charges.

CLINIC

Mayo Code	CPT Code	History and Physical	Medical Decision Making	Counseling/ Coordination of Care *
PHYSICIAN REQUESTED (P) CODES *(requires documentation of requesting physician & reason)*				
P6	99245+99354	Comprehensive - Prolonged	High	>1 hr. 50 min.
P5	99245	Comprehensive	High	1 hr. 20 min.
P4	99244	Comprehensive	Moderate	60 minutes
P3	99243	Detailed	Low	40 minutes
P2	99242	Expanded Problem Focused	Straightforward	30 minutes
P1	99241	Problem Focused	Straightforward	15 minutes
NON-PHYSICIAN REQUESTED				
New Patient (N) codes *(have not been seen in the department in last three years)*				
N6	99205+99354	Comprehensive - Prolonged	High	1 hr. 30 min.
N5	99205	Comprehensive	High	60 minutes
N4	99204	Comprehensive	Moderate	45 minutes
N3	99203	Detailed	Low	30 minutes
N2	99202	Expanded Problem Focused	Straightforward	20 minutes
N1	99201	Problem Focused	Straightforward	10 minutes
***Established Patient (E) codes* *(seen in the department within the last three years)*				
E6	99215 +99354	Comprehensive - Prolonged	High	1 hr. 10 min.
E5	99215	Comprehensive	High	40 minutes
E4	99214	Detailed	Moderate	25 minutes
E3	99213	Expanded Problem Focused	Low	15 minutes
E2	99212	Problem Focused	Straightforward	10 minutes
E1	99211			5 minutes
Confirmatory Consult (CC) codes *(second opinion request of patient or third party payer)*				
CC5	99275	Comprehensive	High	
CC4	99274	Comprehensive	Moderate	
CC3	99273	Detailed	Low	
CC2	99272	Expanded Problem Focused	Straightforward	
CC1	99271	Problem Focused	Straightforward	
***Follow up (F) codes* *(report visits/counseling)*				
F6	99215 +99354			1 hr. 10 min.
F5	99215			40 Minutes
F4	99214			25 Minutes
F3	99213			15 Minutes
F2	99212			10 Minutes
F1	99211			5 Minutes

Codes — Key Components (see reverse) — or — Time

REFERENCE "I have reviewed the history and examined the patient. Agree with findings as documented by (Name) on (date)."

TEACHING PHYSICIAN RULE

When referencing a resident note, staff must also document the relevant findings of the history and exam, and involvement in medical decision making.

All billable services require evidence of a face-to-face encounter.

BILLING ON TIME - DEFINITIONS

*Counseling: discussion with a patient and family concerning one or more of the following areas: diagnostic results, impressions and/or recommended diagnostic studies; prognosis; risks and benefits of treatment options; instructions and follow-up; compliance management; risk factor reduction and patient/family education. Staff and Resident/AHP time is not additive when coding on time.

Outpatient (face-to-face time) - billing physician time spent face-to-face with the patient.

Inpatient (unit/floor time) - billing physician time spent on the Unit/Floor in counseling/ coordination of care (related to the patient).

*The encounter may be coded on time if greater than 50% of the total time spent with patient was counseling/coordination of care. When coding on time, the total time spent with the patient and the topics discussed must be documented.

*Must meet/exceed the selected requirements for 2 of 3 key components (history, exam, and medical decision making).

HOSPITAL

Mayo Code	CPT Code	History and Physical	Medical Decision Making	Counseling/ Coordination of Care *
Initial Hospital Care *(once per admission by admitting service)*				
IH5	99223	Comprehensive	High	1 hr. 10 min
IH4	99222	Comprehensive	Moderate	50 minutes
IH3	99221	Comprehensive or Detailed	Low/Straightforward	30 minutes
***Subsequent Hospital Care* *(once per day)*				
SH3	99233	Detailed	High	35 minutes
SH2	99232	Expanded Problem Focused	Moderate	25 minutes
SH1	99231	Problem Focused	Low/Straightforward	15 minutes
Hospital Discharge Services *(final day, multiple day stay)*				
DD	99238	Discharge Day		≤ 30 minutes
DDM	99239	Discharge Day		> 30 minutes
Outpatient Observation Care				
OC5	99220	Comprehensive	High	
OC4	99219	Comprehensive	Moderate	
OC3	99218	Comprehensive or Detailed	Low/Straightforward	
OCD	99217	Discharge Day		
Initial Inpatient Consultations *(once per service per admission)*				
IC5	99255	Comprehensive	High	1 hr. 50 min.
IC4	99254	Comprehensive	Moderate	1 hr. 20 min
IC3	99253	Detailed	Low	55 minutes
IC2	99252	Expanded Problem Focused	Straightforward	40 minutes
IC1	99251	Problem Focused	Straightforward	20 minutes
***Follow-up Inpatient Consultations*				
FC3	99263	Detailed	High	30 minutes
FC2	99262	Expanded Problem Focused	Moderate	20 minutes
FC1	99261	Problem Focused	Low/Straightforward	10 minutes
Critical Care Codes				
KK	99291/99292	Document Total Time		
Admission-Discharge Same Day (inpt or obsv care)				
SAD5	99236	Comprehensive	High	
SAD4	99235	Comprehensive	Moderate	
SAD3	99234	Comprehensive or Detailed	Low/Straightforward	

Codes — Key Components (see reverse) — or — Time

FIGURE 7-7 continued

second nature in no time. What will continue to be thought provoking and gratifying in the clinic are your patient interactions. There is never a dull moment in the diverse day of a family physician. That is what keeps us sharp. Our commitment to providing quality, integrated primary care keeps us focused. Your outpatient clinic will be your welcome "home base" for growth and development as a family physician.

REFERENCE

1. American Medical Association: Graduate Medical Education Directory. Chicago, American Medical Association, 1998-1999, p 68

8

HOSPITAL ROUNDS

Harvey D. Cassidy, M.D.

Hospital rounds are an integral part of family medicine training and family practice. The practice of ''rounds'' or hospital bedside rounds is thought to have originated around the turn of the 20th century with Sir William Osler, the dean of the nation's first medical school at Johns Hopkins University in Baltimore, Maryland.[1] The process allowed a systematic approach to patient care and served as a tool to teach medical school students. Each patient's case represented a wealth of medical information to be learned and the physical examination allowed hands-on training at the patient's bedside. This time-honored tradition has continued to this day and is the most commonly used technique to examine and treat hospital patients on a daily basis while at the same time teaching medical students, residents, and fellows in academic institutions (Fig. 8-1).

PROGRESS NOTES

Family practice rounds, as with other specialties, consists of seeing patients in the hospital in the morning on a daily basis. Typically, the patient's chart, laboratory results, and progress during the preceding 24 hours are reviewed and the patient is examined. Further treatment, if needed, is determined and ordered. A complete, concise, and legible progress note is placed on the patient's chart and is required of every physician involved in the patient's care. Test results are noted from the previous 24 hours and new orders for that day are written and recorded, providing explicit instructions to nursing and paramedical personnel involved in the patient's care.

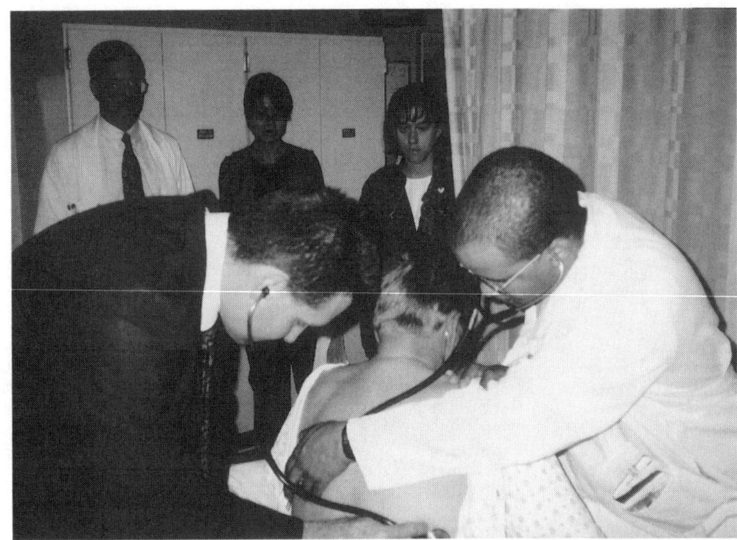

FIGURE 8-1
Bedside teaching remains an important aspect of residency training in family medicine.

A typical hospital progress note should consist of the following.

Subjective: This represents a notation of the patient's complaints and concerns and (in the patient's words) a general description of what has taken place in the last 24 hours.

Objective: This notation consists of collections of data and may include the patient's vital signs, fluid status, physical examination, and any laboratory or test results that are pertinent and available.

Assessment: This represents the examiner's list of conditions or diagnoses that are pertinent to the patient's care and other active factors that may impact the diagnosis.

Plan: This represents an updated detailed plan encompassing laboratory tests, diagnostic procedures, or other specific tests or therapy that may be included in the patient's care.

Although there are many ways to structure a progress note, in most cases, a problem-oriented assessment and plan is best because it details a logical, focused plan of action (a road map) that other physicians and paramedical staff can follow easily. A thorough and concise progress note, legibly written, significantly improves chances for good communication among attending physicians, consultants, and paramedical staff and efficient appropriate medical care.

"The hospital should be a refuge to which the sick might go for relief as they went before our Savior, . . ."

—William J. Mayo

HOSPITAL ROUNDS DURING RESIDENCY

Family physicians typically must balance hospital rounds with a busy office practice and, therefore, rounds generally begin quite early in the morning (eg, 6 AM), depending on the number of patients to be seen. Fewer interruptions occur during these early morning hours, and rounds tend to be more efficient. However, delay in receiving laboratory results can be a problem, and timely availability of these results may need to be worked out with your laboratory or nursing staff.

In most teaching institutions, family practice residents begin their rounds at 6:00 to 6:30 AM, to complete their "work rounds" before the attending staff physician arrives. Work rounds consist of interviewing and examining the patients, reviewing their progress and laboratory test results, and developing a treatment plan that can be presented to the attending staff during formal rounds. The resident responsible for the patient's care should document thoroughly via the progress note the findings during these work rounds. The resident should then be prepared to communicate these findings to the attending staff and colleagues during later rounds.

"The sooner patients can be removed from the depressing influence of general hospital life the more rapid their convalescence."

—Charles H. Mayo

Supervising staff rounds at most teaching institutions begin at about 8:00 to 8:30 AM. These more formal hospital rounds include review of established inpatients as well as new patients who have been admitted to the hospital service in the past 24 hours (Fig. 8-2). All admissions must be reported to staff immediately on admission to the hospital and discussed thoroughly so that an appropriate diagnostic and therapeutic plan can begin without delay. In addition, the staff physician can serve as an information resource for the resident. If the patient is unstable, the supervising physician is given the opportunity to evaluate the patient personally. During formal hospital rounds with supervising staff, new admissions are generally evaluated first and residents are expected to present these admissions in a clear, concise and

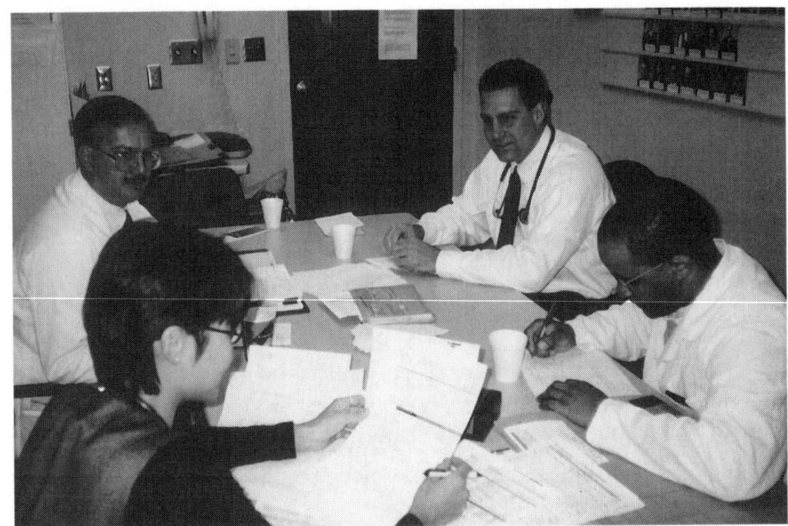

FIGURE 8-2 Morning hospital rounds typically begin with a round-table discussion of new admissions from the preceding day.

organized manner. In addition, established patients are discussed and reviewed with staff and examined, if necessary, by the attending physician.

Residents may at times find hospital attending rounds stressful and intimidating, particularly when attending staff ask various and sometimes difficult questions in an attempt to evaluate a resident's performance. To prepare yourself for these anxiety-provoking times, it is always an excellent idea to read about the patient's diagnosis before presenting the patient so that questions regarding differential diagnosis and management can be answered easily. As the Boy Scout motto says, "Be prepared." Your thorough preparation and comprehensive management of the patient not only impress your supervising staff and make that job easier but also make rounds much more efficient, increasing the time available for teaching.

RESIDENT RESPONSIBILITIES

Residents should also be good consultants. Always communicate with the patient's primary care physician that the patient has been admitted to the hospital and give a brief update regarding diagnosis, management plan, and the patient's status. A periodic courtesy call to the primary care physician is always appreciated, as is a call when the patient is dismissed from the hospital. A complete dismissal summary outlining the patient's diagnosis, hospital course, medications, test results, abnormal laboratory results, and follow-up plans should be completed by the resident caring for the patient and forwarded to the patient's primary care physician as expeditiously as possible.

In most institutions and in private practice, family physicians complete their rounds in the morning and return to their offices to see patients in the outpatient setting. Likewise, family practice residents may spend 3 to 4 hours each morning seeing patients before they return to their respective outpatient rotations in the afternoon to see patients. Generally, depending on volume of admissions, the first-year resident is responsible for admitting all patients and writing most of the patient's progress notes on a daily basis. A second-year resident may also participate in this process and is available to assist the first-year resident with questions or concerns. The third-year resident may also assist and, in addition, is expected to teach lower-level residents and medical students and oversee patient care administered by this team. The attending staff physician assumes ultimate responsibility for the patient's care, oversees the combined efforts of the rounds team, and is responsible for the organization of the educational component during rounds.

CONSULTATIONS

Consultations involving various specialists are ordered by the resident physician in charge of the patient after approval by attending physicians, and information obtained from these consultations must be reported to the rest of the team, including the staff physician. To ensure that residents have a working knowledge of each patient on the service, it is mandatory that they take the responsibility for locating test results and results of consultations in a timely manner. Although this may at times seem tedious and trivial, it is vital that the resident and attending staff have all necessary information available to make informed and appropriate decisions regarding the patient's care.

HOSPITAL CENSUS

The family practice inpatient service varies from day to day and may change depending on the time of year. Generally, winter months are busier than summer months and holidays may be extremely busy. In most institutions, the family practice service census ranges from 5 to 15 patients, but this can vary considerably. During a 24-hour period, residents can generally expect 2 to 6 admissions; however, there may be days and nights on call when there are no admissions or nights when admissions seem endless. Typically, a first- or second-year resident is expected to manage 3 to 10 patients on the service at a time, and the third-year resident is expected to ensure that admissions are distributed fairly and in a manner that is not overwhelming.

TEACHING DURING ROUNDS

Quality education is a key to good teaching rounds. Teaching on the inpatient service is expected of staff and senior level residents. Informal bedside rounds are typical and may include discussions of physical findings, differential diagnoses, and proposed treatment. More formal teaching may take place in the form of "coffee talks" during which articles relevant to the patient's case are supplied and discussed by staff or are assigned to an upper level resident for presentation to the team (Box 8-1). Minilectures can be given

BOX 8-1 COFFEE TALKS

Coffee talks are often an important educational tool for residents during their inpatient or outpatient rotations (Fig. 8-3). In most cases, a supervising staff physician will sit down (often over coffee) and informally present an article or topic that is relevant to a patient's care. Resident physicians often are asked to research specific articles or topics concerning their patients and present them during coffee talks. This form of teaching allows the students to learn about their patients in an informal and relaxed environment. Take advantage of these opportunities to ask questions and discuss relevant issues or concerns.

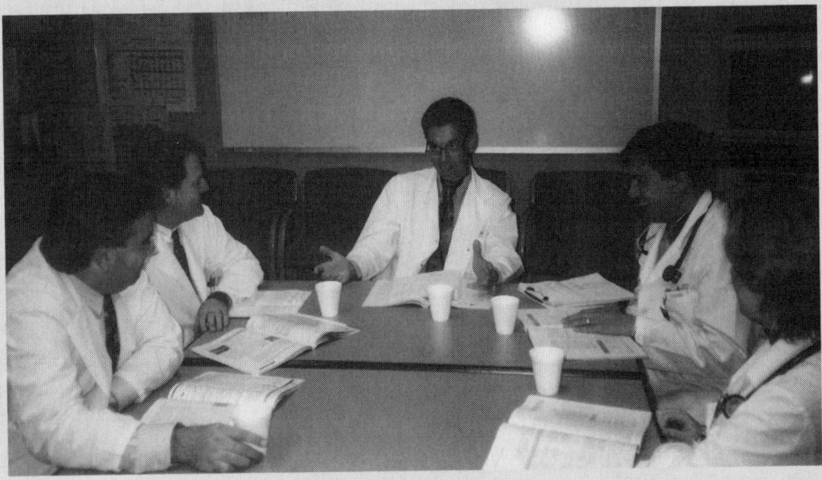

FIGURE 8-3
Coffee talks are typical teaching methods used by staff physicians when resident physicians rotate on the family medicine hospital service.

by staff or fellow residents on the service as interests and time allow. Unfortunately, in some cases, daily formal teaching is not practical because of either a heavy patient load or extended rounds caused by severity of illness or discussions with patients' families. Recognize that this is an integral part of the teaching process and much can be learned from discussions of the patient's progress with specialists, paramedical staff, or the patient's family. Interactive skills, not generally taught in medical schools, can be developed and finely tuned during these interactions.

TELEPHONE CALLS

Telephone calls sometimes seem to be the bane of the resident's existence. These may occur during hospital rounds, while the resident is in the clinic seeing patients, or while the resident is on call. It is vital that the resident develop an organized system for dealing with questions and messages. These calls may arrive from various sources, including nurses on the floor, nursing homes, physicians at other sites who may wish to transfer patients, and from individual patients requesting information or advice. Although often disruptive, these calls are an important part of our practice. Remember that if you are perplexed or uncomfortable with a patient's condition as outlined during a telephone call from the patient or family, it is best to refer the patient to your outpatient clinic or emergency department for evaluation. There is a great risk involved with treating patients over the telephone from a medicolegal standpoint, and many times the history obtained from either the patient or the family is confusing or inadequate. Thus, in many cases, it is entirely appropriate to refer those patients for further evaluation to ensure appropriate medical care. In addition, the practice of telephone medicine requires accurate and timely documentation. All interactions with patients while the resident is on call should be documented thoroughly and discussed with appropriate staff in a timely fashion. Always err on the conservative side—try not to treat patients over the telephone.

TIPS FOR HOSPITAL ROUNDS

Performing well on hospital rounds is often quite similar to performing on a stage. There is a script (a description of the patient's diagnosis and progress) and an audience (consisting of the staff physician, other residents, and paramedical staff). The resident must recognize that the audience requires

BOX 8-2 TIPS FOR HOSPITAL ROUNDS

1. Maintain a professional appearance
2. Be positive or optimistic and humble (even when overworked)
3. Be concise
4. Be organized
5. Be efficient
6. Do not be late
7. See all admissions first; write orders and return to write histories and results of physical examinations when faced with multiple admissions
8. Read about your patients
9. Do not read from your notes
10. Be confident but always seek help if unsure
11. Review all tests, consultations, and radiographs before going home or to bed
12. Make time when you can relax
13. Avoid disruptions or distractions
14. Report all admissions or dismissals to the patient's primary physician
15. Inform attending staff of a change in a patient's condition or a death
16. Be a team player
17. Never eat or drink in front of patients
18. Remember always that the patient's interest comes first
19. Know your patients inside and out
20. Be a constructive influence and avoid complaining

a comprehensive, timely, and efficient performance (Box 8-2). Attention to detail is certainly necessary, but this should not be carried to extremes. Pertinent information presented in an organized fashion is key to quality hospital rounds. Always try to anticipate questions and respond in a focused and organized manner. Unnecessary detail wastes time and can be quite distracting. Certainly, every detail and laboratory test cannot be memorized by the resident, and appropriate notes can and should be used. Make effective use of these notes, but don't rely on them solely. Notes and laboratory slips have an uncanny way of disappearing just before we need them for presentation. Keep a global picture of the patient's course and treatment in mind, highlighted with pertinent data that you can communicate to colleagues and staff. Always examine radiographs yourself and do not rely on written reports or reports by colleagues. Read and research every aspect of your patient's care and communicate this information to your staff and colleagues. Even a brief 1- or 2-paragraph review of your patient's problem found in many textbooks will enable you to more appropriately and efficiently care for your patient.

When interacting with consultants, be precise in what you are asking them to do. (For example, radiologists generally do not have the luxury of examining the patient and, therefore, may miss a subtle finding if appropriate history is not provided.) Consultants need to be clear as to the questions we are asking them to address. This leads to improved quality of care and uses their time in an efficient, cost-effective manner. In addition, it will help to establish rapport with our consultant colleagues. Be meticulous about documentation. This is required for medicolegal reasons, improves communication among consultants, and impresses your attending staff. Always look presentable. An unshaven or disheveled resident who performs rounds in wrinkled scrubs that have been worn for 24 hours does not engender a sense of organization, competence, or professionalism in either patients or staff. Your presentation reflects on your performance. Always maintain a level of professionalism and optimism, even if you are feeling stressed, you have not slept in days, or times are difficult. Never hesitate to discuss problems or frustrations with your Residency Director or attending staff. They are an invaluable resource for you in resolving personal or professional problems. Always try to carve out time for yourself, family, or others important to you, and understand that you have earned it. These seemingly simple hints will serve you well and will not only enhance your performance but increase your enjoyment of medicine as you proceed through your career.

REFERENCE

1. Schneeweiss R: Morning rounds and the search for evidence-based answers to clinical questions. J Am Board Fam Pract 10:298-300, 1997

9

PROCEDURES

Jerry W. Sayre, M.D.

The challenge for each Family Practice residency program is to produce residents capable of practicing competent, quality medicine. Each resident must be prepared with the medical knowledge, the clinical exposure and experience, the communication skills, and the procedural skills necessary for the anticipated practice area. Each resident has unique practice goals, and each must be competent at a basic level and still have the option to acquire additional training based on anticipated future practice needs. Physicians in practice must often seek training for procedures they wish to perform.

As technology and medical advances progress, diagnostic and therapeutic procedures are becoming less specialized and more available to the practicing family physician. Family physicians often are encouraged by their association with managed care organizations to provide a wider range of diagnostic and therapeutic procedures. Other benefits to increased procedural competency include a better understanding of patients' pathologic conditions and disease process, a more active role in treatment, and the additional financial rewards.

Many older and more experienced family physicians with strong procedural training and skills are retiring, and the number of Family Practice residencies that have such skills programs is limited. It has become clear, therefore, that for American family physicians to compete in the current medical marketplace, residency programs must train residents and practicing physicians in the appropriate use of procedures. In response, the American Academy of Family Physicians created a Task Force on Procedures in 1993. This task force identified, in 1995, the procedures being taught and currently being performed by family physicians (Tables 9-1 and 9-2).

TABLE 9-1
PROCEDURES BEING TAUGHT BY *MOST* FAMILY PRACTICE RESIDENCY PROGRAMS*

OUTPATIENT PROCEDURES	% OF RESPONDING PROGRAMS	INPATIENT PROCEDURES	% OF RESPONDING PROGRAMS
Cerumen/foreign body removal from ear	98.0	Lumbar puncture	97.0
Electrocardiogram interpretation	97.7	Vertex delivery	97.0
Skin lesion excision/biopsy	97.2	Episiotomy (incise and repair)	96.7
Flexible sigmoidoscopy	96.5	Low-risk obstetrics	96.5
Joint aspiration	96.0	Venipuncture	96.5
Toenail removal	96.0	Arterial puncture	95.7
Casting	95.7	Fetal monitoring	95.7
Paronychia incision and drainage	95.7	Thoracentesis	95.0
Colposcopy	92.9	Electrocardiogram	94.5
Thrombosed hemorrhoid incision and extraction	89.9	Vaginal laceration repair	94.2
Endometrial aspiration/biopsy	89.4	Neonatal circumcision	94.0
Aspiration of breast cysts	88.7	Endotracheal intubation	93.7
Endometrial sampling	87.9	Paracentesis	92.7
Spirometry	87.9	Manual removal of placenta	92.4
Proctosigmoidoscopy	85.4	Labor induction	91.4
Lumbar puncture	84.4	Subclavian venous catheter/venous cutdown	91.4
Epistaxis treatment/nasal packing	82.9	Arterial line placement	90.2
Reduction of uncomplicated dislocations	82.1	Advanced cardiac life support	86.6
Venipuncture/start intravenous line	81.1	Chest tube placement	86.6
Low-risk obstetrics	79.3	Bladder tap	85.9
		Fecal impaction removal	84.6
		Joint aspiration	80.6

Continued

HOW TO ACQUIRE TRAINING

Residency Core Program

A basic level of clinical and procedural skills is taught in every residency program, although some programs have a greater emphasis on skills than others. Some residency programs have created a wide range of skills clinics or workshops to give residents additional exposure. The average residency core program generally provides the resident with 80 percent of the skills

TABLE 9-1 Continued

OUTPATIENT PROCEDURES	% OF RESPONDING PROGRAMS	INPATIENT PROCEDURES	% OF RESPONDING PROGRAMS
Indirect laryngoscopy	76.3	Umbilical catheter placement	75.6
Advanced cardiac life support	73.3	Forceps delivery	70.3
Fecal impaction removal	72.3	Flexible sigmoidoscopy	69.5
Vasectomy	70.3	Swan-Ganz catheter management	65.5
Slit lamp exam	69.8	Proctosigmoidoscopy	65.0
Neonatal circumcision	67.8	Skin lesion	64.2
Exercise treadmill testing	55.7	Swan-Ganz placement	63.7
Fetal monitoring	53.7	Epistaxis and nasal packing	62.5
		Dilation and curettage	61.0
		Cerumen/foreign body removal from ear	59.4
		Bone marrow biopsy	58.9
		Aspiration of breast cysts	57.2
		Casting	57.2
		Paronychia incision and drainage	55.4
		Spirometry	53.7
		Endometrial sampling	53.7
		Reduction of uncomplicated dislocations	52.9
		Endometrial aspiration	51.6
		Thrombosed hemorrhoid	50.1

*>50% of programs.
n = 397.
From Norris TE, Felmar E, Tolleson G: Which procedures should be taught in family practice residency programs? Fam Med 29:99–104, 1997. By permission of the journal, published by the Society of Teachers of Family Medicine.

necessary for future practice. In addition to these workshops there are many references (eg, *Procedures for Primary Care Physicians*) that can assist a physician in learning new techniques. However, as the old saying goes, ''See one, do one, teach one.'' There is no substitute for hands-on training.

Subspecialty Clinic

The resident and the advisor may determine, based on the future practice plans, that procedures are needed in addition to those taught in the basic

TABLE 9-2
PROCEDURES BEING PERFORMED BY *MOST* PRACTICING FAMILY PHYSICIANS*

OUTPATIENT PROCEDURES	% OF RESPONDING PHYSICIANS	INPATIENT PROCEDURES	% OF RESPONDING PHYSICIANS
Cerumen/foreign body removal from ear	96.9	Lumbar puncture	70.0
Paronychia incision and extraction	92.6	Venous puncture	70.0
Electrocardiogram	93.6	Advanced cardiac life support	68.4
Skin lesion excision/biopsy	91.9	Arterial puncture for blood	58.9
Joint aspiration	87.4	Endotracheal intubation	58.1
Toenail removal	87.1	Neonatal circumcision	56.4
Thrombosed hemorrhoid incision and extraction	78.9	BORDERLINE†	
Venous puncture and intravenous catheter placement	75.2	Proctosigmoidoscopy	49.4
Epistaxis treatment/nasal packing	73.3	Reduction of uncomplicated fractures	49.5
Casting	71.6	Spirometry	48.1
Reduction of uncomplicated dislocations	70.5	Thoracentesis	50.0
Spirometry	69.3		
Fecal impaction removal	66.9		
Proctosigmoidoscopy	62.6		
Aspiration of breast cysts	62.3		
Advanced cardiac life support	60.7		
Flexible sigmoidoscopy	60.5		
Lumbar puncture	60.3		
Endometrial sampling	58.6		
Endometrial aspiration/biopsy	57.7		

*>50% of practicing family physicians.
†Because of the ±2.2% sampling error, those procedures near 50% were included as borderline.
From Norris TE, Felmar E, Tolleson G: Which procedures should be taught in family practice residency programs? Fam Med 29:99–104, 1997. By permission of the journal, published by the Society of Teachers of Family Medicine.

core program. These skills may be mastered either in training sessions focused on a particular skill or as a more extended rotation within a subspecialty clinic. For example, special training can be arranged for procedural competence in treadmill testing or endoscopy or for a more extensive subspecialty rotation in cardiology or gastroenterology. In addition, family practice residents need to remember that other specialists, such as anesthesiologists and pathologists, possess a wide range of valuable procedural skills such as vascular access or bone marrow biopsy. Residents may seek procedural teaching from subspecialists based on their individual interests.

Family Practice Faculty

Family practice faculty possess a range of procedural skills, and no one faculty member can be proficient in all. A resident may find that a visiting community family physician may have a higher level of clinical experience in a desired skill or may possess extensive clinical experience in desired skills not covered in the residency core curriculum program. In addition, the American Academy of Family Physicians has created training programs for faculty in endoscopy, suturing techniques, and fetal monitoring. Conversations with other residents and inquiries with nursing staff often assist the resident in evaluating faculty procedural teaching skills.

> *''We live in proportion to our ability to respond to and correlate ourselves with our environment.''*
>
> —Charles H. Mayo

Continuing Medical Education

Many professional organizations, medical schools, hospitals, and industry groups provide workshops, seminars, and hands-on experience for the teaching of procedures. These courses vary widely in quality. Seminars sponsored by professional organizations are preferred to those from industry. For example, each year the American Academy of Family Physicians offers procedural courses on endoscopy, treadmill testing, colposcopy, and fetal monitoring. Also, as part of continuing medical education, a growing number of videotapes, computer programs, and interactive simulations are available.

Once a level of clinical competency is achieved, the resident or physician in practice must continue to practice the skill. Individual physicians have varied motor and spatial skills and learn at different rates. As you measure your results against other physicians, continue to scan the literature for changing indications, risks, and benefits. By evaluating your own performance, you will continue a lifelong practice of honing valuable skills. The proctoring of resident physicians in training programs by the family practice residency faculty helps validate this performance-based evaluation. Physicians in practice may validate their competence by approval from a physician proficient in the procedure to be learned or by peer-review boards (eg,

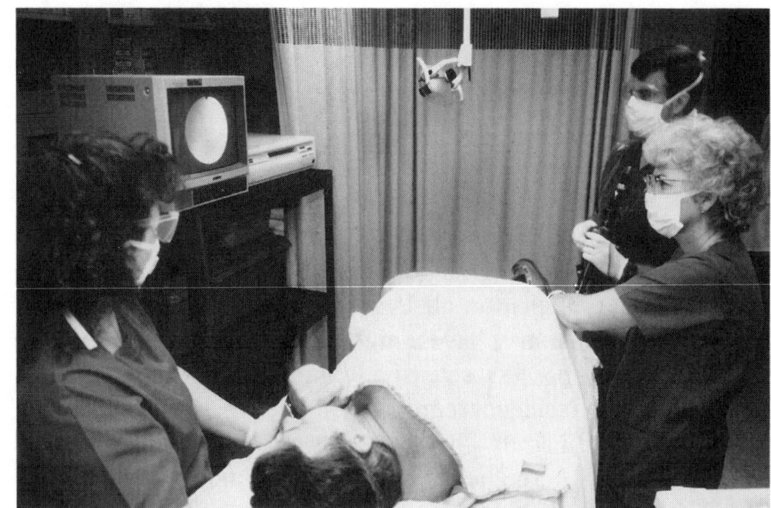

FIGURE 9-1 Flexible sigmoidoscopy is a common procedure performed in family physicians' offices and in Family Practice residency training programs.

hospital procedure committee). A performance-based evaluation is probably of more clinical value than merely counting the number of procedures performed, although credentialing committees of hospitals and professional and specialty organizations often ask for these numbers.

CREDENTIALING AND HOSPITAL PRIVILEGES

The American Academy of Family Physicians, the American Medical Association, and the Joint Commission on Accreditation of Healthcare Organizations stated that delineation of privileges should be determined on individual merit, based on practice, experience, training, and current clinical competence. The various specialty organizations disagree as to the number required in training to achieve clinical competence. For example, the range for flexible sigmoidoscopy (Fig. 9-1) is from 10 to 25 procedures, with the number for esophagogastroduodenoscopy ranging from 7 to 100. For credentialing purposes, be sure to document all procedures and retain operative or procedure notes (Fig. 9-2). Residents in training should obtain documentation with a letter from the program director attesting to their clinical competence.

PROCEDURAL CAVEATS

A decision to include a specific procedure in your office practice should reflect the need for this procedure in your medical community and the

Mayo Clinic Jacksonville
Family Medicine Residency
Procedure Log

Patient Name: ______________________

MCJ Clinic #: ______________________

Date of Procedure: ______________________

Location: ______________________

Diagnosis: ______________________

Procedure: ______________________

____

Level of Responsibility:
1. Did with Staff MD assistance
2. Assisted Staff MD

Consultant: ______________________

____
Signature of Consultant

____
Signature of Resident

FIGURE 9-2
Physicians should always record the number of procedures performed and save the information. Many credentialing boards require this documentation before granting privileges to perform procedures.

economic feasibility of including it in your practice (Fig. 9-3). The despecialization of procedures and the reduced costs for endoscopic, colposcopic, and pulmonary function equipment translate into a rapidly increasing use of procedures by family physicians (Fig. 9-4). However, with increased clinical exposure and technical skills comes increased professional liability exposure and higher professional liability premiums. For example, if performing therapeutic or surgical endoscopy or colposcopy would move you into a higher risk insurance class and your practice volume could not support the increased insurance premiums, then you might wish to limit your procedures to diagnostic only. If you plan on performing obstetrics and assisting on your surgical patients, then, in many cases, no additional coverage would be necessary because both require insurance coverage for operative (high-risk) procedures. Practice patterns tend to be fluid and dynamic; therefore it is essential that

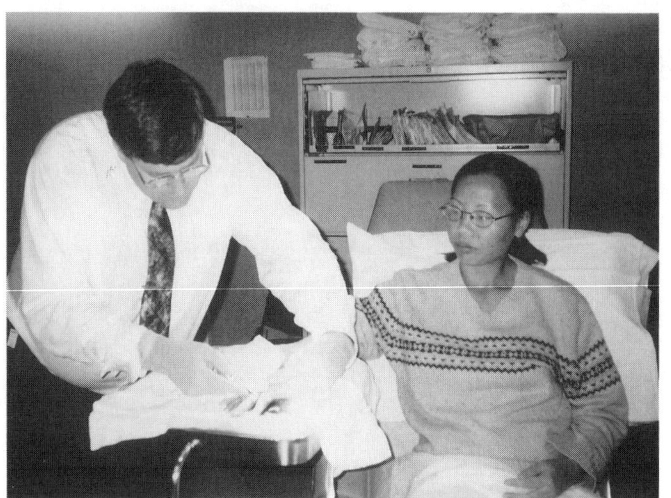

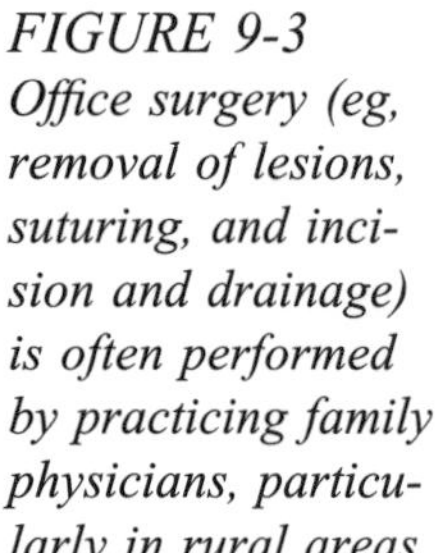

FIGURE 9-3
Office surgery (eg, removal of lesions, suturing, and incision and drainage) is often performed by practicing family physicians, particularly in rural areas.

you discuss this and any future plans for additional procedures with your professional liability insurance carrier.

> *"Experience is the great teacher; unfortunately, experience leaves mental scars, and scar tissue contracts."*
>
> —William J. Mayo

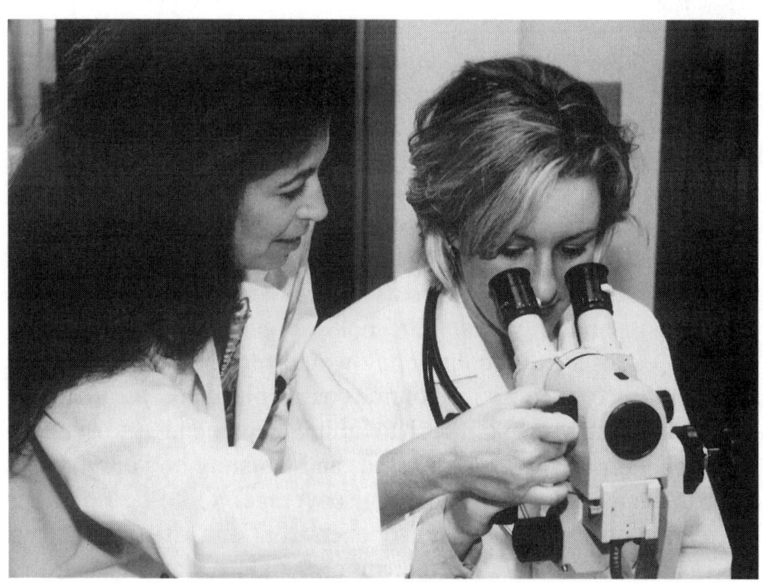

FIGURE 9-4
Most family practice residency programs offer training in basic colposcopy.

Although the increased procedural income may offset the decreased reimbursement for cognitive skills, we must always remember the words of Dr. Will Mayo, "The best interest of the patient is the only interest to be considered" (Commencement address, Rush Medical College, University of Chicago, June 15, 1910. Collected Papers of Saint Marys Hospital, Mayo Clinic, 1910, ii, p 561). If the needs of the patient would be better served by another physician more skilled in performing and interpreting an indicated procedure, then referral is obviously the correct decision.

MANAGED CARE

Managed care has affected the performance of procedures. Conflicts with specialists may arise when medical directors from managed care organizations attempt to hold down costs by influencing primary care physicians to

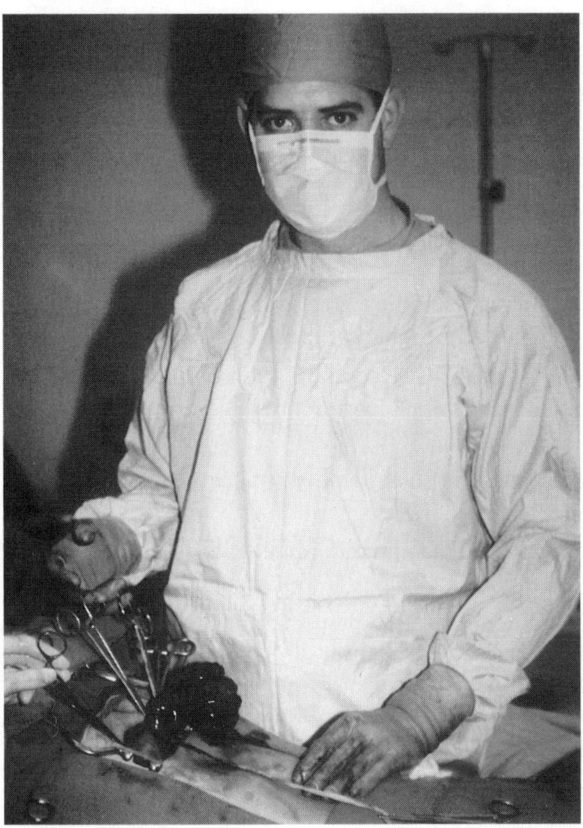

FIGURE 9-5
A few family physicians still do surgery and some assist in surgery. As residents, family physicians rotate on surgical services and focus on the presenting symptoms associated with surgical problems and perioperative management of surgical patients.

perform procedures themselves rather than referring patients to subspecialists. Although the improved status of family practice physicians is certainly welcome and appreciated, new practitioners need to remember that an intensive procedural schedule can create anxiety, stress, and increased time demands. Occasionally, best medical practices dictate that we coordinate consults rather than perform procedures. In other words, ''A man just has to know his limitations'' (Clint Eastwood in the movie Dirty Harry).

The medical student or resident evaluating potential residency programs needs to consider which residency program provides the best preparation for the individual's unique practice goals (Fig. 9-5). If a particular program is right in every way except for strength in a particular procedural skill, then there are many ways the necessary skills can be acquired. Ultimately, each resident is responsible for apprising the residency director of the resident's practice goals. For physicians in practice, it is important to delineate certain procedures that are applicable and necessary for their patients. Training for a wide range of procedures is generally readily available and should be sought. There are situations in which a patient may be better served by a specialist, and it is important for family physicians to know and understand their limitations. With this in mind, most family physicians can master certain procedural skills that will eventually make their practice of medicine more enjoyable.

BIBLIOGRAPHY

Ackerman RJ: Performance of gastrointestinal tract endoscopy by primary care physicians: lessons from the US Medicare database. Arch Fam Med 6:52-58, 1997

Felmar E, Carty-Kemker K, Haynes DG, Hocutt JE, Norris TE, Rodney WM, Susman JL, Varma J: Board of Directors Report D to the 1995 Congress. AAFP Task Force on Procedures, 1995

Musallam LS: Privileges, credentialing, and liability. Primary Care 22:491-498, 1995

Norris TE, Felmar E, Tolleson G. Which procedures should be taught in family practice residency programs? Fam Med 29:99-104, 1997

Rodney WM: Flexible sigmoidoscopy and the despecialization of gastrointestinal endoscopy: an environmental impact report. Cancer 70 Suppl: 1266-1271, 1992

CONSULTATION AND REFERRAL

10

Jan M. Larson, M.D.

One of the most important skills gained in residency training programs is the art of communication. Much time is spent teaching young physicians to communicate properly with patients concerning their individual needs. Unfortunately, less time is spent helping them to develop these same communication skills with their consultant colleagues. Patients expect that their health care providers are working together effectively to enhance their health care and are not fragmenting it into unorganized chaos. Unfortunately, in some cases, poor communication leads to disruptions in continuity of care, delayed diagnoses, unnecessary testing, and iatrogenic complications. In most successful situations, the family physician coordinates the patient's care so that the resources of medicine and society can be used for the benefit of the patient in an efficient manner.[1] This sounds easy enough, but it is indeed an art and requires continual practice.[2]

DEFINITIONS

Before proceeding, definitions are necessary for a few terms. *Consultation,* according to Stedman's Medical Dictionary,[3] is ''the meeting of two or more physicians [or surgeons] to evaluate the nature and progress of disease in a particular patient and to establish diagnosis, prognosis, and therapy.'' A *consultant* is ''a physician or surgeon who does not take actual charge of a patient, but acts in an advisory capacity, deliberating with and counseling the personal attendant.'' On the other hand, a *referral* is ''a request for the services of another person (physician or otherwise) including a permanent or temporary transfer or sharing of responsibility for a patient's care.''[4] Because a referral implies the transfer of responsibility for some aspect of the patient's care, the division must be clearly defined to allow the primary physician, the specialist, and the patient to understand who is responsible in each area.[5]

> *"The definition of a specialist as one who 'knows more and more about less and less' is good and true."*
>
> —Charles H. Mayo

REFERRAL

A referral implies a transfer of responsibility for some aspect of the patient's care. A careful division between the responsibility of the referring physician and that of the specialist must be specified clearly. Referrals are generally based on divisions of responsibility between the referring physician and the specialist. These include interval referral, collateral referral, cross referral, and split referral.[6]

Interval Referral

Interval referral, as the name implies, is for a limited interval of time and involves transfer of the patient for complete care. An example is a referral and transfer of a patient to a coronary care unit for accelerating angina and future coronary artery bypass surgery (Fig. 10-1). In this situation, the

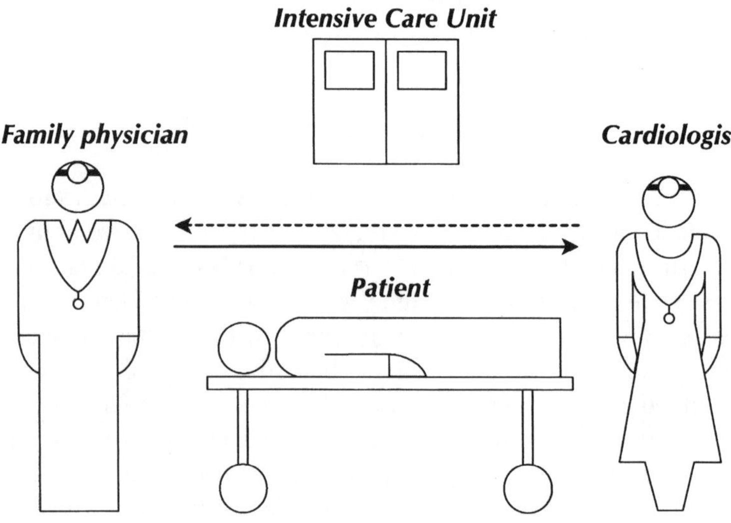

FIGURE 10-1 Interval referral. The patient's complete care is transferred for a limited time.

specialist assumes care of the patient once the patient is transferred to the coronary care unit and remains as the patient's primary physician until the patient is transferred back to the primary care physician. In this case, the family physician usually keeps informed about the patient by reviewing the chart and visits to the patient or by talking to the specialist for updates and comments concerning the patient's condition. In this circumstance, the family physician usually does not write orders for the patient unless asked to do so. The specialist may ask the family physician to act as a consultant if a problem arises that is not in the specialist's area of expertise.

Collateral Referral

Collateral referral is often used for specific problems such as ongoing diabetic eye problems or glaucoma handled by an ophthalmologist, specific orthopedic problems (eg, recent hip operation), abnormal Papanicolaou smear further evaluated by a gynecologist, or psychological problems that may involve a psychologist or psychiatrist (Fig. 10-2). The referring physician still main-

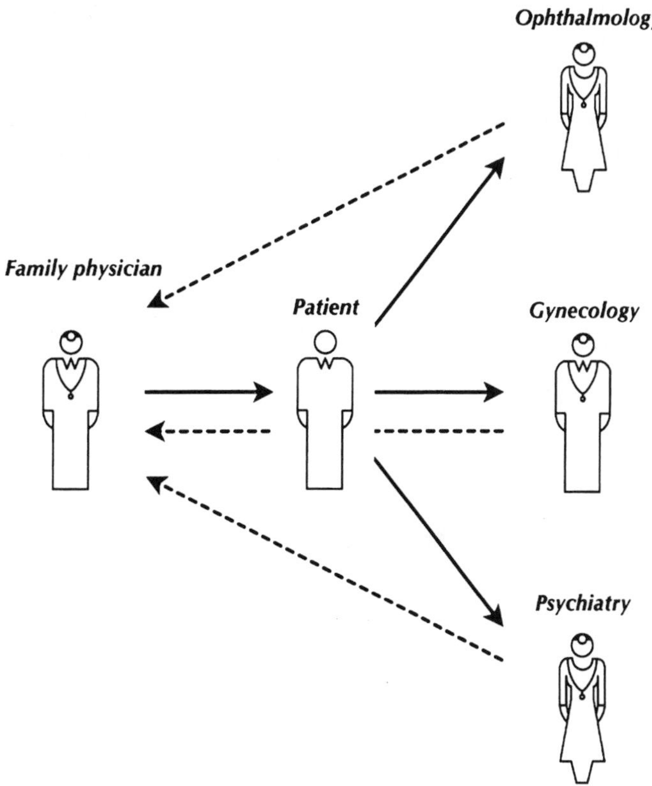

FIGURE 10-2 Collateral referral. Multiple physicians may be involved in patient's care.

tains overall responsibility for the patient; however, the patient's health is enhanced by the expertise of a specialist in an individual area of the patient's care.

Cross Referral

Cross referral occurs rarely in family medicine. Occasionally, there is a loss of confidence in the relationship between the primary care physician and the patient. The patient may self-refer to a different family physician, or the family physician may elect to refer the patient to another family physician for total care and accepts no further responsibility (Fig. 10-3). As is understandable, this can be difficult for both the patient and the physician and is rarely used except when moral or ethical values have been breached. Occasionally, for insurance reasons, a second opinion is required concerning a patient's problem. For example, if two surgeons must be consulted to determine if a hysterectomy is needed, one specialist may refer to another for a second opinion. The first surgeon should, of course, let the referring primary physician know about the second opinion before making any referral. Another example might include a family physician's referral to another family physician who has an interest and expertise in sports medicine when the first physician encounters an athletic injury that has failed to heal. In all of these cases, a patient is referred to another physician within the same specialty.

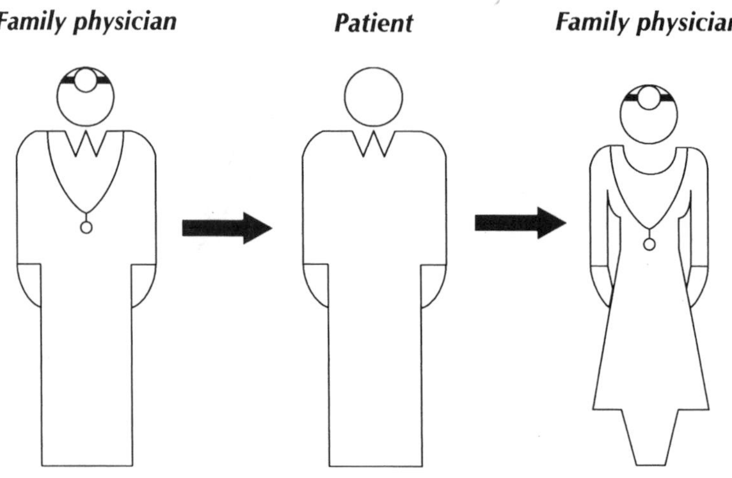

FIGURE 10-3 Cross referral. Patient's care is transferred to another physician within the same specialty.

Split Referral

Split referral occurs in a multispecialty practice or in job shares, in which the responsibility is developed more or less evenly between 2 or more physicians. An example would be a female patient who elects to see a gynecologist for Papanicolaou smears, breast examinations, or other female-related concerns, a cardiologist for cardiac-related concerns, and an endocrinologist for diabetic care (Fig. 10-4). As is obvious from the example, it is quite difficult to determine who is responsible for the overall care of the patient, and this makes coordination of care extremely difficult for the primary care physician.

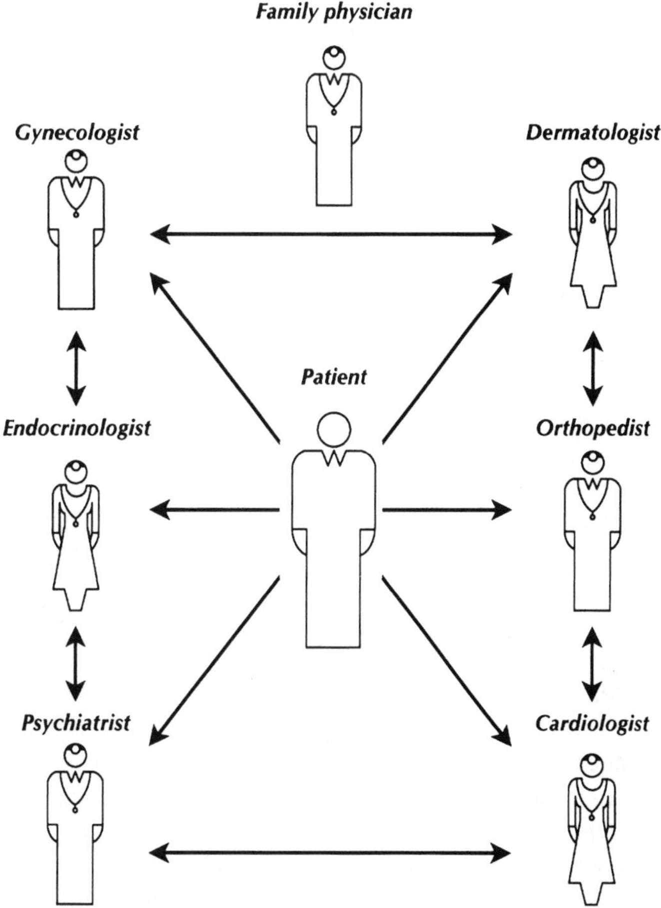

FIGURE 10-4
Split referral. Patient care responsibility is developed evenly between 2 or more physicians.

Family Physician Responsibilities

As a family physician it is important to remember that you have been vested with the often difficult role of coordinating a patient's care so that all the resources of medicine and personnel are used in an efficient manner for the benefit of the patient. This means that decisions being made about the patient's management have to be made with the clear understanding of who is responsible for them. In the setting of multiple physicians caring for a patient, primary care physicians should communicate to the patient who to contact if the patient or family has questions concerning medical care. In most circumstances, the family feels most comfortable addressing their questions to the primary care physician and expects the family practice physician to be abreast of all the medical issues involving the patient. Because of this, the consultation is used more than the referral.

> *"Of all the symptoms for which physicians are consulted, pain in one form or another is the most common and often the most urgent. Properly assessed, it stands pre-eminent among sensory phenomena of disease as a guide to diagnosis."*
>
> —Charles H. Mayo

CONSULTATION

Informal Consultation

In a consultation, the physician responsible for the patient continues to care for the patient. There is no time when the patient is transferred to the care of the consultant. The consultant only offers an opinion about the patient and then allows the primary care physician responsible for the patient to determine if the plan is the best course to follow. The consultation may be formal or informal.

Informal consultations are a part of the daily communication in medicine. They occur as you discuss a patient with a colleague. They may occur on the telephone, in the hallway, or even in the elevator during hospital rounds. Don't develop the bad habit of treating these informal consults in a casual manner. For residents in training it is important to discipline yourself to organize each presentation and formulate treatment plans given to your consultants, colleagues, and staff physicians. This developed communication skill will enhance your reputation for quality care throughout your career.[7] The key is to envision your desired outcome for the patient. Envision the patient's improved health. Ask yourself, as the primary physician, what reponsibilities you have in the allocation of both the financial resources and consultant care. At different stages of your training and practice, these variables will be different.[4] In fact, physicians with less experience tend to consult more than experienced physicians. During your residency training, you are trying to learn as much as possible in as short a time as possible. A great deal can be learned by watching the consultant interact with the patient. What is the thought process? What area of the examination is emphasized? Later in your career, you may not have the luxury of taking time away from your busy day to see a patient with the consultant. Therefore, try to learn as much as possible now during your training from a specialist's consultation.

Formal Consultation

Formal consultation, in contrast to informal consultation, is necessary and expected in the important areas of patient care and medical management. The physician requesting the consultation should communicate directly with the consultant. In most cases, this is done either by letter or note in the hospital chart or, if urgent, by telephone. Often, both a telephone call and a letter from the primary care physician are used and include the purpose of the consultation, the history of the present illness, pertinent points of the past medical history or a copy of the last complete history and physical examination from the patient's chart, medications, and, particularly in the managed care setting, what is expected of the consultation visit. The patient should always be aware of why a consultant is being seen and of the consultant's recommendations. This is the responsibility of the family physician. Unfortunately, not all consultations are helpful. Pitfalls for effective consultations may include differences between physicians, unrealistic desires and expectations of the patient, and limitations imposed by insurance companies or the patient's ability to pay.[8]

Family Physician Responsibilities

A primary physician's consultation request should include the following specific points.[9]

A. Referral physician information
   Your name, your office telephone number and address, and your home telephone number or beeper number

B. Patient information
   1. Problem to be addressed by the consultant
   2. History of present illness: An outline of the medical problem as well as what diagnostic tests have been ordered thus far and any treatments that have already been applied
   3. Past medical history: Important medical history that could relate to the medical problem to be addressed by the consultant
   4. Family history: Pertinent family medical history that could relate to the condition
   5. Social history: Psychological history and matters that might affect the illness and whether or not the patient was involved in the referral procedure
   6. Remarkable physical examination findings (eg, a copy of the results of the most recent examination done in the office)
   7. Differential diagnosis: The working diagnosis or differential diagnosis

C. Expectations for the consulting physician

If the patient is part of the managed care network, further information may be needed, which could include the following.

1. Number of visits allowed
2. Is the consultant allowed to order all tests needed for proper treatment and diagnosis or does this need to be done through the primary care physician?
3. Whom should the patient see in follow-up for discussion of the tests and results of the consultation?
4. What are the expectations for the specialist to communicate back to the primary care physician about the findings and recommendations? Does the primary care physician expect a telephone call after the patient has been seen by the specialist, or is a letter expected?[10]

Once a consultation has taken place, the consultant is expected to reply to the patient's primary physician. This reply should contain:

1. Summary that confirms the patient's course of illness
2. Diagnosis or confirmation of diagnosis
3. Treatment options
4. Advice on treatment options
5. Prognosis for the condition[11]

If the consultant's recommendations do not agree with the patient's expectations or wishes, the primary care physician should review the recommenda-

BOX 10-1 CASE EXAMPLE OF THE FAMILY PHYSICIAN'S ROLE IN REFERRAL

A woman presented to my office for abdominal pain. She was seen in an emergency department the night before. All of her test results were normal. The diagnosis of gastroenteritis was made and she was referred to me for follow-up. After obtaining more history, I noted that she had several episodes of abdominal pain 6 months previously that were not as severe. During my examination, she had no discomfort in the right upper quadrant and was feeling almost 100% improved. However, because of the history of previous episodes, the colicky nature of the attack, age, sex, being overweight and now on a weight reduction diet, I suspected that gallstones were causing biliary spasm resulting in her pain attacks during the last 6 months. I recommended ultrasonography, which was positive for gallstones but not for duct dilatation at this time. Because of her complaints and test results, I referred her to a general surgeon. The surgeon advised laparoscopic surgery, which the patient, after discussion with her husband, refused. The consultant was frustrated with the patient and her husband for not taking the advice. Because I knew the family's situation, it was easier for me to understand her refusal and to help work through the situation. The patient's husband recently had been diagnosed with angina and was reluctant to have coronary artery bypass surgery. His wife was the mainstay in the family and was trying to manage the family business and to take care of her ailing husband simultaneously. I explained the patient's predicament and assured the surgeon that I would try to work out the arrangements with the family. After meeting with the patient and her husband, we agreed to arrange additional help for the office and I further explained the surgical procedure and the expected recovery time and arranged home health care for them during the time she was recovering from surgery. After my lengthy explanation and discussion, she consented to surgery. In this case, it is evident the family physician's role was critical in ensuring proper treatment and referral for the patient.

tions and either confirm and support these to the patient or possibly seek another opinion about the possibility of other options. An important lesson for the resident and the family practice physician is that all physicians, even the best specialists in a given field, may be misinformed, may need more information, or may be wrong. In addition, there may be situations that require delicate negotiation so that the patient receives appropriate treatment (Box 10-1).

> *''Given one well-trained physician of the highest type he will do better work for a thousand people than ten specialists.''*
>
> —William J. Mayo

HEALTH INSURANCE ORGANIZATIONS

Other added variables are health maintenance organization (HMO), preferred provider organization, and managed care contracts. It is important to understand the difference between one patient's preferred provider organization coverage and another's HMO and associated co-payment constraints. Is the specialist a physician on contract for the patient's insurance carrier? In other words, does the consultant agree to see all of the HMO's patients for this particular specialty for one set cost. In these circumstances, many specialists are often willing to talk with the primary care physician about appropriate management and treatment. In fact, they often require telephone consultations before actually seeing the patient. It is important to know the consultants and the quality of their work and to make sure that the same standards are being followed regardless of insurance payment arrangements so that the patient receives the same quality of care as someone who pays a fee for service. An example is a gastroenterology group that receives a fee for service and performs colonoscopies on all hemoccult-positive stool specimens except for their contracted HMO patients, for whom they repeat the hemoccult tests to see if the results continue to remain positive. In addition, if the patient is a member of an HMO in which the consultant's fee comes from the monthly fee paid to the primary care physician and the consultant isn't willing to discuss the case but insists on seeing every patient and ordering an expensive work-up, this is not a consultant to be used for a quality, cost-effective medical practice.

Therefore, it is important in the managed care setting to outline clearly your expectations of the consultant. Also, provide all the pertinent information to improve the effectiveness of the consultation and make sure that the tests that you have already performed are not repeated. In a managed care model, it is even more important not to divest yourself of your duty and authority for overall management of the patient, and, at times, it becomes necessary to ask further questions to ensure efficient and cost-effective care for the patient.

ETHICAL ISSUES ASSOCIATED WITH MANAGED CARE

Ethical issues of managed care and reimbursement incentives may drive behavior in different directions, but the family practice physician has to balance treating the individual patient and respecting the needs and resources of the entire insured population. Much work is being done at present to develop standards of medical necessity and to demonstrate efficacy of various treatment protocols. The goal is, and always will be, to base the decisions on the potential benefit for the patient rather than on financial factors. If the potential benefit is minimal compared with the cost and the treatment or testing is not approved, an unpopular decision may have to be explained to the patient by the primary care physician. Examples of this are the nonspecific

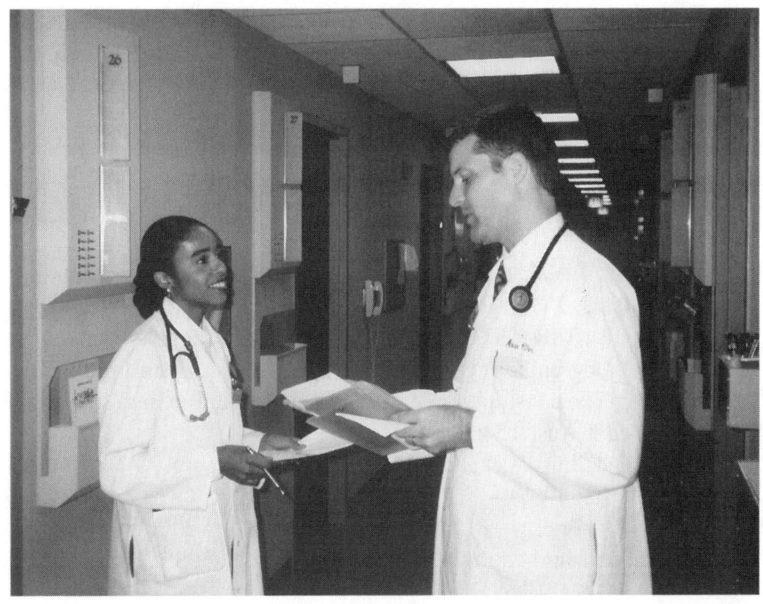

FIGURE 10-5
Consultation and referral are active processes that take place on a daily basis for family physicians.

use of a prostate-specific antigen test in a 70-year-old man and bone density scans in postmenopausal women, regardless of hormone therapy or the number of risk factors for osteoporosis. On the other end of the spectrum, the family physician needs to challenge managed care decisions that limit medically necessary care and always to act as a patient advocate.

CONCLUSIONS

The consultation and referral processes are common tasks for family physicians in practice and in training (Fig. 10-5). Handled effectively, with adequate communication and with the patient's best interest in mind, the processes can substantially enhance the care of your patients—even in today's environment of managed care medicine.

REFERENCES

1. Epstein RM, Beckman HB: Health care reform and patient-physician communication. Am Fam Physician 49:1718-1720, 1994
2. Epstein RM: Communication between primary care physicians and consultants. Arch Fam Med 4:403-409, 1995

3. Stedman's Medical Dictionary. Twenty-fourth edition. Baltimore, Williams and Wilkins, 1982, p 315
4. Brock C: Consultation and referral patterns of family physicians. J Fam Pract 4:1129-1137, 1977
5. Emanuel LL, Richter J: The consultant and the patient-physician relationship. A trilateral deliberative model. Arch Intern Med 154:1785-1790, 1994
6. McWhinney IR: An Introduction to Family Medicine. New York, Oxford University Press, 1981, pp 166-173
7. McCue JD, Beach KJ: Communication barriers between attending physicians and residents. J Gen Intern Med 9:158-161, 1994
8. Geyman JP, Brown TC, Rivers K: Referrals in family practice: a comparative study by geographic region and practice setting. J Fam Pract 3:163-167, 1976
9. Barrand J: The consultation in general practice. 2. Problem solution and management. Med J Aust 154:741, 1991
10. Bradley D: Clinical decision-making in managed care. AAFP Home Study Audio 212:8-11, Jan 1997
11. Nutting PA, Franks P, Clancy CM: Referral and consultation in primary care: do we understand what we're doing? J Fam Pract 35:21-23, 1992

11

THE ART OF TEACHING

R. John Presutti, D.O.

The foundation of medical practice is the understanding that every day is filled with learning and teaching. Physicians spend a career teaching and learning from patients, nurses, and colleagues (Fig. 11-1). As learners we are faced with a seemingly endless stream of facts and comparisons. As teachers, we are sometimes frustrated by our efforts and effectiveness, wondering if today's message reached the learners. Most physician educators hope for more than a lifetime of presenting boring lectures. Indeed, the most effective teachers are able to stimulate creative thought and motivate their students into independent learning.

Every teacher, whether a medical student giving a presentation, a resident physician teaching other residents (Fig. 11-2), or a faculty staff member teaching a resident (Fig. 11-3), develops a personal method of teaching based on past experience as a learner. Most physicians can recall positive and negative role models who helped to shape their own expectations of what it means to be an effective physician educator. We tend to pattern our own teaching on what we judge to have been helpful or detrimental during our own education. Most physicians believe their teaching methods are effective, even though they may have no objective proof. The key to effective teaching is the willingness to try new ideas in education. Even the most experienced physician preceptors need to modify their teaching style continuously as medical practice changes. Advancing medical technology has opened new frontiers in education, which present a continuing challenge. The abundance of research information released daily requires educators and learners to become selective in choosing sources of new knowledge. We must now become efficient learners so that we can become better teachers.

Circles of Influence

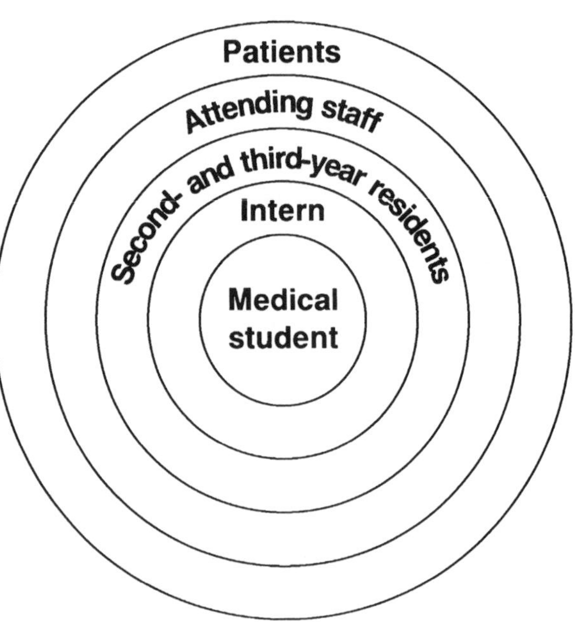

FIGURE 11-1
Circles of Influence. Learning in medicine is shaped by many circles of influence, which interact and overlap with each other. Medical students, interns, and second- and third-year residents as well as attending physicians can all learn from each other as well as from the patients.

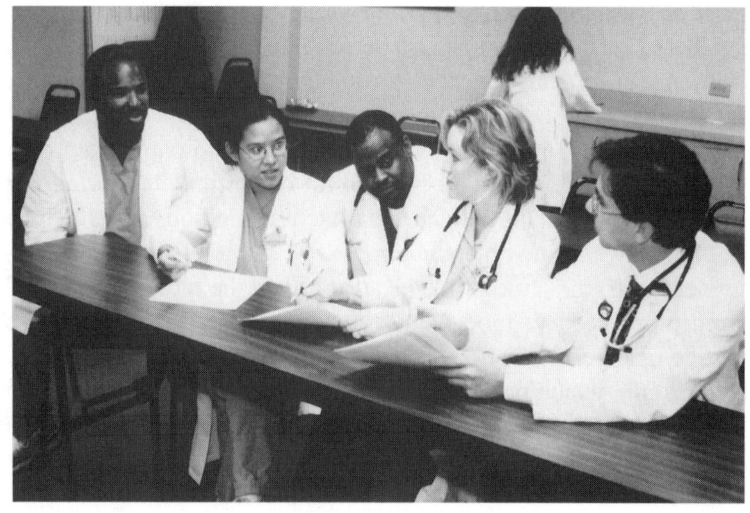

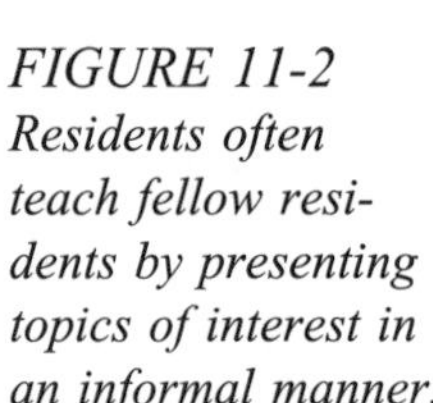

FIGURE 11-2
Residents often teach fellow residents by presenting topics of interest in an informal manner.

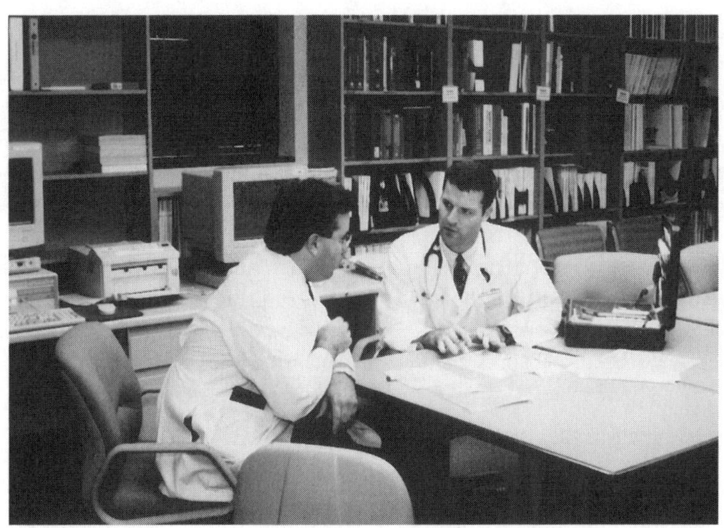

FIGURE 11-3
Attending physicians in many cases provide one-on-one teaching to residents who see patients in the outpatient setting.

> *''One of the chief defects in our plan of education in this country is that we give too much attention to developing the memory and too little to developing the mind . . .''*
>
> —William J. Mayo

In this era of reduced reimbursement, diagnosis-related groups, health maintenance organizations, and managed care, the greatest threat to quality teaching is time. New governmental restraints on reimbursement for teaching, combined with increasing pressure for clinical productivity, have made academic medicine a high-cost item within health care.[1] Teaching must be efficient and precise yet provide quality information and foster new ideas within the student's mind. Family medicine is a unique specialty in that the limited precepting time is usually the principal contact between residents and the seasoned family practitioners they would like to become.[2]

GENERAL COMMENTS ON TEACHING

Do not be misled that lectures are the best way to learn. Medical students and interns require a basic amount of didactic information, but variation is important in keeping the learner's attention and sparks new interests. When possible, it may be helpful to incorporate activities such as journal clubs,

BOX 11-1 CREATIVE TEACHING TECHNIQUES

The Department of Family Medicine at Mayo Clinic Jacksonville, under the direction of Dr. R. John Presutti, has developed a creative teaching tool. Annually, before the American Board of Family Practice board examination, the 3 classes of residents (6 in each class) pair into teams. Each team produces 10 board-format multiple-choice questions with complete references. Those questions are edited, randomly ordered, and presented in an electronic format. Teams are asked questions and compete in a round-robin fashion, 1 point for each correct answer, until all teams have had 3 opportunities to gain points. The 3 leading teams then compete in an elimination round. Overall winning teams are awarded prizes. This interactive teaching tool provides a fun and competitive way to prepare for the board certification and inservice examinations.

debates, and games into the curriculum (Box 11-1). Try to keep the 3 parts of learning (fact, rethinking, usage[3]) in mind when designing activities. Make learning challenging but enjoyable.

When teaching lectures are necessary, there are some valuable points to consider. First, ask yourself what key points you need to make. A 45-minute lecture should have no more than 5 key points. Next, build the talk around these key points. Repeat the key points in at least 3 different ways throughout the talk.[3] Be respectful of the audience's time. Make slides simple and easy to follow. Expensive, complicated slides do not increase the value of your information. Strive to make your conclusions simple and easy to remember.

TEACHING MEDICAL STUDENTS AND INTERNS

Medical students and interns are discussed together because their learning is highly interdependent, especially in the hospital setting. Medical students often feel they receive the most valuable component of their education from house staff.[4] Frequently, the intern's first attempt at teaching is directed toward a medical student after identifying a lack of knowledge in a particular area. Interns frequently sacrifice a significant amount of time and energy to teach medical students, even though they are usually the most overworked members of the team. Whenever possible, an intern's efforts at teaching should be recognized and appreciated.

For medical students, their first interaction with patients begins under the guidance of a physician educator. Frequently, medical students are nervous and rarely have a substantial understanding of how to get the most from their clinical rotations. Interns, however, have most basic examination skills learned, but they need guidance on the big picture of differential diagnosis and management. As an educator, do not allow your students to learn in the dark.[3] Set goals and expectations early to alleviate any confusion. Make sure that basic skills are stressed with medical students and interns. A perfect moment to improve basic examination technique is at patient's bedside. Here the teaching environment becomes a greater challenge.

''The educator has assumed almost full charge of medical education.''

—William J. Mayo

The patient's bedside is an excellent place to demonstrate elements of the physical examination, but there is also great anxiety surrounding bedside teaching. Students are distracted by the fear of appearing ignorant to unexpected questions. Alternatively, some students may become bored on rounds. Involve everyone when possible. Have a plan of action for what you will discuss while in the patient's room. To lessen anxiety, discuss key areas of the physical examination before entering the room. There is no benefit in humiliating the learner. Humiliation makes the patient uncomfortable, resulting in a breakdown in the physician-patient relationship, and the teacher becomes less effective. Also remember that post-call is not a good time for learning.[1,3]

Group time is expensive.[1] Learners become frustrated if they have tasks to perform and no time to complete them. Maintain the focus on teaching during rounds. Demand the students' attention and make their time with you worthwhile. Learning together is valuable. Identify a disease, condition, or physical finding that deserves further discussion. Admit, ''we all need to learn more about this.'' Involve yourself in the reading and discussion. It is comforting to an intern that the attending physician does not know everything. This fosters the idea of continuous learning from an experienced family physician.

As a related issue, time management should be stressed to interns. The internship year is ideal for developing habits and organizational skills that will simplify the remainder of residency. Attending physicians should share their organizational patterns that were particularly helpful during residency. Also stress prioritizing activities. This is especially necessary for interns having difficulty completing work rounds. Keeping a list numbered for priority can be a dramatic step in efficiency for a new intern.

BOX 11-2 FAMILY MEDICINE CORE CURRICULUM

Conferences are an important part of any family medicine residency program. The American College of Graduate Medical Education makes recommendations for Family Medicine teaching staff as well as residents to participate in delivering conferences throughout the residency. In addition to lectures given within the Department of Family Medicine, the educational experience should be supplemented by conferences during specialty and subspecialty rotations. Attendance at these conferences must be recorded and is an integral part of program accreditation. Staff physicians are strongly encouraged to attend these lectures. There should be a forum for evaluations of the lectures so that modifications of the core curriculum can be made.

The Graduate Medical Education Directory,[5] which is published annually, provides a description of specific core curriculum requirements. Human Behavior and Mental Health, Maternity and Gynecologic Care, Care of the Surgical Patient, Sports Medicine, Emergency Medicine, Pediatrics, and Care of the Older Patient are only a few of the areas addressed (Fig. 11-4). Family Medicine Residency Directors use the requirements from the American College of Graduate Medical Education to help formulate their own core curriculum and to ensure an appropriate cross section of didactic, structured education. Most curriculum lectures are given during noon conferences, and many residency programs attempt to provide lunch for their residents during those conferences. Minimum attendance requirements are usually set forth by the program director. Typical minimum attendance requirements are 50 percent for PGY-1, 70 percent for PGY-2, and 80 percent for PGY-3. In addition to traditional didactic presentations, most residency programs have a monthly morbidity and mortality conference to review the prior month's admissions and deaths. This allows a forum for feedback among the Family Medicine residents and attending physicians.

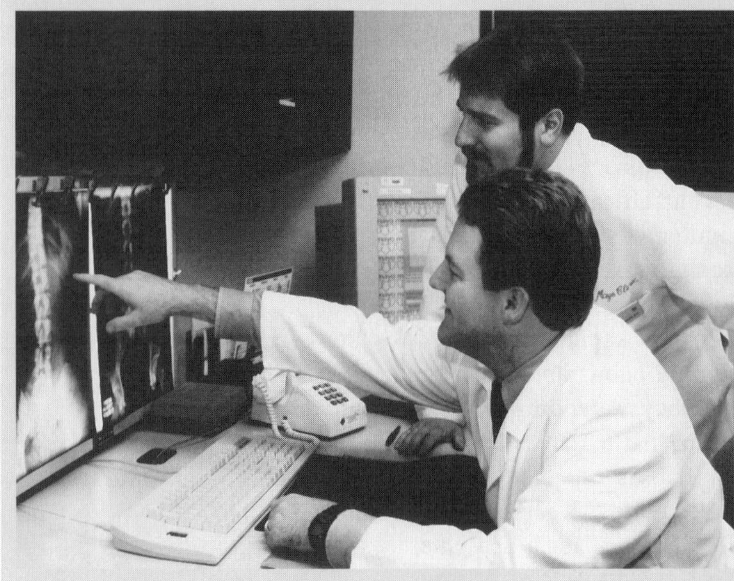

FIGURE 11-4 *Comprehensive care, which may involve multiple fields of medicine, is a hallmark of residency training in family medicine.*

TEACHING JUNIOR AND SENIOR RESIDENTS

As family practice residents move into their second and third years, the emphasis shifts to micromanagement and long-term outcome. Differential diagnosis skills should be well developed. It is during this time that residents can refine their skills in all areas from patient communication to procedures. This is also a transition time for residents who soon will be facing their new positions as family medicine attending physicians.

Junior and senior residents frequently are called on to teach but rarely receive formal training in education techniques. Emphasize goal setting with these residents. Have senior residents express early on what they will expect from their subordinates. Encourage senior residents to recognize performance and give positive feedback immediately. Likewise, provide negative feedback in a timely manner on a one-to-one basis. Residency programs should be encouraged to make teaching programs available for their residents (Box 11-2). The Stanford Faculty Development Program is one such example of a nationally known program designed to help residents and staff physicians improve their teaching and communication skills. Other programs include the ''Five-Step 'Microskills' Model''[2] and modifications of that program.[6]

BEING A GOOD MENTOR

Medical education is a journey to the top of one totem pole, only to fall off and land at the bottom of the next. All physicians have this experience through medical training. However, at no point in the journey are we without the challenge of being role models. The premedical college student gazes on the first year medical student thinking ''I'll be there some day.'' The new intern watches a third-year family medicine resident running a code blue hoping someday to have the same level of confidence. But above all, every move of the attending physician will be observed for clues on how to master the art of family medicine.

As a mentor, compassion is a valuable tool and a cornerstone of family medicine. Patients and families look to their family practitioner for compassion. Residents watch and learn how to deliver that compassion. Families become devoted to a physician who displays genuine concern for the patient. Effective role models learn the value of compassion and communication skills early in medical training.

When residents and medical students were asked what specific traits made

BOX 11-3 ADVISORS IN FAMILY MEDICINE RESIDENCY

At the beginning of a Family Medicine residency, the new intern is assigned to a staff physician who serves as the resident physician's advisor during the 3 years of training. The advisor-resident relationship is important to the growth and develop ment of family medicine residents in training (Fig. 11-5). In most cases, the advisor serves as a mentor and confidant for the resident physician. Career plans are discussed, as are rotation evaluations. Problems encountered during residency, whether

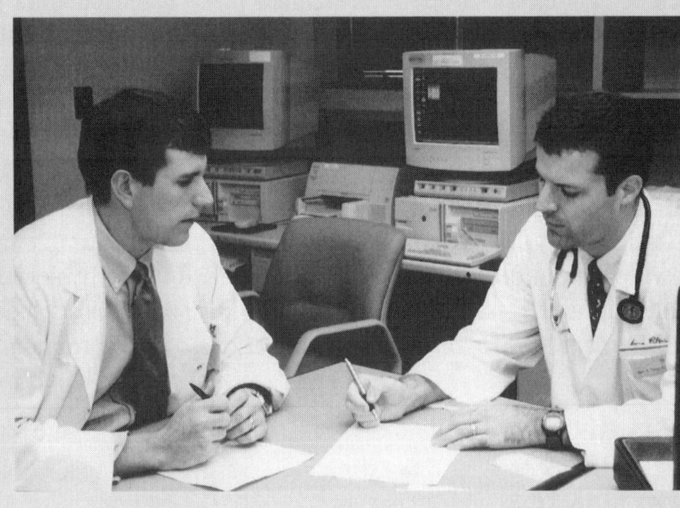

FIGURE 11-5
Supervision by staff physicians allows family medicine residents to enhance their educational experience.

an individual stand out as a role model, they answered with the following (adapted from[7,8]).

Attitudes toward residents and students

Communication skills

Compassion for patients and families

Enthusiasm

Integrity and objectivity

Patience

Proficiency as a diagnostician

Ability to explain difficult subjects

BOX 11-3 Continued

personal or related to residency training, are often discussed. Typically, the advisor and resident meet quarterly to discuss resident's progress and to identify any areas of weakness that need to be focused on in the educational development of the resident physician (Fig. 11-6). Lasting relationships may develop, and further recommendations for employment or hospital privileges may be obtained from staff advisors.

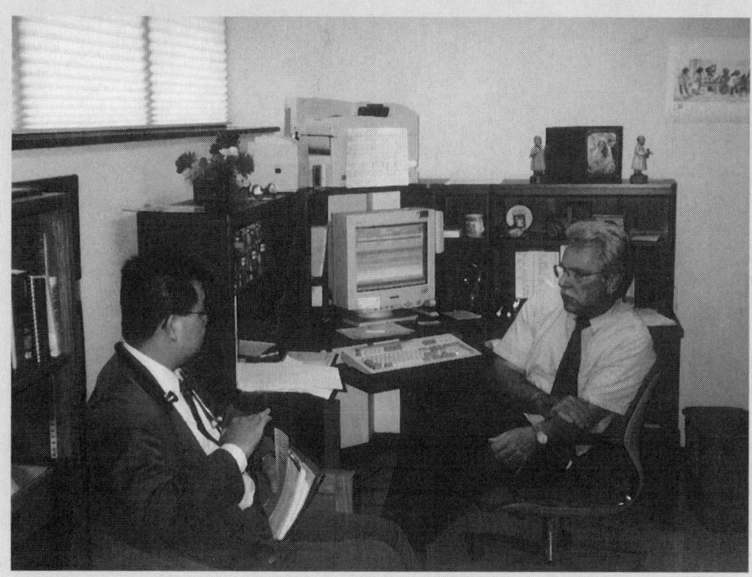

FIGURE 11-6
Resident physicians meet regularly with their advisors to discuss career plans, performance on rotations, and any problems that arise during residency.

To master all of these traits would be an arduous task. An excellent mentor develops a teaching style that projects equality and positive values among these key traits (Box 11-3).

CONCLUSIONS

Medical education always will be rewarding to those educators who strive to ignite the learner's spirit. Understand that the variation in presenting knowledge can sometimes be the key to continued interest from your learners

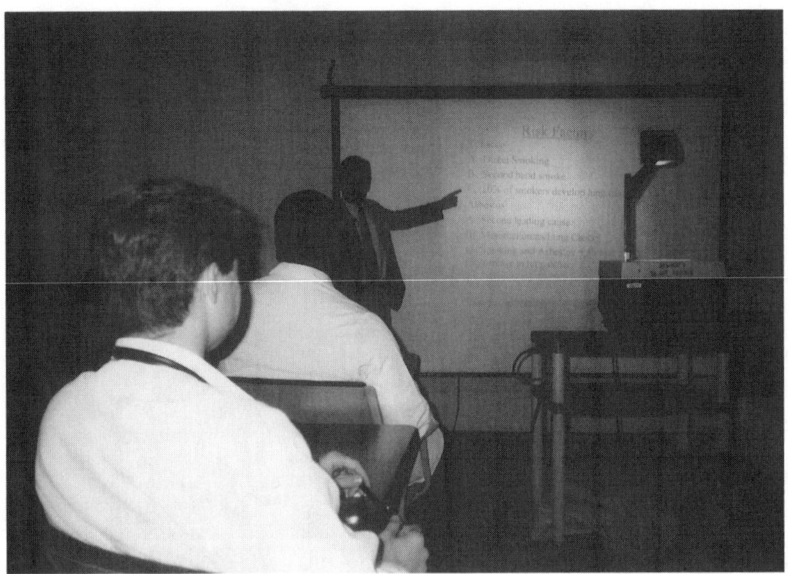

FIGURE 11-7
Break-out sessions are a good method for teaching residents in training.

(Fig. 11-7). Always set goals for the learners and be sure they know what is expected of them from the beginning. Use time efficiently. Become a good learner yourself by always asking questions, and you will become a great educator.

Some particularly valuable references are listed below. ''Bedside Teaching''[1] is a concise description of the problems and solutions surrounding bedside teaching. The ''Five-Step 'Microskills' Model''[2] is an excellent blueprint to begin an educational development program in a residency program. Finally, Hurst's book *The Bench And Me*[3] is an easy-to-read overview of all aspects of teaching and learning for physicians.

REFERENCES

1. Kroenke K, Omori DM, Landry FJ, Lucey CR: Bedside teaching. South Med J 90:1069-1074, 1997
2. Neher JO, Gordon KC, Meyer B, Stevens N: A five-step ''microskills'' model of clinical teaching. J Am Board Fam Pract 5:419-424, 1992
3. Hurst JW: The Bench and Me: Teaching and Learning Medicine. New York, Igaku-Shoin, 1992
4. Gunderman R: The unrecognized medical educator (letter). Acad Med 72:472, 1997

5. American Medical Association: Graduate Medical Education Directory 1998-1999. Chicago, American Medical Association, 1998
6. Wipf JE, Pinsky LE, Burke W: Turning interns into senior residents: preparing residents for their teaching and leadership roles. Acad Med 70:591-596, 1995
7. Wright S: Examining what residents look for in their role models. Acad Med 71:290-292, 1996
8. Wright S, Wong A, Newill C: The impact of role models on medical students. J Gen Intern Med 12:53-56, 1997

12

TIME USE MANAGEMENT

Mark S. Schwartz, Ph.D.

No one has enough (time), yet everyone has all there is!
—R. Alec Mackenzie, *Teamwork Through Time Management: New Time Management Methods for Everyone in Your Organization*

Without a written plan, you are likely to fall prey to putting out fires or to working on someone's agenda other than your own.
—Edward A. Charlesworth and Ronald G. Nathan, *Stress Management: A Comprehensive Guide to Wellness*

What is the best use of my time right now?
—Alan Lakein, *How to Get Control of Your Time and Your Life*

Time use is a major problem for all health care professionals and especially for family physicians and many of their patients. Unfortunately, poor use of time is often a major factor in causing or worsening depression, anxiety, anger, insomnia, headaches, and other psychophysiologic symptoms. Poor use of time also contributes to interpersonal problems, marital and other family problems, and reduced effectiveness at work. Achievements, in medicine or in our personal lives, are compromised or never accomplished when there is frequent and repeated poor time utilization.

Better use of time can help you:

Reduce time pressures and the feeling of being overwhelmed

Meet deadlines successfully

Increase time to do what you want and need to do

Reduce wasted time

Stop trying to do too much

Increase control over your schedule and activities

Prevent or manage procrastination

Stop feeling like you are always behind

Reduce interruptions

Reduce or avoid feeling pulled in several directions

Increase time for relaxation therapies

Increase time for family and friends

Increase your time with self-care healthy behaviors

Reduce symptoms such as fatigue, anxiety, insomnia, depression, headaches, psychophysiologic symptoms, and chronic pain

With these in mind, the family physician or resident in training may benefit from higher job satisfaction and a more enjoyable personal life (Fig. 12-1).

There always will be some wasted time. Even as highly regarded physi-

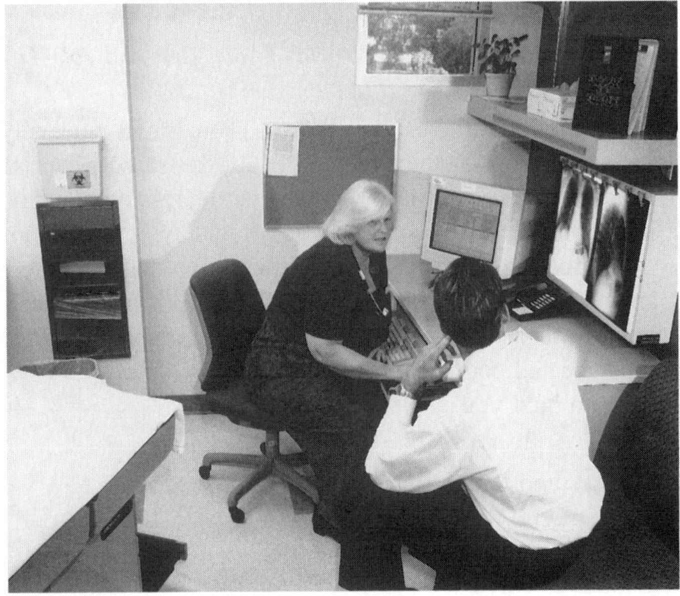

FIGURE 12-1
Time efficiency is an important part of being a successful family physician.

cians who obviously have managed to complete the rigors of medical school, you will never be perfect or nearly perfect in your time use. The questions to ask yourself are:

How much time do I waste?

How often do I waste time?

How long does procrastination or other time wasting last?

How much does it interfere with my life?

Thus, what does the wasted time cost me?

With this introspection, the astute physician can identify areas that need improvement and further attention.

SELECTED GUIDELINES FOR IMPROVING TIME USE MANAGEMENT

This chapter provides comments and recommendations for family medicine residents in training and others in managing or making substantial improvements in the use of time in various situations. There are many discussions of the causes of poor use of time and many suggestions for managing and resolving valuable wasted time. If readers want more information, consider one or more of the books listed at the end of the chapter that are devoted entirely to time use management.

In general, there are exercises that can be followed to improve time management. Many are simple and can be incorporated into your workday.

> *"We must bear in mind the difference between thoroughness and efficiency. Thoroughness gathers all the facts, but efficiency distinguishes the two-cent pieces of non-essential data from the twenty-dollar gold pieces of fundamental fact."*
>
> —William J. Mayo

General

Do your thinking, planning, scheduling, and revising on paper or computer. Include long-term, short-term, and intermediate-term goals. Make the goals specific, realistic, moderately demanding, achievable, and flexible. Consider listing your goals under topics such as: career, health, material and financial, personal growth, personal relationships, family, recognition, recreational, social, community, and spiritual. Your short-term career goals are currently consuming a huge amount of your time. You might perceive that there is barely any time for added goals under several of these categories. However, try to include some items under all of the categories. Even a short time spent on some can be rewarding and can increase the chances of fulfillment in the future. Learn guidelines for completing a goal list and priorities. Set priorities and plan objectives to attain them. Carry this with you. Plan and set priorities for each day.

Allow time for variety, balance, and goal-related activities. Leave open time for unexpected tasks and add about 25% to your first estimate of time needed for objectives. Commitments always seem to require more time than what was originally expected.

Schedule quiet intervals a few times per week to review and revise your objectives and goals. Actions that help you prepare for long-range goals are as useful as direct action toward those goals (Moskowitz's ''Rule of Readiness'').[1] In other words, a good plan with regular reevaluation helps to accomplish goals.

Make *waiting* time a useful *gift of time.* Use the time to apply relaxation techniques, read journal or other articles, do some planning for a project, edit part of a paper you are writing or editing for someone else, and make notes about tasks to be accomplished. Keep and use a list of tasks you can do in 5 minutes or less. Complete simple tasks in these periods to prevent wasted time.

Schedule healthy activities such as recreation, exercise, relaxation therapy, social time, and perhaps even intimate time with your mate. This is similar to *paying yourself first* or putting some money into savings and investments *before* paying bills. Try combining activities. For example, talk with your spouse or mate, children, colleagues, or friends during walking exercise. This is particularly useful for the busy family physician who has to juggle family life.

Many physicians feel compelled to complete all tasks themselves. Obviously, this can be a poor use of time. When possible, delegate tasks at home and at work. Sources of this common time waster include believing you can do it better, anxiety about the other person making mistakes, fear of losing control of the project or task, a perceived need for perfection in more tasks than is necessary, a lack of confidence in others, and a false sense of efficiency. Work on changing these. It can simplify your life and help eliminate unnecessary time commitments.

When you delegate, select a responsible person, make your instructions clear, give needed authority and resources, remain available for help as needed, and get regular follow-up reports for quality control. With these guidelines you can greatly increase your productivity and better use your time.

Medical Practice Time Wasters

The practice of family medicine has many potential time wasters. Determine where you are wasting time and where you can spend less time without losing effectiveness.

Patients We all have patients who are verbose, ramble, or perceive a need for extra social attention from the family physician. Of course, listening time is crucial. However, family physicians can and indeed must control the use of the limited time available. Many patients do not understand and many are uncomfortable with time constraints. Verbal behaviors to keep sessions moving and to end sessions are beyond the scope of this chapter, but examples of specific nonverbal behaviors to end a session include:

Closing your pen or turning off your computer in clear view of the patient when you are done

Putting your hands on the arms of your chair *as if* ready to get up

Standing up and remaining by your chair for a few moments

Taking one or more steps toward the door if needed

Interruptions *Hi, got a minute?* One of the biggest time wasters at work is interruptions by colleagues, allied health professionals, and secretaries. "Got a minute" is never just one minute. It takes much longer than the interruption time. It also takes the time you need to regain your focus and momentum. When a colleague or other employee comes into your office and you do not have time or do not want to take time with them, consider:

Standing up and remain standing

Asking them to walk with you wherever you are going

Handling the question, if the topic is brief or urgent

Setting another time for a more convenient appointment with them

Asking who else they asked or proposing other persons for them to consider

Encouraging or urging them to work on a solution; review in a day or so if needed

A major source of interruptions is an open-door policy. It may be wise to avoid this. The trick is to be accessible to those who need you and to be able to keep your door closed, when appropriate. Use this private time for writing, dictation, telephone calls, and time to think. At home, seek out a quiet time and place to complete tasks and ask family and friends to avoid interrupting you.

Nearly everyone understands that you have limited time. In most cases you can be frank with patients, friends, and colleagues. In the end, they will respect you and your time together.

Telephone Calls at Work and at Home Pager and telephone interruptions at work are often time wasters. Do you answer every page? Do you answer almost every telephone call at work and at home? How long do you spend on these calls? Remember, telephone calls are not always reasonable demands for your attention. In view of this try:

Blocking out times for making calls

If you are going to call someone back: When will they be available? Explain the reason for your call and request any information needed.

You do not need to answer or return all calls. Do not answer your telephone or pager when your time is more valuable than talking on the telephone. You may even want to consider Caller ID.

Delegate someone to screen your calls and to take messages. Delegate appropriate return calls and give specific instructions for those completing this task.

If you have to take a call, take charge of it. Get to the reason for your call quickly and effectively. Avoid long conversations. You will not offend the caller if you keep the call short. Phrases to help keep telephone calls short include:

Before I let you go

I know you are busy, so I will wrap this up quickly

I was just walking out the door

I only have a minute

I have someone in my office, so I need to be brief

Paper

First, clear your desk often. Organize your work areas on a regular basis. Get rid of clutter. Use the TRAF[2] method of handling paper: throw it, refer it, act on it, or, file it. Throw away anything you don't need.

Looking for papers often wastes time. There are many systems for organizing your files. Find and use a system that works for you. Consult references for ideas. It is never too late to develop or revise a system. You do not need to organize all your files, but make an attempt to organize most of them.

Another common paper source of wasted time is magazines, newspapers, and journals. How many news magazines, medical journals, and other references do you subscribe to and need? Many represent unnecessary paper that gets stacked up and only clutters your office. Be selective—save the ones you need and throw the rest away.

If you must read a newspaper every day or on many days, then do so. However, ask yourself how high on your priority list this is. With Internet news services, you can use keywords to select news stories with any topic or keyword. Then, you can check the latest news on only the topics you want or need. This takes less time than newspaper and news magazine page turning and handling. However, there are times and places to do this kind of reading and reviewing. Examples include waiting in line, sitting on an airplane, and certain other sitting activities.

Journals appear more important, and often they are. However, if you subscribe to several, you will review many journals and articles that are of limited value to you at the time you receive and review the journal. Then, there is the issue of storage and organizing the journals. Consider subscribing to the fewest number of journals you can. When you need to research a specific topic, computer reference searches and abstracting services can be more time efficient. You can do the search with your computer or you can delegate the task to someone else with specific instructions.

SAYING NO AND ATTEMPTING TOO MUCH

Family physicians and many others driven by the need to accomplish commonly attempt to do too much at work, to do too many work-related projects such as speaking engagements, and to do too much at home and elsewhere. Being extremely busy and refusing to turn down requests are often major sources of wasted time, because they often take time from goals and tasks higher on your priority list. Requests to give talks and to write chapters appear flattering and are often difficult to resist. However, they often are far more time consuming than the rewards and satisfaction they provide. Be careful! These requests are tempting. Something else on your goal and priority list will be sacrificed. Consider the following courteous regrets.

> Thank you for inviting me to . . . I gave it a lot of thought and struggled with it.
>
> Unfortunately, this would be very difficult for me to do, especially this year. This was not an easy decision. My other obligations place conflicting demands on my schedule, my other plans, and my energy. These obligations include my clinical and administrative work, trying to find and preserve time for existing long-term and short-term goals and projects, looking after my elderly father, and preserving vacation time for needs I know you understand. When I think about all of these, I realize it would not work easily. I hope that another opportunity will arise for me. Thank you again for thinking of me. Cordially and in friendship,

In many instances, physicians are often asked to *push the envelope as far as it will go*—to see more patients and take on more responsibilities. If you must or choose to do so, then something else in your use of time might need to change. Say *NO* to unnecessary added tasks and requests. Do it politely but assertively. As a courtesy, listen. Say no. Give reasons. Offer alternatives.[3] What is the worst that can occur if you say no? Ask yourself:

1. Will anything bad happen if I don't do this task?
2. Is the task *worth* the time investment?
3. Can you do the task *more efficiently* than others?
4. Do you need to perform the task *perfectly?*
5. Do *you* need to do this task?
6. Can you *refer* this task?
7. Do you need to do the task *now?*
8. If the answer is no, do *not* do it.

What do you say if your supervisor persists in a request? Consider saying:

> Do you want me to stop [project X] until this new project is done?
>
> Do you want me to extend the deadline on project X and give this new project a higher priority? Should I have someone else take over [project X]?

With these tools, it should be easier to avoid overextending oneself.

Perfectionism

Perfectionism is an urge for flawless performance beyond practical purposes. It paralyzes effectiveness. It wastes time and energy. It can lead to depression. Do you often think or make any of these statements?

Either I do it perfectly or not at all.

If I make mistakes, I feel bad. Others will think less of me.

I can't stand it when I am average at something.

I should have done it better.

Very few people live up to my expectations.

Some medical tasks do need to be done perfectly, but most tasks, including many work-related tasks for physicians, do not need perfection. For example, proofreading every word in every document and changing every typographic error and every transcription error are often not needed and use time better spent on other tasks and activities. Ask yourself:

Is there a less detailed yet acceptable and practical way to do a task?

Will trying to do this task perfectly take time from other important tasks and projects?

Can a slightly reduced performance by other people still work adequately?

For text for publication, is there someone who can help me do this (eg, an editor or a proofreader)?

Remember, a gem with a flaw is worth more than a perfect brick.[4]

Procrastination

Chronically or periodically putting off starting or finishing work, home, or personal projects is a common and major source of stress and inefficient use of time. It results in wasted time worrying about the project, and it can be distracting during other activities. Procrastination results in inefficient use of time secondary to added time needed to refresh your memory about details, to find needed items and information, and to deal with the consequences of the delays. Putting off completing tasks and having them build up can interfere with other needed work, family, and social activities.

To avoid procrastination, determine why you procrastinate and analyze your reasons. Among the reasons often given are:

Overwhelming size or complexity of the work

Not being in the mood

Perceived need for perfection

Lack of interest

Perceived lack of time

Perceived need for pressure to work better

Start the process to stop procrastination. Commit yourself to avoid procrastination. Realize that you control much of what you do. Does the task or project really need to be done and done by you? If yes, then set a deadline, write it down, and post it. Consider my favorite method adapted from Burns.[5] Instead of saying, ''I'm not in the mood'' to do something, remember the principle: action before mood[5] (motivation).

If not in the mood, start anyway but just for a few minutes and with very small parts of larger tasks. Getting started is often the most difficult hurdle for many people. Starting almost anywhere, even for only a few minutes, often leads to continuation.

Remember TIC-TOC.[5,6] Say to yourself, ''task-oriented cognitions (TOC).'' These include: I will work on it only for 10 or 15 minutes; I can do that much; If I do small parts every day or most days for ___ days, weeks, or months, it will be done. Replace your task-interfering cognitions (TIC) such as: The task is too big to do now; I need a big block of uninterrupted time; If I am not in the mood, I will not do a good job, so I will wait until I feel like doing it; If I do not have enough time to do it perfectly, I should or will postpone doing it.

Losing and Misplacing Items

Keep items in familiar locations. At home, all items from your pockets should go on one table, desk, dresser, or in one basket. For work, have an organizer bag or case or laptop computer case. Personally, I use a rolling *catalog* case with an accordion fan file and places for pens, business and credit cards, and accessories in which I keep my laptop computer, disks, books, file folders, and everything else I need.

Meetings

Do you really have to go to every meeting? Are you a crucial member of the committee? Can you sometimes explain that you have other tasks you must do? Avoid unnecessary meetings or appoint someone qualified to represent you.

Other Time Wasters to Manage (Crises and Surprises)

Unfortunately, an excellent time use management program only manages about half of most people's busy schedules. Unexpected problems and emergencies intrude periodically. However, thinking and planning for these, at least in general, will make them less disruptive. Have contingency plans in mind for possible unexpected events and crises. Record them to help you remember and guide other people to help you when needed.

Examples of such problems and crises include sudden personnel absences, family crises, extra patients, more complicated than anticipated patients, and computer problems. Have alternative child care arrangements made in case of emergency. Enlist the help of others and know who and when to ask for help.

TIME DIARY. HOW DO YOU SPEND YOUR TIME NOW? A TIME USE LOG

". . . *no one* has a realistic idea of where their time goes without a time log. People are *always* surprised."[3]

Most people, including health care providers, have only a rough idea of how they spend their time. Consider keeping a time diary or log for 3 to 7 typical days. It is the most accurate way to learn how much time you actually are spending on various activities and represents a baseline to help measure change. One option is to list all activities associated with a typical day and estimate the time spent in each.

Include at least these activities: drop-in visitors, telephone calls, looking for lost items, driving others, television without other simultaneous activity, meetings, paperwork, doing work for others, socializing at work, housecleaning, organizing, extra time doing tasks perfectly, shopping, laundry or cleaners, waiting without having useful tasks to do, health care behaviors, and pleasure. Focus on areas that need improvement. Consider repeating the diary once or twice a year.

WHAT IF YOUR GOALS AND PRIORITIES APPEAR OVERWHELMING?

When you view the task before you, it may appear overwhelming and too much to accomplish even with adequate time allowed to complete the task. Reynolds and Tramel[7] provide a wonderful metaphor and viewpoint for this type of situation.

> The giant octopus has eight powerful arms, each provided with two rows of adhesive suckers. Like [*many people*], octopuses live between rocks and hard places most of the time. Suppose you are a giant octopus and you have planted each arm on a different rock; each rock represents an area of your life that is demanding your attention and time. Now, imagine you have mysteriously lost the ability to release your arms. The more you try to pull them back, the tighter they stick. The tighter they stick, the more they pull away from you. Something has to give—and it's not going to be a rock! The moral: Before you plant your arms be sure you are planting them where you want them to be. And be sure you will be able to release them. An octopus uses only two arms to move ahead. While these are alternately planted and released, . . . the other arms flow free much like feelers. Sometimes an octopus stops and gathers all his arms about himself for protection.
>
> You can accomplish everything on your big chart in a normal life span, and perhaps do more, if you know when to plant and when to release, when to feel your way and when to rest.

You can use your time more effectively. You must choose how to use time. After all, you manage your life, or at least a larger portion than you might think, in relation to time. Devote yourself to improving your use of time in specific areas of your life. Once these goals are accomplished, move on to other areas. However, it is important to avoid excessive time use management methods. There are limits. Do not let the "tail wag the dog." A rigid schedule without flexibility may serve only to cause additional stress. Do not feel guilty if you are not perfectly time efficient. Start somewhere, be realistic, and keep practicing. After all, "practice makes perfect."

TOOLS FOR ORGANIZING YOUR LIFE

Becoming better organized goes a long way to improving time use and reducing stress.[8] Consider these references on time management: Eisenberg *Organize Yourself*,[9] Schlenger and Roesch *How To Be Organized in Spite of Yourself: Time and Space Management That Works With Your Personal Style,*[10] Winston *The Organized Executive: New Ways to Manage Time, Paper, People, and the Electronic Office,*[2] and Winston *Getting Organized: The Easy Way to Put Your Life in Order.*[11]

A large (24 × 36 inches) wall calendar with 12 months displayed may help organize the year's events. In addition, there are software programs to help organization. One well-known program is the Day-Timer HomeLife CD-ROM. However, calendars, to do lists, telephone and address lists, lists of credit card numbers, and inventories can be made easily with a simple word processor. Intuit Quicken is a superb personal finance software to help pay bills on-line, keep all financial records, track investments, and more. However, one must consider the time to learn the program and the additional time to enter all the data regularly. Options for electronic work organizers (personal data assistant) include the handheld 3COM Palm III Organizer, the Psion Series 5, the Franklin Rolodex Electronics REX PC Companion, and the Hewlett-Packard 320LX or 620LX Palmtop PC. People comfortable with these high-tech devices can make good use of them. For those unfamiliar with the high-tech option, it might be worth a trial. However, learning and maintenance require added time and must be compared with alternative time management options. If you are truly disorganized, need a lot of help, get desperate enough, and can afford the investment, hire a professional organizer with several years of experience and with satisfied references. Contact the National Association of Professional Organizers at (512) 206-0151.

REFERENCES

1. Moskowitz R: How to Organize Your Work and Your Life. Garden City, New York, Doubleday, 1981
2. Winston S: The Organized Executive: New Ways to Manage Time, Paper, People, and the Electronic Office. Updated edition. New York, WW Norton, 1994
3. Mackenzie RA: The Time Trap. New York, AMACOM, 1990
4. LeBoeuf M: Working Smart: How to Accomplish More in Half the Time. New York, Warner Books, 1979
5. Burns DD: The Feeling Good Handbook. New York, Plume Book, 1989
6. Beck AT, Emery G: Anxiety Disorders and Phobias: A Cognitive Perspective. New York, Basic Books, 1985
7. Reynolds H, Tramel ME: Executive Time Management: Getting 12 Hours' Work Out of an 8-Hour Day. Englewood Cliffs, New Jersey, Prentice-Hall, 1979, pp 6-7
8. Reynolds JE: The 10 best tools for organizing your life (at last!). Money 26:162-163, Aug 1997

9. Eisenberg R: Organize Yourself! New York, Collier Books, 1986
10. Schlenger S, Roesch R: How to be Organized in Spite of Yourself: Time and Space Management That Works With Your Personal Style. New York, New American Library, 1989
11. Winston S: Getting Organized: The Easy Way to Put Your Life in Order. Revised edition. New York, Warner Books, 1991

SUGGESTED READING

Carter J, Carter JD: He Works, She Works: Successful Strategies for Working Couples. New York, AMACOM, 1995

Carter S, Sokol J: Lives Without Balance: When You're Giving Everything You've Got and Still Not Getting What You Hoped For. New York, Villard, 1992

Charlesworth EA, Nathan RG: Stress Management: A Comprehensive Guide to Wellness. New York, Ballantine, 1985

Douglass ME, Douglass DN: Manage Your Time, Your Work, Yourself. Updated edition. New York, AMACOM, 1993

Elliott M, Meltsner S: The Perfectionist Predicament: How to Stop Driving Yourself and Others Crazy. New York, William Morrow, 1991

Klein R: Where Did the Time Go? The Working Woman's Guide to Creative Time Management. Rocklin, California, Prima Publishing, 1993

Lakein A: How to Get Control of Your Time and Your Life. New York, New American Library, 1974

Mackenzie RA: Teamwork Through Time Management: New Time Management Methods for Everyone in Your Organization. Chicago, Dartnell, 1990

Mayer JJ: Time Management for Dummies. Foster City, California, IDG, 1995

McGee-Cooper A, Trammell D: Time Management for Unmanageable People. New York, Bantam Books, 1994

Roesch R: The Working Woman's Guide to Managing Time: Take Charge of Your Job and Your Life While Taking Care of Yourself. Englewood Cliffs, New Jersey, Prentice Hall, 1996

13

COMPUTERS IN FAMILY PRACTICE*

John W. Bachman, M.D.

The "computer age" is here. Computers are being used increasingly for just about any task. Medicine, in many respects, is leading the way in new technology, which will eventually improve health care to our patients. From advances in radiologic imaging to medical record keeping and billing, the explosion of computer technology has improved our practice of medicine (Box 13-1). Advances in the future even involve evaluating and treating patients with videoconferencing capabilities, with the patient or physician never leaving the comforts of home (Fig. 13-1). With these drastic technologic changes, the family physician will continue to be the leader in the delivery of primary care, but first we must enter the world of computer technology. This chapter outlines rules for the computer novice who is interested in diving into the deep pool of information technology.

RULE 1: BUY A LAPTOP COMPUTER

You need to own and use a laptop computer and it must be connected to the Internet. Owning a laptop computer and being connected to the Internet encourages you to be a part of the information age. As a physician who wants to be current, the only acceptable way of doing this is with a portable computer. The barriers to computer use are cost and fear. Currently, you can purchase a high-quality laptop computer that meets your needs for less than $1,600. If you feel you can not come up with the money, you can borrow the money or lease the computer. The investment in this electronic

*Nothing in this chapter implies that Mayo Foundation endorses any of the products mentioned in this chapter.

BOX 13-1 COMPUTERS AT MAYO CLINIC

The Departments of Family Medicine at all 3 locations (Rochester, Jacksonville, and Scottsdale) currently are implementing advanced computer-based systems that will improve productivity and the quality of care to our patients. Like most family physicians' offices, scheduling and billing via computer-based programs have been in place for several years.

Newer advances in Jacksonville have computerized the medical record, including radiographs and scanned images of such things as electrocardiograms, pulmonary function tests, audiograms, and old records. By doing this, the entire Mayo Clinic Jacksonville is paperless, relying on the printed page only for backup if there is a complete power failure preventing existing computer-based backup programs from functioning.

In addition, Mayo Clinic is experimenting with a videoconferencing-based computer system that allows a physician to examine a patient face to face by computer while the patient remains at home. Variables such as blood pressure, weight, oxygen saturation, auscultation of heart and lung sounds, and electrocardiograms can be assessed.

In the future, electronic dictation, which transcribes the physician's dictation of a patient encounter, will be developed and used, drastically reducing the overhead costs of a typical family physician's office.

The explosion of technology has affected every aspect of our lives. To date, we have witnessed only the "tip of the iceberg." Although change is always difficult and sometimes slow to come, the use of computers eventually will make the practice of family medicine more enjoyable and profitable for the family physician.

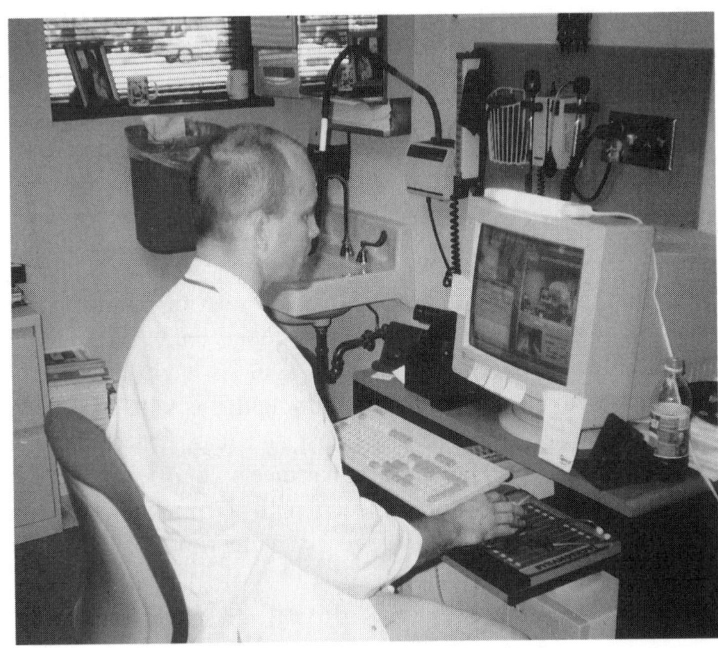

FIGURE 13-1 Telemedicine applications are being used to see and evaluate patients via a computer link without the patient leaving the comforts of home.

device will pay you back many times. It is like comparing someone who rides a horse to someone who rides in an automobile. Fear is an emotion resident physicians and physicians in practice deal with frequently. Overcome fear with constructive action. Buy the laptop computer and you will no longer fear the decision.

Some physicians see the computer as a mystical device, which is incomprehensible to them. Other physicians fail to see the application of the computer in daily practice because few individuals can mentor and teach them. A final group feels that computer technology is moving so fast that they are concerned the investment they make will be obsolete in a few months. These are not valid reasons to avoid computers. After reading this chapter, the physician will see the fallacy in these positions.

> *"I have been surprised to note the readiness with which high-grade young men, graduates from medical institutions which are models for our time, yield to the temptation of machine-made diagnosis."*
>
> —William J. Mayo

If you have a laptop computer and carry it with you, you have a device that has the capability of improving the quality of your interactions with patients and colleagues. By being hooked up to the Internet via any telephone port, you have a vast warehouse of information at your fingertips. Furthermore, if you own a computer, you rapidly learn about computer limitations. Some people expect equipment perfection. Unfortunately, this is not the case. In fact, computers break down and send erroneous messages on a regular basis. Learning to cope with the glitches and bugs is a part of being a knowledgeable user. Owning a laptop computer gives you the freedom to solve your own problems and become a better user of the latest technology.

RULE 2: BUY A LAPTOP COMPUTER THAT SUPPORTS Windows

There may be better systems in the world than that produced by Microsoft. The problem is that Microsoft dominates the market so much that in the long run it is better not to fight the giant. The office package that can be purchased with your computer should include Word, a word processing program with self-correcting features that may improve your grammar and spelling; Excel, an electronic data spreadsheet; and PowerPoint, a presentation program. The typical personal computer also will have Microsoft Exchange and Explorer for dealing with e-mail and using the Internet. If there is an innovation Microsoft will more than likely provide it to you quickly.

One valuable tool if you choose Microsoft Office is Camcorder. This program is free and can be downloaded from Microsoft's Web site. The Camcorder program records your activity performed on the World Wide Web. If you wish to make a presentation that features Web activity you can go to the Web and record it. At future presentations, you can play it back without the need for Internet connections.

RULE 3: LEARN A FEW COMMANDS

The typical screen of a computer program such as Word or PowerPoint bears a striking similarity to the screen and the control panel of a Boeing 747! In Word 97 there are 71 icons and 110 items in the pull-down menus. In Word developed in 1992, there were only 211 commands in the whole program. Now there are more than a thousand. It is so complex that when Microsoft surveyed its customers to find out what they wanted in the next package, 40% of the items requested were already in the program!

One of the reasons for purchasing a laptop computer is to begin learning the basics so you can prepare yourself for the future. There are some Microsoft-based commands that are nice to know and extraordinarily useful. The first commands have to do with using the clipboard. When you are in a Windows program you may copy material to a clipboard and paste it (move it) to another application. For example, if a paragraph is needed somewhere else in a presentation, one can highlight the paragraph with the cursor and type CTRL-C (control copy it). Then you can remove the paragraph by typing CTRL-X (control x it) and paste the paragraph anywhere the cursor is located with CTRL-V (control view it). There are icons for this function but these 3 commands from the keyboard will save you a great deal of time. Other useful commands are CTRL-TAB, which allows you to move between programs, and ALT F4, which closes programs for you.

There are lots of shortcuts or tricks of the trade. A simple way of learning how to get around is to get a program and a book that tells you how to use it. The best books for novices are the short, concise books that have many pictures. As the old adage goes, "A picture is worth a thousand words." You can purchase these at local bookstores or through the Internet at sites like Amazon.com (a computer-based bookstore that allows the ordering and purchasing of books over the Web).

RULE 4: USE PowerPoint FOR PRESENTATIONS

PowerPoint is relatively easy to use and has a tremendous impact on the way you perform needed tasks. A physician is often asked to give multiple presentations. PowerPoint is presentation software. To begin the program, click the PowerPoint icon or program. You will see a screen. Choose the option that states, ''blank presentation.'' Another screen will appear that looks like a group of slides. You will now learn a universal rule about computers. If you have a screen that asks if something is ''ok'' and you have no idea what to do, click on the ''ok'' button. The screen you will see is a little odd, so look to the bottom and find an icon that says, ''outline view'' (holding the cursor over each icon for a few seconds results in a box appearing to tell you what the icon is). Click the outline icon. You then can type an outline of what you want to present. Click on the icon that looks like a slide and you will see that your outline is in a slide format. You may enter a template (this colors the slide). If you want to enhance your presentation, you may try inserting clip art or music on a compact disk. If you get stuck, press the ''help'' button or purchase a book on PowerPoint.

There are courses on the Internet that will instruct you for a small fee. Residents may wish to begin with a presentation on hospital rounds. As you become more sophisticated, try a residency conference and ultimately a staff conference. Make up a presentation for your patients about things you want them to know. If your residency has a Web site, your presentations can easily be placed for all to see. As you develop your skills, you will find that almost all lecture rooms have devices for projecting from a laptop computer, and you will never need to have slides. With each presentation try something new: sounds, animation, and special effects. At major meetings you will be able to rearrange your talk based on what has been presented at the meeting, and if someone has a presentation you really like, you can ask them to download it into your computer. Remember, PowerPoint also produces handouts.

RULE 5: DO YOUR EXAMINATIONS WITH Shorthand

The strength of a computer is that it does the same thing over and over again (this is also its weakness). Shorthand is a product that creates templates. Eighty percent of your written work as a physician can be changed to templates. You can download Shorthand from the Internet for less than $30. You can locate Shorthand at http://www65.pair.com/lim/shorthand. After you download it, you may begin constructing a template for your physical examinations. An example follows.

PAST MEDICAL HISTORY

Hospitalizations (none or input them)

Trauma (none or input them)

Significant Events Past Year (none or input them)

Immunizations: Diphtheria and tetanus (input year); Measles, mumps, rubella (input year); Hepatitis B (input year); Tuberculin (input year); Hepatitis A (input year); Influenza (input year); Pneumococcal (input year)

Shorthand would bring up this template when you wish to record the patient's past medical history and prompt you for responses. You then press ''type it'' and a Past Medical History is typed into Word. Files you can create include history and physical examinations, prevention guidelines, well-child information, and anything that you do that is repeated. Shorthand is a fantastic tool. You can easily see the benefits of a laptop computer. You can make the templates. Your examinations can be thorough and performed quickly, and the results are typed. In my practice, the nurse uses Shorthand to obtain the patient's history, thus saving me a great deal of time.

RULE 6: E-MAIL SHOULD BE USED

Electronic mail (e-mail) is a wonderful way to communicate with patients and colleagues (Fig. 13-2). More than 50 million people already use it. It is fast and inexpensive. The disadvantage is that it is not secure. The way to help your patients understand this lack of security is to compare e-mail to a postcard. In the future, e-mail may have many new applications once security is achieved. Patients may elect to use e-mail to communicate their concerns to you. You, in turn, can send reminders and laboratory results. Academically, e-mail will allow you to exchange information with other physicians about patients and colleagues. Hotmail, Lycos, and Yahoo all have an e-mail-related program that is free. It is located at http://www.hotmail.com/ or at Yahoo and Lycos sites. A nice feature of this service is that you can have periodicals and newspapers (eg, *USA Today*) sent to your e-mail address for you to open!

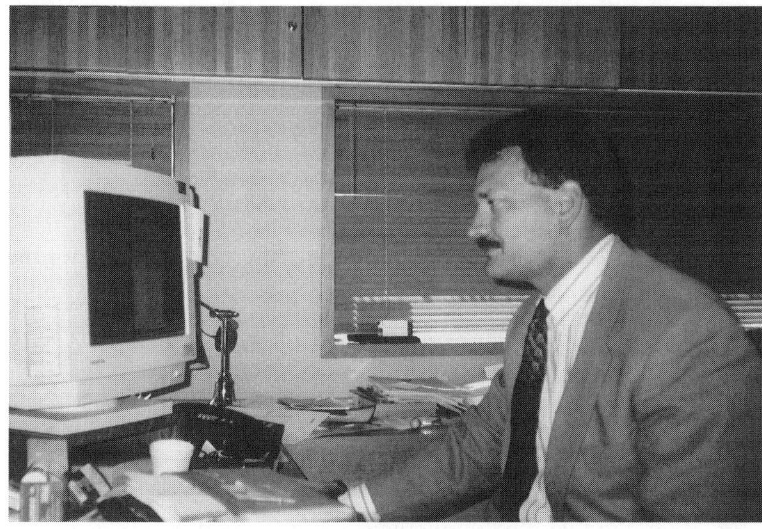

FIGURE 13-2
Residents and physicians in practice spend many hours in front of the computer, performing research, reviewing patients' charts, and communicating via electronic mail.

". . . the highly scientific development of this mechanistic age had led perhaps to some loss in appreciation of the individuality of the patient and to trusting largely to the laboratories and outside agencies which tended to make the patient not the hub of the wheel, but a spoke."

—William J. Mayo

RULE 7: USE THE WORLD WIDE WEB ON A DAILY BASIS

The Web is a wonderful resource for residents and physicians in practice to provide education to their patients. The following are some outstanding resources to get you started.

Patient Education Sites

1. Mayo Clinic Health Oasis (http://www.mayohealth.org/) is an incredible site for patient information. The reference for the site is the Mayo Clinic Health Letter's back issues and the Mayo Clinic's patient education publications.
2. KidsHealth (http://KidsHealth.org/) is a user friendly site.
3. Healthfinder (http://www.healthfinder.gov/) is the information site of the US government.

4. Coastal Medical (http://users.aol.com/renmed/Pat_Ed_Resources.html) has a list of patient education sites.
5. Ethnomed (http://healthlinks.washington.edu/clinical/ethnomed/) has patient education resources in different languages.

Resident Sites

1. MedConnect (http://www.medconnect.com/) has several resources for the resident physician.

General Medical Sites

1. Check out Yale University's Internet Resources (http://info.med.yale.edu/library/sir).
2. John G. Faughnan has a nice site entitled ''A Family Physician's Web Starter'' (http://dragon.labmed.umn.edu/~john/bookmark.html).
3. Wheeless' Textbook of Orthopaedics (http://medmedia.com/med.htm) is a must site for family physicians.

Finding information on the web requires learning how to use a Search Engine. There are numerous engines you can use. An excellent site that has links to search engines is http://www.dreamscape.com/frankvad/search.html. The beauty of this site is its description of the various engines and what they do. Cliniweb International at http://www.ohsu.edu/cliniweb/ is a medical search site that is useful. To ''surf the web'' you need to use search engines. One piece of advice to know is how to modify your search so that it is narrowed to the information you want. The following are common methods of doing this.

PLUS: A + sign in front of the word requires that the word be included in the search

MINUS: A − sign in front of the word requires that the word not be in the search

QUOTATION MARKS: This requires the search to find a phrase

AND: This requires the words linked by ''and'' be included in the search

OR: This requires that either of 2 words linked by ''or'' be included in the search

CAPITALIZATION: This requires words to be capitalized in the search. Lowercase will find words in either uppercase or lowercase

RULE 8: USE COMPUTERS FOR ROUTINE REPETITIOUS ACTIVITY

Computers work well for any activity that is repetitious. Examples are call backs for laboratory results. Use of e-mail or voice mail is excellent. In our program, we use Lab Talk for voice mail. A demonstration of this program can be accessed by calling 1-800-882-8772. Lab Talk has methods of contacting patients with surveys and appointment reminders. Another useful device is a Palmtop or PalmPilot. These handheld devices can hold e-mail, access your schedule, and remind you of important things. There are many programs you can download from the Web to help with your productivity as a busy family physician. Physicians Online (http://www.po.com/), an Internet site for physicians, is an excellent reference for such programs.

RULE 9: INITIATE INTERACTIVE HISTORY TAKING BY COMPUTER

The details of this application can be found at http://www.medicalhistory.com/. Patients can use a computer to provide medical information to the physician. One such program, Healthlink, allows patients to sit in the lobby and answer questions about prevention and then receive education (Fig. 13-3). The staff can then review the output and update the patient's prevention

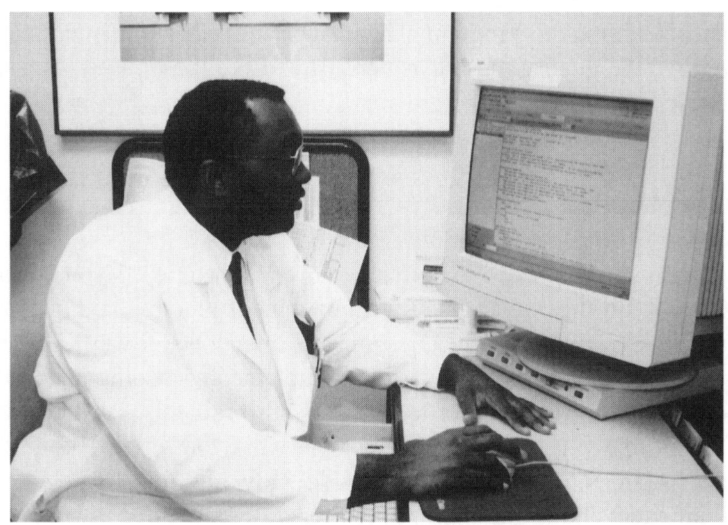

FIGURE 13-3
Patient records are completely computerized at Mayo Clinic Jacksonville, which allows the physician to review various consultations, prior visits, and laboratory results at the click of a mouse.

profile at that visit. The more sophisticated program, Instant Medical History, has more than 15,000 possible questions for patients. The system is reliable and readily used by patients. One of the assets of the system is that it provides many objective scales to summarize your data. For example, the Zung Depression Scale is an excellent way of monitoring depression. A patient can answer the questions on a laptop computer and you can monitor the improvement in an objective manner.

RULE 10: TRAINING, TRAINING, AND MORE TRAINING

As a resident you will find that many on your faculty are computer illiterate. As a practicing physician you may find that your partners are uneducated when it comes to computers. Many times you will feel isolated in your pursuit of computer-based technology. There will be pressures on you to avoid the use of a computer. Time constraints may prevent the learning process—but work on your computer skills. Find the time! In the long run, it will make your life much easier. Learn about software that helps you do a better job more efficiently.

For example, QMR is a relatively expensive program for listing differential diagnoses. What an extraordinary tool. You can enter symptoms and it will provide differential diagnoses and possible questions to ask to define the correct diagnosis. It also indicates inexpensive and expensive tests that can be ordered. Imagine being able to determine that a patient needs a simple urine test instead of an expensive blood test and to cite the literature that not only is it less expensive but the sensitivity is 50 percent improved. A few hours spent learning this program will enhance your education or practice and can improve the quality of your patient care. Take the time to learn to use the tools.

CONCLUSIONS

How many hours do you work in a week? How much time do you spend asking how can I do this well? Quality improvement requires taking time out of your schedule and asking the question, "Is there a better way?" Once a better way is found, training needs to be implemented. Computers are, and will continue to be, the answer to many of our problems. Productivity is not the hours of work that are done but the work that can be done in those hours. Physicians and staff need to do only high-level integrated thinking. Computers should do dull, routine repetitious tasks.

14

REFERENCES FOR FAMILY PHYSICIANS

Robert L. Bratton, M.D.

Susan L. Wickes, M.D.

The specialty of family medicine encompasses the comprehensive, continuous care of patients of all ages. It is composed of a body of information that crosses many specialty boundaries and allows the family physician to approach the patient as a whole being rather than as a specific organ system or disease. With this comprehensive approach to patient care, the family physician must call on a broad knowledge base. It would be impossible to become an expert in every field, but as family physicians we can become experts in the care of our patients. During medical school and residency, we acquire a solid knowledge base. We continually build on this during our years of patient care. To assist us with our care of our patients, we need references that cover the spectrum of medical care. With time pressures in the office and in the hospital, practical information for our day-to-day practice must be readily available. The following chapter focuses on references that are helpful to both the practicing family physician and resident in training (Table 14-1).

> *"To books we turn to learn of the past, opinions of the present, and prognostications of the future."*
>
> —William J. Mayo

TEXTBOOKS

Family Practice

In 1973, 4 years after the official recognition of family practice as the 20th medical specialty, the first family practice textbook was published entitled

TABLE 14-1
REFERENCES FOR FAMILY PHYSICIANS

REQUIRED TEXTS
Harrison's Principles of Internal Medicine (Fauci et al.),[1] *Cecil Essentials of Medicine* (Andreoli et al.),[2] or *Scientific American Medicine* (Rubenstein and Federman)[3]
Nelson Textbook of Pediatrics (Behrman et al.)[4]
The Harriet Lane Handbook: A Manual for Pediatric House Officers (Barone)[5]
Williams Obstetrics (Cunningham et al.)[6]
Textbook of Family Practice (Rakel)[7] or *Family Medicine: Principles and Practice* (Taylor and Buckingham)[8]
The Merck Manual of Diagnosis and Therapy (Berkow)[9]
Washington Manual, *Manual of Medical Therapeutics* (Orland and Saltman)[10]
The Sanford Guide to Antimicrobial Therapy (Sanford et al.)[11]
Physicians' Desk Reference[12]
RECOMMENDED TEXTS
Drugs in Pregnancy and Lactation: A Reference Guide to Fetal and Neonatal Risk (Briggs et al.)[13]
Guide to Clinical Preventive Services: Report of the U.S. Services Task Force[14]
Textbook of Primary Care Medicine (Noble et al.)[15]
Primary Care Medicine: Office Evaluation and Management of the Adult Patient (Goroll et al.)[16]
Saunders Manual of Medical Practice (Rakel)[17]
Procedures for Primary Care Physicians (Pfenninger and Fowler)[18]
Essentials of Musculoskeletal Care (Snider)[19]
Color Atlas and Synopsis of Clinical Dermatology: Common and Serious Diseases (Fitzpatrick et al.)[20]
Neurology for the House Officer (Weiner and Levitt)[21]
Conn's Current Therapy (Rakel)[22]
University of Iowa: The Family Practice Handbook (Graber et al.)[23]
Report of the Committee on Infectious Diseases (1998 Red Book)[24]

Family Practice.[25] For 25 years this textbook has served as one of the premier resources for family physicians. No family physician library should be without it. The text covers various areas that involve the specialty of family practice. One of the biggest advantages is that the text provides an approach to the patient from the family physician's perspective.

In 1978, the second family practice textbook was published entitled *Family Medicine: Principles and Practice*.[8] Similar in scope, this text also approached the care of the patient from a family physician's perspective. The text is now in its fifth edition and is an excellent reference.

Internal Medicine

No physician's office is complete without a comprehensive textbook of internal medicine. *Harrison's Principles of Internal Medicine*[1] *and Cecil Essentials of Medicine*[2] are detailed references that outline the knowledge base for the practice of general adult medicine. Some may find the texts at times burdensome and too detailed for quick review during a patient's office visit; however, they remain excellent resources for the diagnosis, pathophysiology, and treatment details of your patients' diseases. These texts do not give a cookbook approach to managing a disease and do not give medication dosages, but they definitely will broaden your knowledge of the entire disease process.

One disadvantage of any textbook is that it is often outdated by the time it is published. For this reason, many find *Scientific American Medicine*[3] a useful substitute for the standard text of internal medicine. This publication comes in 3 large binders or CD-ROMS, with the same type of material that is in your standard internal medicine textbook. The key difference is that updates are sent out quarterly on different sections, so that the text is being updated continually.

A practical general medicine text is *Primary Care Medicine: Office Evaluation and Management of the Adult Patient,*[16] because it is organized by symptom. It is a quick and easy reference to consult when there is a patient waiting in the office. In addition, *Griffith's 5 Minute Clinical Consult*[26] is another practical reference to use in the office setting. Information is organized in outline form with basic information, differential diagnosis, and guidelines for treatment. Later, when time allows, additional, more detailed information can be reviewed from an internal medicine text.

Pediatrics

Nelson Textbook of Pediatrics[4] is a helpful textbook for any family physician. The text is a comprehensive reference for any physician who cares for pediatric patients.

The care of pediatric patients often requires multiple calculations for medication dosages. Of all the pediatric resources available, perhaps the most useful is Johns Hopkins Hospital, *The Harriet Lane Handbook: A Manual for Pediatric House Officers.*[5] This book has an easy-to-use table that outlines dosages for commonly used pediatric medications. The book contains numerous facts that are germane to the care of pediatric patients.

The "Red Book," *Report of the Committee on Infectious Diseases*[24] from the American Academy of Pediatrics, is a practical and easy-to-use guide to pediatric infectious diseases. If you cannot remember the incubation period for chickenpox, use this book.

> *"Books become friends that never fail; . . ."*
>
> —William J. Mayo

Obstetrics and Gynecology

For family physicians who practice obstetrics, *Williams Obstetrics*[6] is suggested. This is a comprehensive reference for the care of the obstetric patient.

One of our most frequently used obstetrics books in the office has been *Drugs in Pregnancy and Lactation: A Reference Guide to Fetal and Neonatal Risk.*[13] This is an essential reference for any physician who needs to know what drugs are safe for the pregnant or breast-feeding patient.

Another common task for family physicians is managing patient use of oral contraceptives and their side effects. Perhaps one of the most comprehensive and easy to use references is *Managing Contraceptive Pill Patients,*[27] which is loaded with easy-to-read charts and facts concerning the use of oral contraceptives.

Psychiatry

Every day family physicians see patients with underlying psychiatric disorders. It has been estimated that as many as 25 percent to 50 percent of all patients seeking medical care have an underlying psychiatric problem or disorder. In view of this, the family physician must have an understanding of the signs and symptoms of various psychiatric disorders. Perhaps the most well-recognized text for psychiatry has been the *Diagnostic and Statistical Manual of Mental Disorders,*[28] which is now revised to its current 4th edition. The text provides a list of criteria for diagnosing psychiatric illnesses. For the purpose of defining certain psychiatric illnesses, the text does an excellent job; however, the frequent revisions may render your edition out of date. In addition, there are no treatment options given for those affected with a particular diagnosis. Because of this, many family physicians do not find the text useful in their everyday practice. The textbooks on family practice and internal medicine usually provide adequate information on both the presenting signs and symptoms and the treatment of most psychiatric illnesses.

Surgery

Family physicians are trained to do many procedures in their offices, from lesion removal and laceration repair, to toenail procedures, to vasectomy. Perhaps the most useful text on surgical procedures is *Procedures for Primary Care Physicians.*[18] This text focuses on outpatient procedures and is recommended for all family physicians who perform office surgery.

Depending on where they practice, family physicians may assist in surgery, but the days of family physicians doing major surgery in the operating room are almost nonexistent. Legal issues and the explosion of specialists have almost eliminated every opportunity. Nevertheless, it is helpful to have a broad understanding of surgical procedures to share with your patients, especially because family physicians still provide preoperative and postoperative care. A comprehensive text on general surgery is not generally necessary for a family physician's office, but for those with a special interest, *Principles of Surgery*[29] by Schwartz et al. may be helpful.

Orthopedics

All family physicians see orthopedic conditions and must have an adequate knowledge base in orthopedics. One of the most helpful references for family physicians is *Essentials of Musculoskeletal Care.*[19] This book possesses a wealth of information concerning the evaluation and treatment of common orthopedic problems encountered in a family physician's office. The text is organized by the joint affected and also includes a special pediatric section. Another reference is *Physical Examination of the Spine and Extremities,*[30] which remains a favorite among family physicians in practice. Both texts are excellent and either will suffice. Additionally, an easy-to-use text for common problems is *Ramamurti's Orthopaedics in Primary Care.*[31] *The Team Physician's Handbook*[32] is a well-organized text for those interested in sports medicine.

Dermatology

Dermatology references are an absolute requirement in a family physician's office. Always select a reference with many photographs. Perhaps one of the most useful is *Color Atlas and Synopsis of Clinical Dermatology: Common and Serious Diseases.*[20] This book provides an easy-to-use reference source for those in family practice. It offers concise text that describes the etiology and treatment recommendations for the various dermatologic diseases.

Neurology

Neurologic problems often are seen by family physicians in hospitalized patients and in the clinic setting. A solid understanding of neurologic disorders and nerve innervation helps in establishing the diagnosis. Perhaps one of the most used texts in our office is *Neurology for the House Officer.*[21] This text covers the basics of neurology and presents the information in a practical and clinically relevant way. Such important topics as headache, cerebral vascular accidents, and nerve root distribution are covered. In addition, *Mayo Clinic Examinations in Neurology*[33] is an excellent reference source for patients with neurologic complaints.

Ophthalmology

Every family physician should know how to treat common eye complaints. Although family physicians do not always have access to a slit lamp, they should be skilled with an ophthalmoscope, a Snellen eye chart, and a fluorescein eye examination. A good reference for eye complaints often encountered by family physicians is *General Ophthalmology.*[34] The common ophthalmologic problems are covered in the family medicine and primary care books, making a separate ophthalmology text optional.

Hospital Care

Without a doubt, one of the most important references used in the hospital setting is the *Manual of Medical Therapeutics,*[10] also referred to as the ''Washington Manual.'' The spiral-bound text provides comprehensive information concerning the care of hospital and clinic patients. Because of its size, it can often fit into a laboratory coat pocket. It provides practical and specific information that aids in writing orders and managing your hospital patients.

Another reference commonly used in the hospital setting is the extremely helpful *The Sanford Guide to Antimicrobial Therapy.*[11] This pocket-sized book describes acceptable and appropriate antibiotic therapy for many diseases and organisms. Every year the text is updated and pharmaceutical companies distribute complimentary copies.

Interpretation of electrocardiograms is another important task in caring for hospital patients. Unfortunately, many residency programs do not have formal classes that teach the art of reading electrocardiograms. In view of this, many of us are self-taught. *Rapid Interpretation of EKG's: A Programmed Course*[35] is the best-known resource that teaches the physician interpretation of electrocardiograms in a structured and organized manner. The book is easy to read and teaches the fundamentals of interpretation. In addition, there are quick reference sheets that can be cut out and carried in a laboratory coat pocket for easy reference.

Although the *Physicians' Desk Reference*[12] is a required text for every family physician's office, it is extremely heavy. Fortunately, it is found in most hospital nursing stations, so drug information is easily accessible in the hospital setting. Two easy-to-use pocket references are the *1998 Tarascon Pocket Pharmacopoeia*[36] and *Handbook of Commonly Prescribed Drugs,*[37] which list hundreds of commonly prescribed medications and appropriate adult dosages. Like the Sanford guide, complimentary copies of the *Handbook of Commonly Prescribed Drugs* often are available. Others may choose to subscribe to the *Monthly Prescribing Reference,*[38] which reviews new medications and provides a reference for more commonly prescribed medications.

Laboratory Test Interpretation

As medicine becomes more and more advanced and the number of tests to detect disease increases, physicians are inundated by thousands of laboratory tests. Unfortunately, no one can know the significance of every test. When uncertainty arises, one of the best references is *Bakerman's ABC's of Interpretive Laboratory Data,*[39] a pocket-sized reference that provides a differential diagnosis based on the outcome of common laboratory tests.

General Texts

The Merck Manual of Diagnosis and Therapy[9] is an excellent reference that does not take up much room on the bookshelf but nevertheless remains comprehensive for the practice of general medicine. *Conn's Current Therapy*[22] is celebrating with its recent 50th anniversary edition. Although a little bulky to carry around, this text provides an excellent reference for the practice of clinical medicine. In addition, the book's editor, Robert Rakel, is a well-known family physician who displays a family practice approach to clinical practice. Another longstanding text related to physical diagnosis and examination is *DeGowin & DeGowin's Diagnostic Examination.*[40] This book covers important physical findings and is an asset in any family physician's library.

Family physicians need to stay up to date on prevention and screening for diseases. The *Guide to Clinical Preventive Services: Report of the U.S. Services Task Force*[14] is a good practical reference outlining the general consensus on the evidence for a multitude of screening tests. When you are trying to decide what screening tests to perform on patients of different ages, this reference details the data for and against different recommendations in easy-to-use charts.

JOURNALS

Physicians depend on journals to keep up to date with medical advances. For family physicians, this is especially true, because their care covers many different areas. The following journals are often used by family physicians to stay current in the medical field.

American Family Physician

This is the most recognized journal for the specialty of family practice. The journal is filled with review articles that emphasize important problems encountered in a family practice setting. The journal is clinically oriented and often gives a problem-focused approach to the care of patients. In addition, as the official journal of the American Academy of Family Physicians, this monthly periodical provides important information concerning continuing medical education (CME) courses, national conventions, and political updates relevant to family physicians. The journal is peer-reviewed.

The Journal of the American Medical Association (JAMA)

Every physician, regardless of specialty, should have some knowledge of this journal. Published weekly by the American Medical Association, this journal contains important studies that often determine clinical treatment. The national media often report on studies published in *JAMA,* which prompts many patients to present to your office with questions concerning the latest studies. It is helpful to review this journal on a regular basis, not only to stay abreast of new advances in medicine but also to be able to respond appropriately to patient questions.

The New England Journal of Medicine

Published weekly by the Massachusetts Medical Society, this nationally recognized journal also publishes important studies that lead to improved patient treatment. In addition, it contains experimental research advances. Much like *JAMA,* it is reported on in the national media and many patients may have questions regarding the studies published in this journal. Our advice is to read all the abstracts and only read the full articles when they are relevant to your practice. The review articles are thorough, and many are applicable to primary care.

Archives of Family Medicine

This is an academic journal that provides the results of experimental studies as well as editorial topics. The journal is produced by the American Medical Association, which also publishes *JAMA.*

The Journal of Family Practice

Endorsed by the Society of Teachers of Family Medicine, this monthly journal contains family medicine-based research, along with clinically based review articles.

The Journal of the American Board of Family Practice

Published every 2 months by the American Board of Family Practice, this journal contains research articles relevant to the practice of family medicine and editorials concerning the specialty, in addition to important board news concerning certification, recertification, and certificate of added qualifications examinations.

Mayo Clinic Proceedings

Traditionally thought of as a subspecialty journal, the *Mayo Clinic Proceedings* has changed in recent years to be more clinically oriented toward primary care. In fact, there is now a special section devoted to primary care physicians. The journal also has a resident clinic section, which describes an interesting and sometimes challenging case. The section leads the reader through the presentation, evaluation, and treatment.

Family Practice Management

Published monthly by the American Academy of Family Practice, this journal focuses on the business side of family practice, including discussions on managed care, coding, and billing.

Family Practice Recertification

This journal has multiple clinically related articles and a section of questions and answers that simulate board-type questions. It is most helpful for preparing for Board examinations and practicing test-taking skills.

> *''Reading papers is not for the purpose of showing how much we know and what we are doing, but is an opportunity to learn''*
>
> —William J. Mayo

Postgraduate Medicine

Published monthly by McGraw-Hill, this peer-reviewed journal is filled with review articles that cover problems commonly seen in family physician offices. The journal is easy to read and can be used as a quick reference in the office setting.

Morbidity and Mortality Weekly Report

This is prepared by the Centers for Disease Control and distributed by the Massachusetts Medical Society. It gives national statistics on the incidence of reportable infectious diseases and case reports and guidelines regarding a wide range of infectious diseases. In addition, regular supplements provide the latest recommendations regarding immunizations and other public health issues. The major reports in this weekly are also published in *JAMA,* so a separate subscription is not necessary. For those interested in more detailed statistics and reports, this weekly is interesting reading.

Many journals are available to the family physician. Over the course of a week, a stack of journals may arrive in your mailbox, both journals you have subscribed to and journals mailed to you because you are on a physician list somewhere. Do not try to read them all, but instead concentrate on only those journals most relevant to your practice. There are not enough hours in the day to keep up with the vast amount of information published daily. Because of this, one must limit the resources to review based on interest and practice style. To form a foundation, the journals mentioned in the preceding sections may be used as a guideline. In addition, *Journal Watch,* a publication from the Massachusetts Medical Society, reviews many of the leading journals, including other specialty journals, and summarizes the important findings. By using this resource, one can reduce the number of journal subscriptions and quickly review a multitude of important studies. The *Journal Watch* approach seems to expand continually, with Journal Watches for specific areas, such as *Journal Watch Women's Health, Cardiology,* and *Infectious Diseases.*

There are also newsletters published on drug information. *The Medical Letter on Drugs and Therapeutics* (published by the Medical Letter, Inc.) historically has been a good, unbiased review of new drugs on the market, comparing them in effectiveness and cost with drugs already available. *The Medical Letter* periodically has an excellent table on the drugs recommended for treatment of parasitic infections—an important resource in this era of international travel.

MISCELLANEOUS REFERENCE SOURCES

In addition to textbooks and journals, there are numerous other references available to the family physician (Box 14-1).

Family Practice Home Assessment Course

The American Academy of Family Practice produces this study course. Each month those who have subscribed to the course are sent a workbook that covers a clinically oriented problem, with both a pretest and a posttest. In addition, there is a cassette tape included, which also covers another topic commonly encountered by family physicians. The tape is accompanied by a written outline that allows the listener to follow along. Physicians are required to return test questions to the American Academy of Family Practice to receive CME credit.

BOX 14-1 FAMILY DOC: THE MAKING OF A FAMILY PRACTITIONER

Perhaps one of the most enlightening books concerning the daily trials and tribulations of a family practice resident is *Family Doc: The Making of a Family Practitioner*[41] (Fig. 14-1). This book tells the true story of Dr. Robert E. Brown, a family practice resident, during his 3-year residency program at the fictional Peabody Clinic. Physicians in practice as well as residents in training can identify with many of the stories told. From the first day of residency to the day of graduation, the reader gets a first-hand view of what can be expected during family practice residency training.

As quoted by Dr. Robert E. Rakel, Professor of Family and Community Medicine at Baylor College of Medicine, "This book is a well-written and spellbinding account of [Dr. Brown's] experiences as a family practice resident. Once started, I could not put it down . . . . This book colorfully describes the joy and excitement of residency training . . . ."[41]

The paperback edition can be ordered from Parthenon Publishing Group (New York, London) ISBN 1-85070-969-6 (176 pages) at (800)-735-4744 or by contacting www.amazon.com or your local bookstore. The price is $17.95.

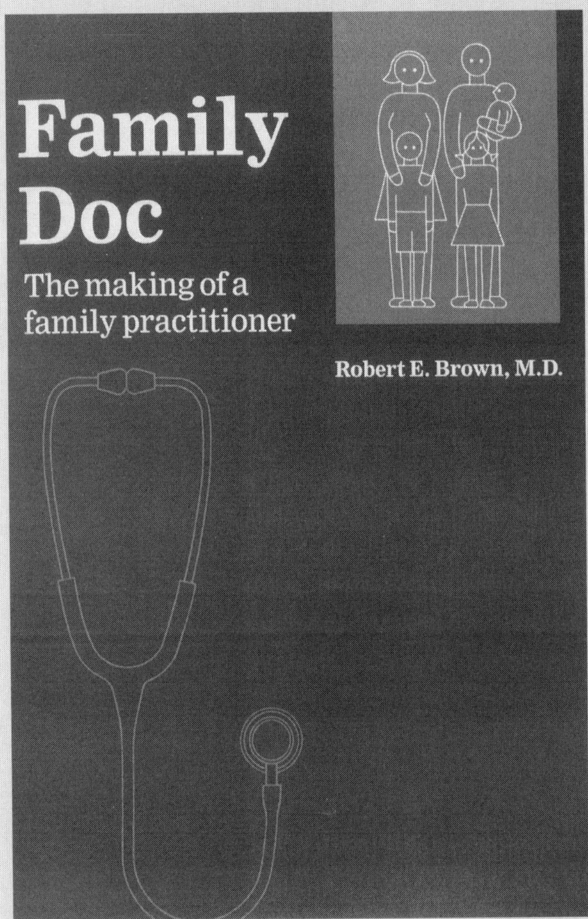

FIGURE 14-1
From Brown RE: Family Doc: The Making of a Family Practitioner. New York, Parthenon Publishing Group, 1998. By permission of the publisher.

CME Courses

Every board-certified family physician is required to obtain 150 hours of CME credit every 3 years to maintain board certification status. As a result of this requirement, an enormous number of courses have been developed. In almost every location in the world, family physicians can enroll in CME courses that cover every aspect of medical care. To ensure proper credentialing and a quality conference, one may want to talk to colleagues who have participated in the conferences or to contact the American Academy of Family Practice or the American Board of Family Practice for more information. The American Academy of Family Practice Annual Scientific Assembly, held every fall, has become an excellent resource for obtaining CME credits, and it also provides an excellent opportunity for networking with family physicians. It is important to keep a record of your CME credit. The American Academy of Family Practice offers members a CME credit reporting service and provides periodic updates on the total accumulated hours.

COMPUTERS

All family physicians should become acquainted with information services available through computer-based systems (Fig. 14-2).

CD-ROM Textbooks

Many of the textbooks mentioned previously are available on CD-ROM.

Computer-Based Programs

Many programs are now available to the family physician that provide differential diagnosis based on presenting symptoms. In addition, there are many programs that review medications and their indications, dosages, and side effects as well as any important drug interactions. Eventually all aspects of medical practice will have computer-based programs to provide important information and assist in the delivery of health care.

Internet Sites

The use of computers to access the World Wide Web is revolutionizing the way information is received. Currently, there are numerous Web sites that

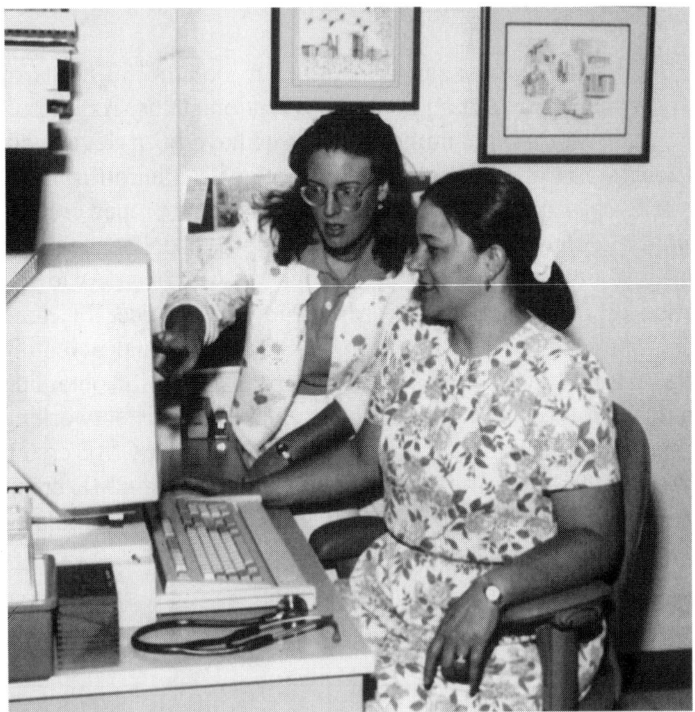

FIGURE 14-2
Computer-based educational resources are increasingly used by family physicians to gather information.

assist family physicians (Table 14-2). Abstracts of some journal articles are available on the Internet. The Centers for Disease Control site covers health recommendations for international travel as well as routine immunization information and *Morbidity and Mortality Weekly Report* recommendations and reports. In addition, there is a wealth of patient education material available on the Internet from reliable sources as well as CD-ROM programs with patient education for use in the office. As the Internet continues to grow and become more user friendly, more and more physicians will rely on the Web as an important resource to gain medical information relevant to their practices.

CONCLUSIONS

Family physicians are challenged to keep up with a vast amount of information from many fields of medicine. In view of this, busy physicians must develop a regular reviewing schedule that efficiently allows them to keep

TABLE 14-2
INTERNET ADDRESSES FOR FAMILY PHYSICIANS

NAME	ADDRESS	CONTENT
American Academy of Family Practice	http://www.aafp.org/	Information related to AAFP *American Family Physican Family Practice Management*
American Board of Family Practice	http://www.abfp.org/	Information related to ABFP, certification Link to *Journal of the American Board of Family Practice* (via http://www.medscape.com/)
American Medical Association	http://www.ama-assn.org/	Information related to AMA *JAMA* *Archives of Family Medicine* Links to: *Journal of the American Board of Family Practice* and to *NEJM*
Centers for Disease Control	http://www.cdc.gov/	*MMWR* Travel information Immunization guidelines Public health information
Mayo Clinic	http://www.mayo.edu/	*Mayo Clinic Proceedings* (table of contents)
Massachusetts Medical Society	http://www.mms.org/	Information on *Journal Watch, NEJM* (subscriptions needed for both)
New England Journal of Medicine	http://www.nejm.org/content/index.asp	Table of contents (subscription needed for full articles)
Mayo Health Oasis	http://www.mayohealth.org/	Patient education

AAFP, American Academy of Family Practice; ABFP, American Board of Family Practice; AMA, American Medical Association; *JAMA, Journal of the American Medical Association; MMWR, Morbidity and Mortality Weekly Report; NEJM, New England Journal of Medicine.*

abreast of important advances in medicine. The ideal schedule will differ for each individual, from several hours per week to an hour or more of reading daily. In addition, a family physician must strategically plan for CME credit by selecting quality CME programs and courses that allow fulfillment of American Board of Family Practice requirements for recertification. With a well-planned schedule that is followed regularly, practicing physicians can remain confident they are keeping up to date with medical advancements and are providing the highest level of care to their patients.

REFERENCES

1. Fauci AS, Braunwald E, Isselbacher KJ, Wilson JD, Martin JB, Kasper DL, Hauser SL, Longo DL, editors: Harrison's Principles of Internal Medicine. Fourteenth edition. New York, McGraw-Hill, 1998
2. Andreoli TE, Carpenter CCJ, Bennett JC, Plum F: Cecil Essentials of Medicine. Fourth edition. Philadelphia, WB Saunders Company, 1997
3. Rubinstein E, Federman DD, editors: Scientific American Medicine. New York, Scientific American, 1998
4. Behrman RE, Kliegman RM, Arvin AM, Nelson WE, editors: Nelson Textbook of Pediatrics. Fifteenth edition. Philadelphia, WB Saunders, 1996
5. Barone MA, editor: The Harriet Lane Handbook: A Manual for Pediatric House Officers. Fourteenth edition. St. Louis, Mosby, 1996
6. Cunningham FG, MacDonald PC, Gant NF, Leveno KJ, Gilstrap LC III, Hankins GDV, Clark SL, editors: Williams Obstetrics. Twentieth edition. Stamford, Connecticut, Appleton & Lange, 1997
7. Rakel RE, editor: Textbook of Family Practice. Fifth edition. Philadelphia, Saunders, 1995
8. Taylor RB, Buckingham JL: Family Medicine: Principles and Practice. New York, Springer-Verlag, 1978
9. Berkow R, editor: The Merck Manual of Diagnosis and Therapy. Sixteenth edition. Rahway, New Jersey, Merck Research Laboratories, 1992
10. Orland MJ, Saltman RJ, editors: Manual of Medical Therapeutics. Twenty-fifth edition. Boston, Little, Brown, 1986
11. Sanford JP, Gilbert DN, Moellering RC Jr, Sande MA: The Sanford Guide to Antimicrobial Therapy. Twenty-seventh edition. Vienna, Virginia, Antimicrobial Therapy, 1997
12. Physicians' Desk Reference. Fifty-second edition. Montvale, New Jersey, Medical Economics Company, 1998
13. Briggs GG, Freeman RK, Yaffe SJ: Drugs in Pregnancy and Lactation: A Reference Guide to Fetal and Neonatal Risk. Fifth edition. Baltimore, Williams & Wilkins, 1998
14. U.S. Preventive Services Task Force: Guide to Clinical Preventive Services: Report of the U.S. Services Task Force. Second edition. Baltimore, Williams & Wilkins, 1996
15. Noble J, Greene HL, Modest GA, Levinson W, Young MJ, editors: Textbook of Primary Care Medicine. Second edition. St. Louis, Mosby-Year Book, 1996

16. Goroll AH, May LA, Mulley AG Jr, editors: Primary Care Medicine: Office Evaluation and Management of the Adult Patient. Third edition. Philadelphia, Lippincott, 1995
17. Rakel RE (editor): Saunders Manual of Medical Practice. Philadelphia, WB Saunders, 1996
18. Pfenninger JL, Fowler GC, editors: Procedures for Primary Care Physicians. St. Louis, Mosby-Year Book, 1994
19. Snider RK, editor: Essentials of Musculoskeletal Care. Rosemont, Illinois, American Academy of Orthopaedic Surgeons, 1997
20. Fitzpatrick TB, Johnson RA, Polano MK, Suurmond D, Wolff K: Color Atlas and Synopsis of Clinical Dermatology: Common and Serious Diseases. Second edition. New York, McGraw-Hill, Health Professions Division, 1992
21. Weiner HL, Levitt LP: Neurology for the House Officer. Fifth edition. Baltimore, Williams & Wilkins, 1994
22. Rakel RE, editor: Conn's Current Therapy. Philadelphia, WB Saunders, 1998
23. Graber MA, Toth PP, Herting RL Jr, editors: University of Iowa: The Family Practice Handbook. Third Edition. St. Louis, Mosby, 1997
24. American Academy of Pediatrics. Committee on Infectious Diseases: Report of the Committee on Infectious Diseases. Twenty-fifth edition. Elk Grove Village, Illinois, The Academy, 1998
25. Conn HF, Rakel RE, Johnson TW, editors: Family Practice. Philadelphia, WB Saunders, 1973
26. Dambro MR, Griffith JA: Griffith's 5 Minute Clinical Consult. Sixth edition. Baltimore, Williams & Wilkins, 1998
27. Dickey RP: Managing Contraceptive Pill Patients. Ninth edition. Durant, Oklahoma, Essential Medical Information, 1998
28. American Psychiatric Association: Diagnostic and Statistical Manual of Mental Disorders. Fourth Edition. Washington, DC, American Psychiatric Association, 1994
29. Schwartz SI, Shires GT, Spencer FC, Daly JM, Fischer JE, Galloway AC, editors: Principles of Surgery. Seventh edition. New York, McGraw-Hill, 1999
30. Hoppenfeld S: Physical Examination of the Spine and Extremities. New York: Appleton-Century-Crofts, 1976
31. Steinberg GG, editor: Ramamurti's Orthopaedics in Primary Care. Second edition. Baltimore, Williams & Wilkins, 1992
32. Mellion MB, Walsh WM, Shelton GL, editors: The Team Physician's Handbook. Philadelphia, Hanley & Belfus, 1990
33. Members of the Mayo Clinic Department of Neurology: Mayo Clinic Examinations in Neurology. Seventh edition. St. Louis, Mosby, 1998
34. Vaughan D, Asbury T, Riordan-Eva P: General Ophthalmology. Fourteenth edition. Norwalk, Connecticut, Appleton & Lange, 1995
35. Dubin D: Rapid Interpretation of EKG's: A Programmed Course. Fifth edition. Tampa, Florida, Cover Publishing Company, 1996

36. Green SM, editor: 1998 Tarascon Pocket Pharmacopoeia. Loma Linda, California, Tarascon Publishing
37. DiGregorio GJ, Barbieri EJ: Handbook of Commonly Prescribed Drugs. Twelfth edition. West Chester, Pennsylvania, Medical Surveillance, 1997
38. Murphy JL (editor): Monthly Prescribing Reference. New York, Prescribing Reference
39. Bakerman P, Strausbach P: Bakerman's ABC's of Interpretive Laboratory Data. Third edition. Myrtle Beach, South Carolina, Interpretive Laboratory Data, 1994
40. DeGowin RL: DeGowin & DeGowin's Diagnostic Examination. Sixth edition. New York, McGraw-Hill, Health Professions Division, 1994
41. Brown RE: Family Doc: The Making of a Family Practitioner. New York, Parthenon Publishing Group, 1998

15

FAMILY PRACTICE ORGANIZATIONS

John M. Wilkinson, M.D.

The field of family practice has a diverse membership: from family physicians who practice in remote rural settings to family physicians who serve as faculty in major academic centers located in metropolitan areas. To inform, educate, and provide cohesiveness to the group, there are organizations within the specialty that assist the members. This chapter reviews the major organizations that play an important role for the family physician; the most prominent are the American Academy of Family Physicians (AAFP), the American Board of Family Practice (ABFP), and the Society of Teachers of Family Medicine (STFM).

The AAFP, located in Kansas City, Missouri, represents the broad interests of the specialty of family practice, emphasizing political, social, and educational areas. The ABFP, located in Lexington, Kentucky, is a separate and autonomous body that acts as the certifying agency for the specialty of family practice. It works with various groups to contribute to the educational process for family physicians. The STFM was founded to respond to the needs of family medicine educators and has a membership of more than 4,600 teachers of family medicine. The STFM administrative offices are housed with the AAFP in Kansas City, enhancing the close relationship between the two organizations. Both the ABFP and the AAFP as well as the STFM work closely toward the common goal of providing better health care through the specialty of family practice. Other organizations of interest include the American Medical Association (AMA) and its component groups as well as the North American Primary Care Research Group (NAPCRG) and the international umbrella organization of family practice groups, WONCA.

"Medicine is a profession for social service and it developed organization in response to social need."

—Charles H. Mayo

AMERICAN ACADEMY OF FAMILY PHYSICIANS

The AAFP is a national association of family physicians. It is one of the largest national medical organizations, with more than 80,000 members. The Academy was founded in 1947 as the American Academy of General Practice; the name was changed in 1971 to reflect more accurately the changing nature of primary health care. Its mission continues to be to "promote and maintain high quality standards for family doctors who are providing continuing comprehensive health care to the public" (http://www.aafp.org/about/300_a.html). In keeping with its mission, the AAFP works to:

Provide health-related advocacy and education for patients and the public

Preserve and promote quality cost-effective health care

Promote the science and art of family medicine

Ensure an optimal supply of well-trained family physicians

Ensure the right of family physicians to perform all procedures for which they have been trained and are qualified

These are just a few of the important services the AAFP provides. The organization is a vital resource for the family physician. Perhaps one of the biggest roles for the AAFP is through its lobbying efforts with the federal government. Through lobbying and education, the AAFP works on behalf of family physicians for fair reimbursement and works to reduce the hassle factors of practicing medicine, both nationally and locally.

At its conception, the founders of the AAFP specified in its bylaws that members must complete a minimum of 150 hours of approved continuing medical education every 3 years to retain membership (resident physician members are exempt). This requirement was a unique idea at the time and it has become the standard for many other medical groups in recent years.

There are also state chapters of the AAFP, which provide programs and

BOX 15-1 GET INVOLVED

Izabela Riffe, M.D. Senior Associate Consultant, Department of Family Medicine, Mayo Clinic Jacksonville, Jacksonville, Florida

Residency is a time-demanding occupation. There are nights on call, clinics, reading, and anything else you want to add to the list. So why look for more obligation? I decided early in my second year to attend a family practice weekend sponsored by the Florida Academy of Family Physicians. I was hooked after the first meeting.

After attending and meeting other residents and family practitioners across the state, I became a program representative for my residency program. The Florida Academy has a regular residency representative meeting at each of the 4 meetings per year, where typically 2 representatives from each residency program in the state attend to exchange ideas and concerns. For me, learning the political process started here. I then ran for the office of Secretary/Treasurer of the residency representatives statewide. The office enabled me to be a board member of the Florida Academy of Family Physicians with full voting privileges.

I had the opportunity to learn, to lead, and to assist in running meetings. I was able to network with other residents across the state. I also attended various committee meetings. For a resident seriously thinking of staying in the state in which you are training, there are distinct advantages of becoming involved in your state's academy. For those of us who naturally have no talent in networking, participating in your academy is a natural way of meeting other practitioners across the state. This is also a safe environment to practice your leadership skills. The board meetings of the Florida Academy are open to all members, so members can keep up on current concerns of practitioners in Florida. I also had the opportunity to attend the Kansas City meeting as a Florida representative to recruit future residents to the state of Florida. Of course, all these activities are usually at resorts and posh hotels, a far cry from the typical call room.

The only disadvantage I encountered is that of time. It took the commitment of my husband and children to travel with me to be able to spend time with each other. We tried to view this as a family activity. It also gave my spouse a chance to meet my colleagues.

I highly recommend becoming involved in your state academy. The effort has to be yours. They are always looking for new leaders and people concerned with the practice of medicine in their state. After attending a Florida Academy weekend, I would feel charged up and could actually see the light at the end of the tunnel.

My academy involvement has not ended. I've had the opportunity to attend the national meeting and plan on attending future state meetings. We all need to become involved at some level and at some point. Your state academy is another resource to enhance the breadth of your residency experience.

services oriented toward local concerns and interests (Box 15-1). Contact the AAFP or the state chapters directly for further information (Fig. 15-1).

Publications of the American Academy of Family Physicians

American Family Physician is the official clinical journal of the AAFP. It is an excellent source of timely articles on a wide variety of clinical topics

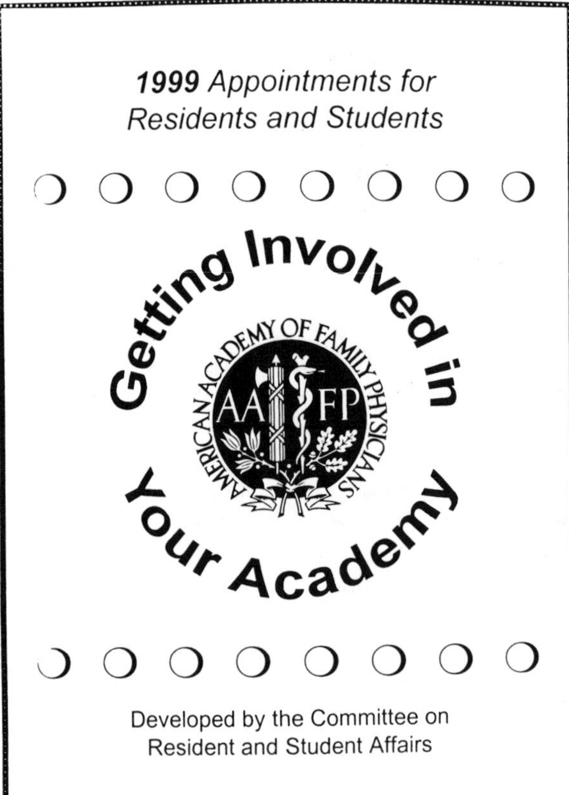

FIGURE 15-1
The American Academy of Family Physicians provides written materials to help physicians, residents, and medical students become involved in the Academy. This publication describes various activities and committees for residents and medical students. (By permission of the American Academy of Family Physicians.)

relevant to family physicians. From the diagnosis and management of low back pain to the treatment of otitis media, the topics reviewed are pertinent to the practicing family physician.

Family Practice Management deals with practice management and socioeconomic issues, all designed to "help family physicians adapt their practices to . . . the changing health care system" (http://www.aafp.org/fpm/). In the constantly evolving environment of health care, this journal is particularly useful for information about the business aspects of family practice.

FP Report is a monthly newsletter and features articles of interest for members of the AAFP. The publication gives a brief synopsis of breaking stories that affect family physicians.

Internet Resources Provided by the American Academy of Family Physicians

The AAFP web site at http://www.aafp.org/ has additional detailed information about the Academy and the specialty of family practice, links to AAFP publications, and excellent links to other sites of interest to family physicians.

General Information

AAFP members have access to additional family practice-related information within the site's member section: *AAFP Online* (http://www.aafp.org/members.html). Membership identification is required for access to the membership database, to view personal continuing medical education files, and to access comprehensive continuing medical education listings.

The *Directory of Family Practice Residency Programs* (http://www.aafp.org/residencies/) is the best source for information on family practice training programs. This directory lists each program in the United States and covers many topics in detail, including faculty, administration, accreditation, size, and salaries.

The *Fellowship Directory for Family Physicians* (http://www.aafp.org/fellowships/) is produced by the AAFP in cooperation with the STFM. It provides up-to-date information on fellowships in Adolescent Medicine, Faculty Development, Geriatrics, Obstetrics, Preventive Medicine, Family Medicine Research, Rural Medicine, Sports Medicine, Substance Abuse, and other fellowships as they become available.

The *AAFP Catalog* (http://www.aafp.org/catalog/) includes various educational services and products for family physicians, including the AAFP Home Study Self-Assessment and *American Family Physician* CD-ROM collections.

Career Opportunities Online (http://www.aafp.org/careers/index.html) is an extensive listing of career openings for primary care physicians from the current issues of *American Family Physician* and *Family Practice Management.*

Practice Management

AAFP Physician Placement Services (http://www.aafp.org/careers/plac indx.html) is available only to family physicians who are members of the AAFP. It provides rapid, up-to-date information on practice opportunities all over the country. It pairs physicians with jobs that meet their individual geographic, demographic, professional, and social criteria. This service is free and pledges to provide no hassles or sales pitches.

> *''Medicine is about as big or as little in any community, large or small, as the physicians make it.''*
>
> —Charles H. Mayo

OPPORTUNITIES FOR MEETING AND NETWORKING

The Annual Scientific Assembly (http://www.aafp.org/assembly/) is the Academy's largest meeting, drawing more than 17,000 physicians and visitors (Fig. 15-2). At this meeting, residents or physicians in practice can talk to exhibitors confidentially in one-on-one interviews. Information on practice opportunities nationwide is available at the Placement Center Databank. Physician Placement Sessions are also offered; these are designed to help improve negotiation and interviewing skills.

The National Congress of Family Practice Residents, sponsored by the Academy and typically held in the summer in Kansas City, presents workshops, business meetings, procedure courses, exhibits, and social events all specifically designed for family practice residents. Residents sharpen procedural skills, meet other family practice residents from all over the

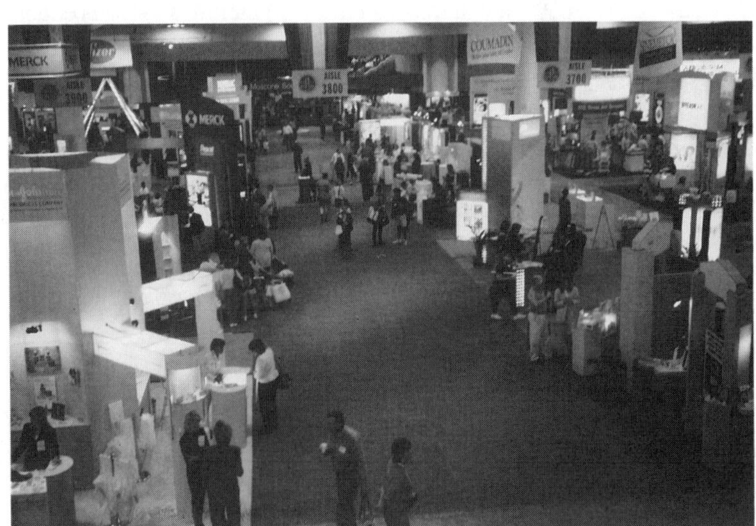

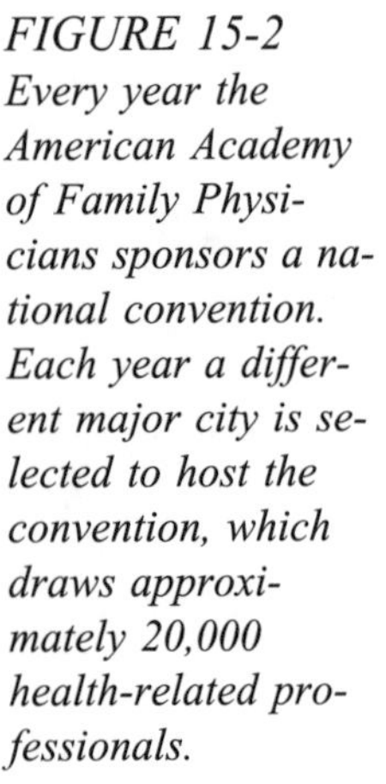
FIGURE 15-2
Every year the American Academy of Family Physicians sponsors a national convention. Each year a different major city is selected to host the convention, which draws approximately 20,000 health-related professionals.

country, talk with exhibitors about potential practice opportunities, and get up-to-date information on practice management and clinical topics.

To contact the AAFP:

American Academy of Family Physicians

8880 Ward Parkway

Kansas City, Missouri 64114

Telephone: (816) 333-9700; (800) 274-2237

E-mail: fp@aafp.org

AAFP web site: http://www.aafp.org

SOCIETY OF TEACHERS OF FAMILY MEDICINE

The STFM was founded in 1967 to respond to the needs of family medicine educators. Beginning with 105 founding members, the STFM has grown to a membership of more than 4,600 teachers of family medicine. The STFM's purpose is to:

Support and promote family medicine as an academic discipline

Maintain and continually improve the quality of family medicine and general medical education

Encourage research and teaching in family medicine

Facilitate the professional growth and development of family medicine educators

Encourage a multidisciplinary and international approach to family medicine education

Provide a forum for the interchange of experience and ideas among its members and other interested persons

Persons training in any approved family practice program, department, or medical school may join the STFM as Affiliate Members. Dues for 1999 were: physician member, $195; active fellow-in-training, $60; resident, $45; and medical student, $15.

Publications of the Society of Teachers of Family Medicine

Family Medicine is the official journal of the STFM. This monthly publication features peer-reviewed clinical and educational research articles that help define the discipline.

The *STFM Messenger* provides a bimonthly update of STFM activities. The STFM also publishes and distributes books, monographs, and videotapes of interest to family medicine educators.

Internet Resources Provided by the Society of Teachers of Family Medicine

The STFM web site is found at http://www.stfm.org/ and has information about STFM membership, events, publications, and other items of interest.

Opportunities for Meeting and Networking

The STFM sponsors several annual conferences that provide participants the opportunity to hear plenary speakers address issues facing academic family medicine and to participate in workshops and informational sessions. Presentations for these meetings are selected through a call for papers and peer-review process. STFM's annual conferences include:

Annual Spring Conference (held in late spring)

Predoctoral Education Conference (held in late winter)

Conference on Families and Health Care (held in early spring)

Conference on Patient Education, cosponsored with the AAFP (held in the fall)

Regional Meetings (held in different geographic regions in the fall)

Faculty Development/Management Skills Workshops (held throughout the year)

As a group, members of the STFM enjoy teaching and sharing knowledge about family medicine and are open and welcoming to new members.

STFM members place a high value on the opportunities provided for communication among individuals with common interests and goals. At any given time, there are 25 to 35 special interest groups (officially named Groups on . . .) operating within the Society. These groups provide an opportunity for residents and others to become involved in areas of special interest and to develop curricula, monographs, meetings, and networks. Membership is open to all STFM members.

STFM groups include the following of particular interest to resident physicians: Adolescent Health Care, Alternative Medicine, Computing, Ethics & Humanities, Evidence-Based Medicine, Family-Centered Perinatal Care, Fellowship Training, Lesbian/Gay Health, Minority Health, Multicultural Health Care & Education, Spirituality, Sports Medicine, Violence Education, and the Women in Family Medicine Network.

The Rural Interest Group is committed to providing a comprehensive source of information needed for those in family medicine education and practicing in rural areas of the United States. For information on current issues facing rural medicine, communications from STFM's Rural Interest Group, and the *Rural Family Doctor* newsletter, visit the Web site at http://www.ruralfamilymedicine.org/. It also contains links to sites about rural America, rural health, community-oriented primary care, and information for rural family medicine educators.

AMERICAN BOARD OF FAMILY PRACTICE

The ABFP was founded in 1969 and is the second largest medical specialty board in the United States (Fig. 15-3). Its purpose is to:

Improve the quality of medical care available to the public by establishing and maintaining high standards of excellence in family practice

Improve the standards of medical education and facilities for training in family practice

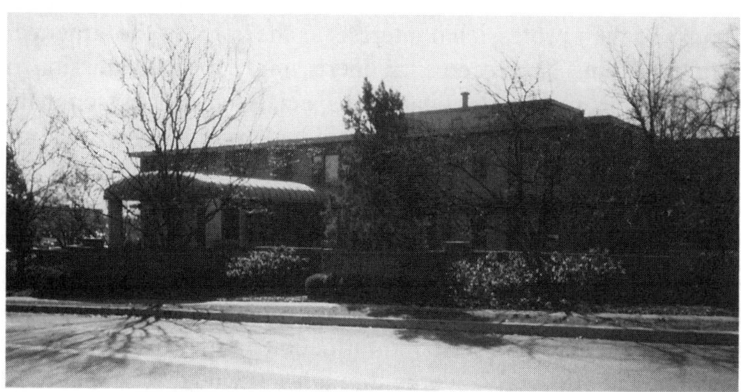

FIGURE 15-3
The American Board of Family Practice, founded in 1969, is located in Lexington, Kentucky.

Determine by written examination the fitness of specialists in family practice and design and conduct these written examinations, grant and issue board certification in family practice, and suspend or revoke certification if necessary

Information about the ABFP is available on-line at http://www.abfp.org. This site contains information about ABFP certification, recertification, board review courses, board examinations, residency training requirements, *Journal of the American Board of Family Practice,* and history of the medical specialty of family practice.

To contact the ABFP:

American Board of Family Practice

2228 Young Drive

Lexington, KY 40505-4294

Telephone: (888) 995-5700 (toll free); (606) 269-5626

Fax: (606) 335-7501; (606) 335-7509

E-mail: general@abfp.org (general information) webmaster@abfp.org (Webmaster)

AMERICAN MEDICAL ASSOCIATION

The AMA was founded in 1847 by a group of physicians concerned about advancing the quality of medical education, science, and practice. Its core purpose is, "To promote the art and science of medicine and the betterment of public health." The AMA attempts to speak for all physicians on matters of public health and their professional interests as the voice of the American medical profession. This has become an increasingly difficult mission in recent years, as physicians have gravitated to specialty groups, which many view as being better able to represent their individual priorities and concerns. Still, the AMA's sheer size, 300,000 members representing about 40% of all US physicians, carries considerable influence at national and state levels, particularly with regard to matters of public health. The AMA's work includes the development and promotion of standards in medical practice, research, and education; advocacy on behalf of patients and physicians; and a commitment to providing accurate and timely information on topics important to the public health. The AMA also works through individual state and local medical associations; membership at these levels is coordinated through the larger AMA.

Publications of the American Medical Association

JAMA began publication in 1883 and is one of the most widely read of all medical journals. The AMA also publishes Archives journals, including the *Archives of Family Medicine,* which is a monthly peer-reviewed journal providing academic and clinical information for family and general physicians.

Resident Forum is a resident's newsletter that appears weekly in *JAMA* and provides information about the AMA-Resident Physicians Section (RPS), current legislative and regulatory activities, and other issues of concern to residents.

Code Blue, which carries socioeconomic and legislative news of interest to resident physicians, is bound into the monthly magazine, *Resident & Staff Physician.*

AMA News is a weekly publication, with information on events and people affecting the practice of medicine.

Internet Resources Provided by the American Medical Association

The AMA web site is located at http://www.ama-assn.org/ and contains information on membership, medical education, press releases, and links to their scientific journals. There are also links to their collection of disease-specific Information Centers (including HIV/AIDS, asthma, migraine, and women's health), a patient information area, and a physician locator.

Opportunities for Meeting and Networking

AMA policy is developed at annual and semiannual House of Delegates meetings. In addition, member special interest groups are an attempt to allow smaller groups to have a greater voice within the larger AMA. There are 9 special interest groups, including the Medical Student Section, the RPS, the Young Physicians Section, Women in Medicine, Minority Physician Services, and others. The Medical Student Section, RPS, and Young Physicians Section each have a structure and organization that mirrors the AMA House of Delegates.

Special groups, including Women in Medicine and Minority Physician Services, provide direct counsel to the AMA Board of Trustees. Resident physicians may participate in these groups to help fashion policies and to suggest new initiatives on health and professional concerns that have particular impact on their constituencies.

The RPS of the AMA is composed of residents and fellows who are AMA members and are in approved training programs. AMA-RPS has approximately 35,000 members and is the largest resident organization in the United States. Its major goals are to educate residents about issues concerning graduate medical education and national health policies and to train young physician leaders. Currently, dues are $45 each year.

The AMA-RPS has played a role in several policy areas.

Resident Work Hours and Supervision—AMA-RPS has worked to implement reform in this area, and the Accreditation Council on Graduate Medical Education now has specific criteria on work hours that are written into the program requirements for each specialty's residency review committee.

Student Loan Deferment and Forbearance—The AMA-RPS played a role in creating regulations that allow medical school loan repayment to be deferred for up to 3 years during residency.

Resident Representation on Residency Review Committees—The AMA-RPS and AMA continue to work on this issue, with the goal of having residents represented on each residency review committee.

AMA-RPS is active in other areas, including physician workforce issues, resident due process and protections, graduate medical education funding, domestic violence, and public health.

For more information on the AMA-RPS, write or call:

Department of Resident Physician Services

American Medical Association

515 North State Street

Chicago, IL 60610

Telephone: (312) 464-4751

E-mail: rps@ama-assn.org

The AMA recently launched a new organizational forum for women physicians. The Women Physicians Congress provides another opportunity to participate directly in the AMA and to influence national health policy and advocacy on important women's health and women physician professional issues. The goals of the AMA Women Physicians Congress include:

Increase the percentage of women physicians in leadership and senior management positions in medicine

Enhance AMA advocacy on women physician policy issues

Facilitate the professional development of women physicians through leadership development, education, and training

Foster collaboration among the AMA, American Medical Women's Association, women physician specialty organizations, national women's health groups, and other organizations with mutual concerns

Increase flexibility within all levels of the profession in balancing professional and family responsibilities

Provide a forum for mentoring, networking, and ongoing communication for women physicians

Monitor trends and emerging issues that will affect women in the profession

Highlight and advance the women's health agenda

Increase the membership and participation of women physicians in their professional societies and the AMA

Membership is open to all AMA members—women physicians, women medical students, and all physicians interested in women's issues. Physicians who are not members can join the Congress on a trial basis for 1 year. There is no charge. An electronic communication network is being established that will link members to each other and to the AMA.

For more information on AMA's Women Physicians Congress contact:

Women in Medicine Services

American Medical Association

515 North State Street

Chicago, IL 60610

NORTH AMERICAN PRIMARY CARE RESEARCH GROUP

NAPCRG is a multidisciplinary organization formed in 1972 to foster the development of primary care research. Although oriented toward family medicine, all primary care generalist disciplines are represented within NAPCRG. In addition, NAPCRG represents members from related sciences, notably epidemiology, behavioral sciences, and health services research. NAPCRG is essentially a binational group, with balanced participation by physicians from the United States and Canada. International membership has been growing, with members from the British Isles, Europe, South America, and Asia.

NAPCRG's accomplishments include fostering:

Development of practice-based research networks

Development of primary care classification taxonomies

Linkages between qualitative and quantitative approaches to research

The NAPCRG web site is found at http://views.vcu.edu/napcrg/. This site contains information about NAPCRG's organization, annual meeting, publications, services, mailing list, and other research-related information.

WONCA

The name WONCA is an acronym made up of the initials of the first part of the name World Organization of National Colleges, Academies and Academic Associations of General Practitioners/Family Physicians. The short name is World Organization of Family Doctors.

WONCA is made up of national organizations concerned with the academic aspects of general family practice. Founded in 1972, WONCA now has 54 member organizations in 51 countries. In all, the total membership of the member organizations of WONCA is about 150,000 family physicians and general practitioners.

The goal of WONCA is to improve the health of the peoples of the world by fostering and maintaining high standards of care in family medicine. WONCA provides a forum for the exchange of knowledge among member organizations and supports the development of academic organizations of general practitioners and family physicians.

For more information concerning WONCA contact:

World Organization of Family Doctors

Locked Bag 11

Collins Street East Post Office

Melbourne, Victoria 8003

AUSTRALIA

Telephone: 61 3 9650 0235

Fax: 61 3 9650 0236

CONCLUSIONS

As health care changes, there will be a need for increasing numbers of family physicians to provide primary care. As the number of family physicians grows, they will need a solid infrastructure that supports the specialty. Many groups currently provide important resources to family physicians in many different arenas, but they will become even more important as the specialty expands in numbers and diversity. By providing multiple services, these groups, and others like them which will surely develop as the need demands, will serve as the foundation and framework for the specialty of family practice.

16

RESEARCH IN FAMILY MEDICINE

Floyd B. Willis, M.D.

"Family practice physicians must study themselves, or all of the studying will be done by researchers outside the specialty, often by groups eager to take over the roles traditionally held by family physicians."

—J. E. Scherger, M.D., & H. F. Young, M.D., *Journal of Family Practice* 46:203, 1998

IS THERE A NEED FOR MORE FAMILY MEDICINE-BASED RESEARCH?

There is currently a major effort under way to increase the research activity within the discipline of family medicine. However, recognition of the importance of the intellectual growth of family medicine extends back to the late 1960s when the specialty was founded and the political and educational organizations were developed.[1] The delivery of health care constantly evolves and, all too often, that evolution is driven by competition for health care dollars. It is important that family physicians help to define their own role in such an environment, lest it be defined by someone else less knowledgeable of the specialty. One way that residents and practicing physicians may help to clarify our importance is to initiate and participate in research projects that apply to family medicine (Fig. 16-1).

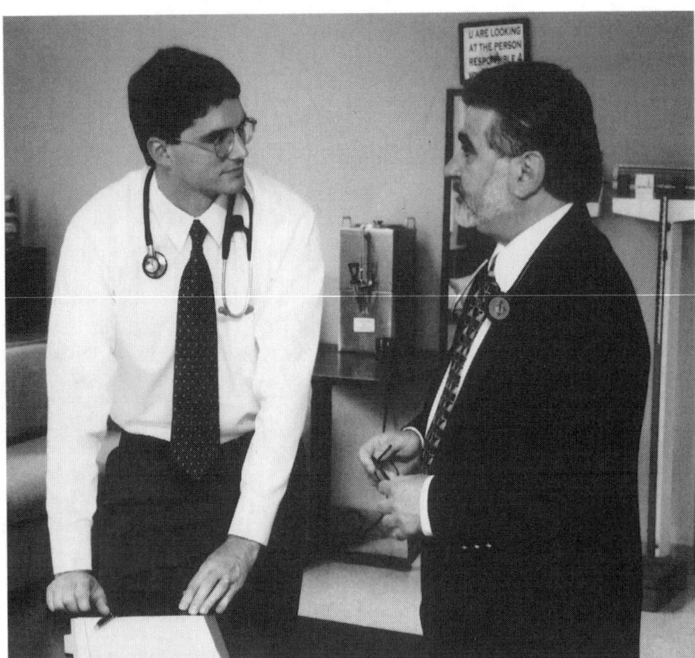

FIGURE 16-1 Family physicians are often involved in many aspects of research. However, clinical research that involves direct patient care is uniquely suited to the practicing family physician.

SHOULD I GET INVOLVED IN RESEARCH?

There are numerous ways to contribute to the continued growth of family medicine. The specialty is strengthened by its constituents' initiatives and leadership in various areas, including education, clinical practice, organized medicine, and research. However, one should strongly consider getting involved in research if you are naturally inquisitive and have persistence enough to lead a project to completion.

Many residents and practicing physicians encounter situations or interesting cases during patient encounters that they consider viable research projects (Box 16-1). Often, these potential research endeavors are abandoned because of difficulties in organizing and launching the project. By following several simple strategies, physicians with a genuine interest in research will likely achieve success at starting and completing research projects. The information presented below is simple advice that might aid a novice to pursue and maintain a budding interest in research.

"The scientist is not content to stop at the obvious."

—Charles H. Mayo

BOX 16-1 FAMILY MEDICINE RESEARCH AT MAYO CLINIC

The Department of Family Medicine at Mayo Clinic Jacksonville, led by principal investigator Dr. Floyd Willis (family physician), is conducting research on dementia in different ethnic groups. These studies involve gathering baseline information on neuropsychological tests and specific genotypes in African Americans, which will help determine this group's risk factors for Alzheimer's disease as the participants are followed over time. Funding, provided by the National Institutes of Health, is used along with the assistance of Dr. Neill Graff-Radford and Dr. Steven Younkin, leading researchers in the study of the genetics of Alzheimer's disease. This is an example of a group approach, combining a family physician's special interest with expertise of benchmark researchers to pursue a project that neither could do alone. This is an excellent example of how family physicians can enhance our specialty and medicine in general by getting involved in research.

HOW DO I GET STARTED?

Choose an Area of Study

Although the specialty of family medicine covers all ages and spreads over a broad range of medical topics, research efforts may be more successful if a focused area of interest is chosen by the potential researcher.

It has been suggested that researchers and clinicians are different in many ways but are much alike with respect to the passion that drives curiosity and the strong desire to solve problems.[2] These similarities should be remembered as you choose an area of interest. A research area in which you have a strong personal interest will likely demand more of your attention and this may translate into successful completion of the project.

Choose a Mentor

Recently published literature verifies that the availability of research mentors is an important characteristic in successful research activity for residents and faculty.[3,4] Most successful researchers can identify one or more mentors from whom they have received direction and advice.

Mentors can be extremely helpful for any person in pursuit of a general long-term goal, and they are particularly important in family medicine research. The rapid pace of the family medicine training program and clinical practice often makes it difficult to navigate through the learning process required to successfully start a research project. An experienced researcher can be invaluable in guiding you along more efficient pathways to your short-term and long-term goals.

Unfortunately, some suggest that family physicians with skills to be senior researchers and mentors number only 50 to 100 in the United States.[1] This means that a mentor might need to be chosen from a discipline other than family medicine. This should not matter as long as the mentor is willing to guide or collaborate in a helpful, cooperative, and unobtrusive manner.

HOW DO I GET ORGANIZED?

Narrow Your Topics

After an area of general interest has been chosen, one must narrow that general topic in one or more ways. The way to focus on a specific area is to decide whether you wish to investigate the epidemiologic and clinical questions, health delivery issues, behavioral issues, or educational issues. Shank[5] developed a table (Table 16-1) that organizes various potential research topics into groups. Such a table may help in focusing your interest on one specific area of research.

Another way to narrow the topics is to choose a specific medical symptom or diagnosis of interest and to use Table 16-1 to identify a major research problem or question area in which you will investigate that medical concern.

Literature Searches

Because any idea one may have may, in fact, have already been studied, it is prudent to investigate previous research on the topic of choice as soon as feasible. This can prevent duplication of previous studies and may help to refine your idea and prevent mistakes encountered in previous similar studies.

The majority of literature searches are now performed via computerized databases. This may be done in the library by the physician or librarian or from the physician's home or office via the Internet and World Wide Web. Virtually all medical libraries have access to computerized databases. There is also inexpensive and even free home access to on-line services that provide entry to MEDLINE and other National Library of Medicine databases.

State the Research Question

The specific research question should be stated clearly and in simple terms. In some instances, a research question may be transformed into a statistical or null hypothesis. The null hypothesis assumes that the results would be the same for an experimental and control group. One collects data to justify rejecting the null hypothesis.[6]

Example:

Research Question: "Does vaccination for measles, mumps, and rubella (MMR) diminish a person's risk of contracting measles?"

Null Hypothesis: "Persons vaccinated for MMR are as likely to contract measles as those not vaccinated for MMR."

Descriptive studies, which may be more appropriate for beginners, do not need a null hypothesis.[6] Nevertheless, the objective of the study should be written in a concise and clear manner. This statement will likely dictate the subsequent design of the study.

Choose the Type of Study

There are usually two basic approaches to a research study: observational and experimental. Experimental studies are designed to manipulate one or more variables in a study that measures change. (An example might be measuring a specific vital sign in a group of people, providing a specific medication to that group, and remeasuring the vital signs at a later point.) Experimental approaches require significant resources, involve ethical considerations, and may be difficult for a resident physician or beginning researcher to organize.

> *"The sciences bring into play the imagination, the building of images in which the reality of the past is blended with the ideals for the future, and from the picture there springs the prescience of genius."*
>
> —William J. Mayo

Observational (nonexperimental) studies are those in which no intervention is made deliberately. A natural course of events is allowed to unfold, and results are documented carefully. Table 16-2 presents the strengths and weaknesses of various observational studies.[2]

(*Continues on page 199*)

TABLE 16-1
RESEARCH AREAS IN FAMILY PRACTICE

PRIMARY RESEARCH AREA	MAJOR RESEARCH PROBLEM AREA
Epidemiologic and clinical research	
Practice studies	
	Content
	Common problems/diseases
	Variation with geographic setting
	Consultation rates
	Changing patterns
Single problem studies	
	Morbidity
	Natural history
	Prevention
	Early diagnosis
	Management
	Case reports/literature review
Clinical decision making	
	General theory
	Specific common problems
Geriatric problems	
Environmental and occupational health problems	
Health services research	
Consumers	
	Health/illness behavior
	Needs/demands
	Consumer participation
	Patient/health education
	Patient compliance
Providers	
	Numbers/distribution
	Efficiency/utilization
	M.D. performance
	Referral patterns
	Record keeping
	Models of primary care
	Paraprofessional studies
	Drug/laboratory procedures

Continued

TABLE 16-1 Continued

PRIMARY RESEARCH AREA	MAJOR RESEARCH PROBLEM AREA
Interface	
	Preventive medicine
	Community health services
	Patient outcome studies
	Cost and incentives
	Cost/benefit ratios
	Facilities and utilization
Behavioral and family research	
Physician-patient relationship studies	
Impact of societal changes on primary care	
Family studies—"family epidemiology"	
	Morbidity
	Prevention
	Crisis prevention
	Role of genetic counseling
Family dynamics	
	Normal/abnormal
	Changing patterns—"the household unit"
	Aspects of the family life cycle
	Teenage problems
	Social problems of aging
Counseling	
	Methods
	Results
Educational research	
Medical student interest in family practice	
Teaching aids for family practice	
Family practice residency programs	
	Educational objectives
	Role of medical unit
	Program costs
	Model clinic costs/revenue
	Self-assessment methods
	Documentation of experience
	Continuing education needs/results

From Shank.[5] By permission of the Society of Teachers of Family Medicine.

TABLE 16-2
STRENGTHS AND WEAKNESSES OF OBSERVATIONAL STUDIES

STUDY TYPE	METHODOLOGY	STRENGTH	WEAKNESS	INTERPRETATION
Case report Case series Population Longitudinal	General observation of the relationship of the disease (variable) and basic characteristics (person, place, time)	Seeks only to describe and have great value in reporting new information	Limits generalization from results; empirically not as much control as more sophisticated methods	Description of what happened
Cross-sectional	Examines the relationship between disease and other characteristics of interest as they exist in a defined population at one time	Quick	No time frame Need large numbers of subjects Existing cases may not be representative of all cases	Prevalence of disease
Case-control (retrospective)	Compares persons with disease and persons without disease with regard to how frequently the attribute was present	Easy (time and money) Few subjects Tests multiple exposure hypothesis No attrition	Cannot measure risk Information collected for other reasons Existent disease only	Comparative frequencies of risk factors of those with and without disease
Cohort (incidence prospective)	Study population is free of disease; attributes of interest are measured and followed over time; development of the disease is measured	Measures relative risk Less biased information on exposed persons	Money and time Attrition Single (few) exposure categories End points difficult to define	Measures the relative attributable risk of disease development

From Holloway and Rogers.[2] By permission of WB Saunders Company.

WHERE CAN I FIND SUPPORT?

Research Networks

Practice-based networks are organizations of primary care clinicians who are drawn together by shared commitment to pursue research. One such organization is the Ambulatory Sentinel Practice Network (ASPN). The ASPN was created in 1978 and entered into an agreement with the American Academy of Family Practice (AAFP) in 1992. It is composed of 122 practices in 40 states and 6 Canadian provinces. This network provides care for more than 1.5 million patients. Additionally, ASPN is working to promote collaboration and research among 20 local and regional research networks in family practice that have developed during the last 5 years. ASPN serves as a clearinghouse for like-minded people and organizations who seek to advance practice-based research through research networks. You may contact ASPN at:

Ambulatory Sentinel Practice Network (ASPN)

1650 Pier Street

Denver, Colorado 80214

Telephone: (800) 854-8283; Fax: (303) 202-1539

Family Medicine Organizations

The AAFP has an organized Commission on Clinical Policies and Research. This commission actively encourages research by family physicians and maintains general information on family physicians' activities and research. They may be contacted at the following address:

Herbert F. Young, M.D.

Staff Executive, Commission on Clinical Policies and Research

American Academy of Family Physicians

8880 Ward Parkway

Kansas City, MO 64114-2797

Telephone: (800) 274-2237 extension 5500

Institutional Committees

Many medical institutions provide peer groups to assist with research endeavors.

Research Committees Most institutions involved in research have active research committees. These committees are generally assigned to review and approve all research projects that operate within their institution. Contacting the chairperson of this committee or requesting to become involved in this committee may provide valuable insight on how to further your own research project.

Institutional Review Boards All institutions that use human subjects in research and receive federal funds must have an institutional review board. Many beginning research designs (chart reviews, surveys) do not require approval of the institutional review board. However, this committee still may be used as a source of information.

HOW DO I GET MY PROJECT FUNDED?

The AAFP actively funds research projects by family physicians. The AAFP also recommends that the Agency for Health Care Policy and Research in Rockville, Maryland, be contacted as a possible source of funding for family medicine research.

Agency for Health Care Policy and Research

2101 East Jefferson Street

Rockville, MD 20852

Telephone: (301) 594-1364

Other sources of funding may include support from local social and civic groups for small projects and support from a physician's hospital or training facility.

In consideration of funding, it is important to make the budget list as detailed as possible. Include items such as time for clerical staff to select patients or charts randomly, clerical support, cost of stamps for mailing, funding for second and third follow-up mailings, cost for computer data entry, cost for biostatistician services, and cost of editorial services for those who publish results.

WHERE CAN I FIND REFERENCES ON SELECTION OF SUBJECTS, STATISTICS, AND BACKGROUND INFORMATION ON RESEARCH?

The publication entitled *Practice-Based Research in Family Medicine*[6] by the AAFP contains an appendix with a good reference list. Also included in this appendix is information on literature-retrieval resources, a glossary of statistical terms, and a research workbook.

CONCLUSION

Those who feel they have any interest in family practice-based research, no matter how small, owe it to themselves and to the specialty of family practice to pursue that interest. Many have been surprised by the level of excitement that is generated when that ill-defined interest begins to blossom into a viable research protocol and project. We must encourage ourselves as well as our colleagues to nourish our research interests, because research may in time become vitally important to our specialty maintaining its rightful place in the health care paradigm.

REFERENCES

1. Culpepper L: Family medicine research: major needs. Fam Med 23:10-14, 1991
2. Holloway RL, Rogers JC: Research methodology. In Textbook of Family Practice. Fourth edition. Edited by RE Rakel. Philadelphia, WB Saunders Company, 1990, pp 1811-1821
3. Mills OF, Zyzanski SJ, Flocke S: Factors associated with research productivity in family practice residencies. Fam Med 27:188-193, 1995
4. Hueston WJ, Mainous AG III: Family medicine research in the community setting: what can we learn from successful researchers? J Fam Pract 43:171-176, 1996
5. Shank JC: Research highlights—a taxonomy for research. Fam Med Teacher Sept/Oct:22-33, 1980
6. Berg AO, Gordon MJ, Cherkin DC: Practice-Based Research in Family Medicine. Kansas City, Missouri, American Academy of Family Physicians, 1986

17

HEALTHY LIVING DURING RESIDENCY

David C. Agerter, M.D.

Most family practice residents experience significant stress during the course of their residency training. From the seemingly endless hours without sleep to the trying task of managing life-threatening conditions, there are a multitude of demands placed on the resident physician throughout training. Currently, there are efforts under way to reduce the number of on-call hours and days per week that are required of residents during their training program. This should reduce at least some of the stress that they may experience. With these stresses in mind, it is critically important that resident physicians spend a sufficient amount of time researching and deciding on which residency program they truly would like to attend. All aspects (eg, salary, call schedule, location, faculty) should be considered. If a resident physician is married and has a family or has a significant other, it is imperative that these individuals be a part of the interview process and decision making. If the resident in training is satisfied with the relocation, but family and loved ones are not, it will likely cause additional unnecessary stress. The following chapter outlines some important coping strategies for dealing with the rigors and stresses of family practice residency training.

RESIDENT IN TRAINING SURVEY

In 1996, a survey was done of Minnesota family practice residents and Resident Program Directors to look at issues related to stress and ways to improve stressful situations for residents in training. The study was conducted by Dr. Monica Myklebust and Dr. Kellie M. Kershisnik (Mayo Clinic Family Practice residents) and published by the Minnesota Academy of Family Physicians.[1]

A survey was sent to 287 residents; 162 responded for a response rate of 56 percent (66 men, 93 women, and 3 not identified). The survey included residents in all 3 years of training. Sixty percent of the residents reported working 60 to 80 hours per week on the average, with 36 percent working more than 80 hours per week. Understandably, fatigue was the most often cited stress-related symptom in 65 percent of the respondents. Twenty-two percent of residents reported suffering from depression during their training. Thirty-nine percent of the residents reported problems with relationships, with 5 percent experiencing divorce or separation during residency training.

From the results of this study, it is quite evident that there are enormous time demands with the family practice residency curriculum, much of which is spent away from family and friends. Although not necessarily proven, it can be assumed that much of the stress and fatigue contributes to depression and difficulties with interpersonal relationships. With this in mind, the successful family practice resident must develop adequate coping strategies.

''Good health is an essential to happiness, and happiness is an essential to good citizenship.''

Charles H. Mayo

COPING STRATEGIES

Various coping strategies are used commonly among family practice residents: regular exercise (Fig. 17-1), healthy eating, and protected time with their family or friends.

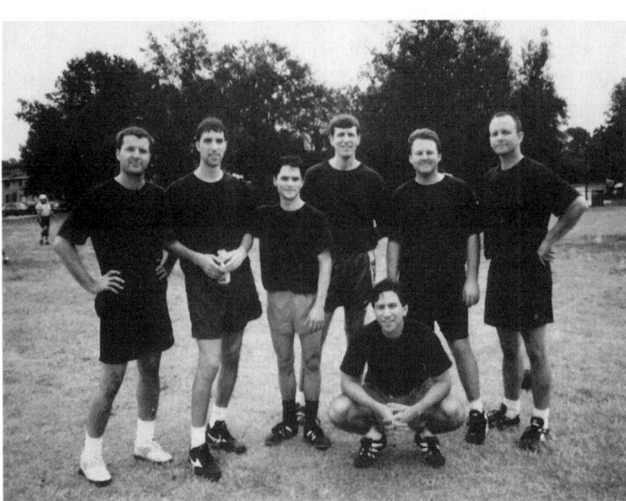

FIGURE 17-1 Participation in recreational activities is important in maintaining a healthy lifestyle during residency training.

Exercise

It is understandable that physicians need to be mindful of their own health because they are at risk for the development of health-related problems. One of the most commonly used and effective coping devices is regular exercise. A personal exercise prescription is really no different than what you might explain to other healthy patients in your practice. When beginning to consider a personal exercise prescription, look at the key components of an exercise session. These should include a warm-up phase of 5 to 10 minutes and an endurance phase of 20 to 30 minutes. The intensity of exercise should be monitored by appropriate heart rate monitoring or ratings of perceived exertion. The frequency of exercise should be 3 to 4 times per week, and there should be an appropriate cooldown phase of 5 to 10 minutes. If you exercise with a friend or family member, you are much more likely to continue the exercise program on an ongoing basis.[2]

Many guidelines exist for heart rate monitoring. Certainly, one can monitor heart rate through an appropriate treadmill exercise test, but other more simplified guidelines are available. For example, determine your heart rate maximum by simply subtracting your age from 220.[3] Many individuals use perceived exertion as a way of monitoring their workouts (Table 17-1).

Certainly, there are many derived benefits of regular exercise: reduction in heart disease, cancer, and stroke. The most important aspect of exercise for many people, including family practice residents, is an improved sense of self-esteem and well-being, an important quality that is essential for the development of a family physician. Numerous studies have shown that individuals who have regular exercise are much less likely to experience periods of acute illness and time away from their jobs.

TABLE 17-1
THE RATING OF PERCEIVED EXERTION SCALE

SCALE	PERCEIVED EXERTION
6–7	Very, very light
8–9	Very light
10–11	Fairly light
12–13	Somewhat hard
14–15	Hard
16–17	Very hard
18–19	Very, very hard

Nutrition

Nutrition also is important. The typical American diet is 40 percent fat and only 45 percent carbohydrates (by calories). Obviously, an increased amount of fat leads to the potential for heart disease and certain forms of cancer, not to mention obesity.

General recommendations should include: carbohydrates 50 to 60 percent (of caloric intake), protein 10 to 15 percent, fats 30 to 35 percent, and alcohol no more than 2 percent. There are additional dietary guidelines that one could follow (Table 17-2).

In the survey conducted by Myklebust and Kershisnik, residents emphasized the need for proper nutrition, especially while they are on call. Avoid heavy, fat-laden meals. Fast food or junk food in place of healthy eating can translate into excessive weight gain and decreased mental alertness. Obviously, there needs to be judicious use of caffeine and other stimulants during periods on call. Alcohol should never be used while on call (Box 17-1). Recreational drugs should not be used.

Set Priorities

It is essential that residents in training set priorities. I believe it is important for residents to do their absolute best to maintain hobbies and interests outside of medicine. Ideally, resident physicians should set aside one evening a week for themselves. This may be a time when resident physicians can pick up a new interest or hobby that will broaden their horizons (Fig. 17-2). I also believe that it is critically important for resident physicians to set aside time that is protected as much as possible to be with their families.

When residents are on call, they should make short periods of time when they can sit down, relax, consume a healthy snack, or call their families. Whenever possible, residents' families should join them for meals. If allowed,

TABLE 17-2
DIETARY GUIDELINES

1. Eat a wide variety of foods
2. Maintain healthy weight
3. Choose a diet low in fat, saturated fat, and cholesterol
4. Choose a diet with plenty of vegetables, fruits, and grain products
5. Use sugars only in moderation
6. Use salt and sodium only in moderation
7. If you drink alcoholic beverages, do so in moderation

BOX 17-1 DRUG AND ALCOHOL ABUSE AFFECTING PHYSICIANS

Residents in training and family physicians in practice are not immune to the problem of drug and alcohol abuse. The current prevalence of alcohol and drug dependence (prescription and illicit drugs) for physicians is similar to that for the general population (5 to 8 percent of the adult population). This means that 30,000 to 50,000 physicians currently have an alcohol or drug problem. Contrary to common belief, performance issues are often the last sign of a substance use problem.[4] Nevertheless, the effects of drug and alcohol abuse are devastating. From poor decision making to difficulties with interpersonal relationships, the effects are many and varied. In many cases, the problem is hidden from those who work around the individual affected until the point when something bad occurs that brings the problem to light. If you suspect you have a drug or alcohol problem, seek help. Untreated, these conditions may lead to loss of your medical license. If unsure, ask yourself the CAGE questions.

C = Have you ever tried to *c*ut down on your drinking?

A = Has anyone been very *a*nnoyed by your drinking?

G = Have you ever felt *g*uilty about your drinking?

E = Have you had an *e*ye-opener (do you drink in the morning)?

Two positive responses might indicate a drinking problem, whereas a positive response for 3 or 4 of the questions likely identifies a drinking problem.

If you suspect a drinking or drug-related problem, a good source of help would be your residency director or advisor. For physicians in practice, your personal physician or in some cases your local medical society may assist you in getting help through several different agencies (eg, Impaired Physicians Group, Alcoholics Anonymous). Many of these organizations can be contacted by simply looking up their telephone numbers in the telephone book. Despite the embarrassment, hassle, and consequences you may endure by seeking help—in the end you will be better off, both professionally and personally. As physicians, we must maintain high standards, not only for our patients but also for ourselves. Approach your problem as an illness and get appropriate medical help before it affects you or, worse, the people around you or your patients.

and it is not necessary to stay at the hospital, take calls from home. The lifestyle of a physician is without a doubt demanding and often doesn't improve once residency has ended. Establish strong family ties whenever time allows.

CONCLUSIONS

Adequate time should be spent sorting through the various family practice residency programs that are available. There are more than 400 residency programs now available in family medicine in the United States. Programs vary and, fortunately, many are outstanding. Know what support mechanisms

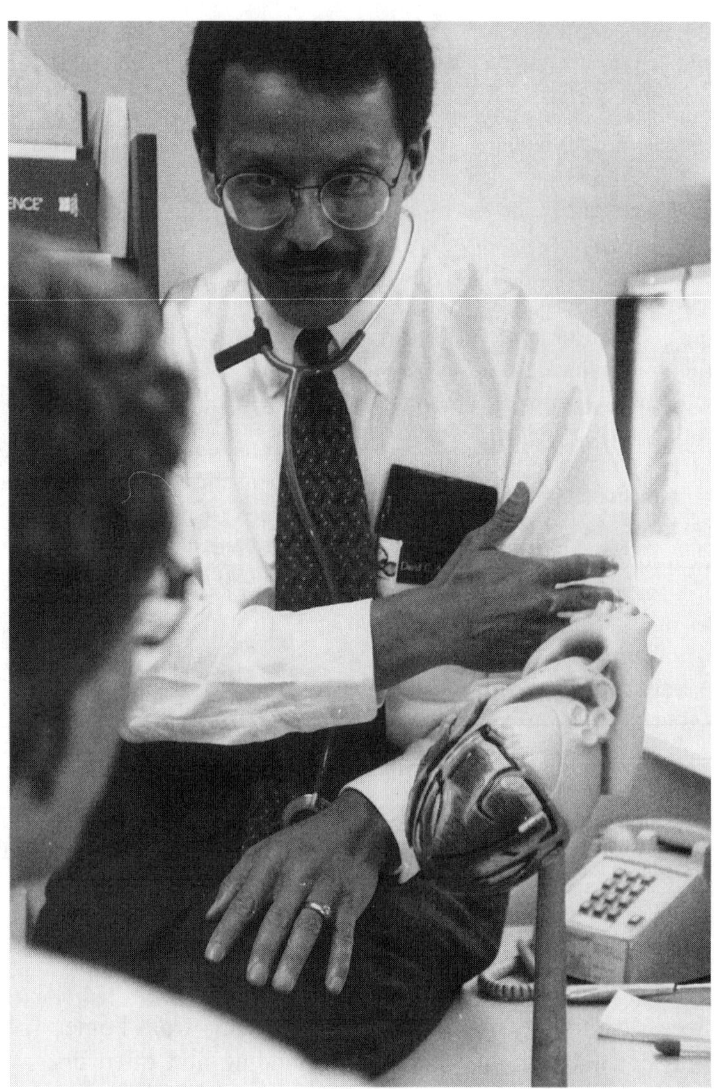

FIGURE 17-2
Remaining fit both physically and psychologically can help set a good example for your patients.

are available in the various programs and how residents feel they are treated. Such support systems may include the appointing of an advisor for each resident who meets regularly to assess the resident's performance and to discuss any problems or concerns. In addition, many programs have a behavioral psychologist who meets regularly with residents to discuss issues such as stress (Box 17-2), coping mechanisms, and time management.

Residents in training will find that it is important to find a mentor—another resident or a family practice faculty member to whom they can relate. If a

BOX 17-2 STRESS MANAGEMENT

Perhaps one of the most difficult tasks as a resident physician or physician in practice is the management of stress. Although it is not entirely possible to alleviate stress, the best way to deal with stress is to avoid it. The following is a humorous approach to avoid stress that can be applied to the teaching and practice of medicine.

How to Swim With Sharks: A Primer

Voltaire Cousteau*

Foreword

Actually, nobody *wants* to swim with sharks. It is not an acknowledged sport, and it is neither enjoyable nor exhilarating. These instructions are written primarily for the benefit of those who, by virtue of their occupation, find they *must* swim and find that the water is infested with sharks.

It is of obvious importance to learn that the waters are shark infested before commencing to swim. It is safe to assume that this initial determination has already been made. If the waters were clearly not shark infested, this would be of little interest or value. If the waters were shark infested, the naïve swimmer is by now probably beyond help; at the very least he has doubtless lost any interest in learning how to swim with sharks.

Finally, swimming with sharks is like any other skill: it cannot be learned from books alone; the novice must practice in order to develop the skill. The following rules simply set forth the fundamental principles which if followed, will make it possible to survive while becoming expert through practice.

*Little is known about the author, who died in Paris in 1812. He may have been a descendant of François Voltaire and an ancestor of Jacques Cousteau. Apparently this essay was written for sponge divers. Because it may have broader implications, it was translated from the French by Richard J. Johns, an obscure French scholar and Massey Professor and director of the Department of Biomedical Engineering, The Johns Hopkins University and Hospital, 720 Rutland Avenue, Baltimore, Maryland 21205.

Rules

1. *Assume unidentified fish are sharks.*—Not all sharks look like sharks, and some fish which are not sharks sometimes act like sharks. Unless you have witnessed docile behavior in the presence of shed blood on more than one occasion, it is best to assume an unknown species is a shark. Inexperienced swimmers have been badly mangled by assuming that docile behavior in the absence of blood indicates that the fish is not a shark.

2. *Do not bleed.*—It is a cardinal principle that if you are injured either by accident or by intent you must not bleed. Experience shows that bleeding prompts an even more aggressive attack and will often provoke the participation of sharks which are uninvolved or, as noted above, are usually docile.

Admittedly, it is difficult not to bleed when injured. Indeed, at first this may seem impossible. Diligent practice, however, will permit the experienced swimmer to sustain a serious laceration without bleeding and without even exhibiting any loss of composure. This hemostatic reflex can in part be conditioned, but there may be constitutional aspects as well. Those who cannot learn to control their bleeding should not attempt to swim with sharks, for the peril is too great.

The control of bleeding has a positive protective element for the swimmer. The shark will be confused as to whether or not his attack has injured you, and confusion is to the swimmer's advantage. On the other hand, the shark may know he has injured you and be puzzled as to why you do not bleed or show distress. This also has a profound effect on sharks. They begin questioning their own potency or, alternatively, believe the swimmer to have supernatural powers.

3. *Counter any aggression promptly.*—Sharks rarely attack a swimmer without warning. Usually there is some tentative, exploratory aggressive action. It is important that the swimmer recognizes that this behavior is a prelude to an attack and takes prompt and vigorous remedial action. The appropriate

BOX 17-2 Continued

countermove is a sharp blow to the nose. Almost invariably this will prevent a full-scale attack, for it makes it clear that you understand the shark's intentions and are prepared to use whatever force is necessary to repel his aggressive actions.

Some swimmers mistakenly believe that an ingratiating attitude will dispel an attack under these circumstances. This is not correct; such a response provokes a shark attack. Those who hold this erroneous view can usually be identified by their missing limb.

4. *Get out if someone is bleeding.*—If a swimmer (or shark) has been injured and is bleeding, get out of the water promptly. The presence of blood and the thrashing of water will elicit aggressive behavior even in the most docile of sharks. This latter group, poorly skilled in attacking, often behaves irrationally and may attack uninvolved swimmers or sharks. Some are so inept that in the confusion they injure themselves.

No useful purpose is served in attempting to rescue the injured swimmer. He either will or will not survive the attack, and your intervention cannot protect him once blood has been shed. Those who survive such an attack rarely venture to swim with sharks again, an attitude which is readily understandable.

The lack of effective countermeasures to a fully developed shark attack emphasizes the importance of the earlier rules.

5. *Use anticipatory retaliation.*—A constant danger to the skilled swimmer is that the sharks will forget that he is skilled and may attack in error. Some sharks have notoriously poor memories in this regard. This memory loss can be prevented by a program of anticipatory retaliation. The skilled swimmer should engage in these activities periodically, and the periods should be less than the memory span of the shark. Thus, it is not possible to state fixed intervals. The procedure may need to be repeated frequently with forgetful sharks and need be done only once for sharks with total recall.

The procedure is essentially the same as described under rule 3—a sharp blow to the nose. Here, however, the blow is unexpected and serves to remind the shark that you are both alert and unafraid. Swimmers should take care not to injure the shark and draw blood during this exercise for two reasons: First, sharks often bleed profusely, and this leads to the chaotic situation described under rule 4. Second, if swimmers act in this fashion it may not be possible to distinguish swimmers from sharks. Indeed, renegade swimmers are far worse than sharks, for none of the rules or measures described here is effective in controlling their aggressive behavior.

6. *Disorganize an organized attack.*—Usually sharks are sufficiently self-centered that they do not act in concert against a swimmer. This lack of organization greatly reduces the risk of swimming among sharks. However, upon occasion the sharks may launch a coordinated attack upon a swimmer or even upon one of their number. While the latter event is of no particular concern to a swimmer, it is essential that one know how to handle an organized shark attack directed against a swimmer.

The proper strategy is diversion. Sharks can be diverted from their organized attack in one of two ways. First, sharks as a group are especially prone to internal dissension. An experienced swimmer can divert an organized attack by introducing something, often something minor or trivial, which sets the sharks to fighting among themselves. Usually by the time the internal conflict is settled the sharks cannot even recall what they were setting about to do, much less get organized to do it.

A second mechanism of diversion is to introduce something which so enrages the members of the group that they begin to lash out in all directions, even attacking inanimate objects in their fury.

What should be introduced? Unfortunately, different things prompt internal dissension or blind fury in different groups of sharks. Here one must be experienced in dealing with a given group of

BOX 17-2 Continued

sharks, for what enrages one group will pass unnoted by another.

It is scarcely necessary to state that it is unethical for a swimmer under attack by a group of sharks to counter the attack by diverting them to another swimmer. It is, however, common to see this done by novice swimmers and by sharks when they fall under a concerted attack.

From Cousteau V: How to swim with sharks: a primer. Perspect Biol Med 16:525-528, 1973. By permission of the University of Chicago.

resident is unable to communicate effectively with the advisor, the resident should have the freedom to seek out a new advisor. If you are faced with this predicament, your residency director should assist you with finding another mentor or advisor.

As resident physicians continue to take care of their patients and families, they will be able to better relate to them if they "practice what they preach," meaning regular exercise and good nutrition. Patients will accept a physician who they know is trying to follow the same healthy lifestyle.

REFERENCES

1. Myklebust M, Kershisnik KM: Stress surveys of Minnesota family practice residents and resident program directors. Minn Acad Fam Physicians June:1–19, 1996
2. Agerter DC: So you want to run a marathon. Talk presented at Scott and White Clinic, Austin, Texas, April 30, 1995
3. Thomas RJ: The Heart and Exercise: A Practical Guide for the Clinician. New York, Igaku-Shoin, 1996
4. Fleming MF: Physician impairment: options for intervention. Am Fam Physician 50:41–44, 1994

18

INTERNATIONAL ROTATIONS

Walter B. Franz III, M.D.

This chapter provides basic guidelines for those family practice residents or family physicians in practice seeking international experience. Most family practice residents will not have had a previous experience because of the relative scarcity of international medical rotations in medical school. This chapter will primarily be aimed toward family practice residents in their second or third year because these residents will likely have the elective time available in their curriculum to explore international possibilities. However, early planning and self-education starting in the first year of residency lead to the best overall experiences on international rotations.

WHY IS INTERNATIONAL EXPERIENCE OR ROTATION IMPORTANT?

The reasons to seek international experiences are as varied as the people who are interested in them. From the humanitarian standpoint, some of my best and most poignant practice experiences have been during international service. Going beyond the obvious interest and pleasure of travel, international rotations offer a broad appreciation of critical world health issues, many of which usually are not seen in great concentration in the United States or covered in your medical school or residency education.

Although they are not the only medical education experience in which to have a broad-based cross-cultural experience, international rotations often immerse the health professional in cross-cultural scenarios. Even if a resident or physician in practice never planned to seek knowledge of international health issues in developing countries, family physicians will likely face international issues. International travel has mandated an understanding of previously thought "exotic" diseases, because any primary care provider will see patients going to or coming from international locations. In my practice at the time of writing this chapter, I saw several patients who were planning international trips for which malaria prophylaxis, immunizations, consideration of water purity, personal safety issues while traveling, and infectious diseases were all germane to the office visit. In addition, our community encompasses a wide spectrum of people from other countries who come to our Family Medicine Department for ongoing care. My international rotations have prepared me to better deal with the cross-cultural and medical needs of these patients.

> *"The problem before us is so to exchange information, and so to educate men through travel that there shall develop a final, cosmopolitan system of medicine which will combine the best elements to be found in all countries."*
>
> —Charles H. Mayo

Because of the great needs in many developing countries, residents may need to focus more on public health issues for international rotations. Because of the pressure of time in many family practice curricula, public health issues may not be covered in depth unless an international rotation is sought. International relief organizations emphasize that an international health curriculum prepares physicians for medical work in areas of resource constraint. Furthermore, international health focuses on the medicine of poverty and stresses both clinical and community problem solving. Therefore, an excellent way to prepare for the public health issues that you are likely to need to master as a family physician is to consider an international rotation.

Many family practice physicians would comment quite appropriately that they already care for patients who suffer from disease found in developing countries in their family practice centers in the United States. In our own family practice program, we care for people who enjoy the longest life span in the United States as well as for people who are indigent and some who have life spans on average but less than those people in developing countries. We stress an ecumenical approach to world health needs to our physicians in training and ask them to seek expertise wherever the opportunity best presents itself. One can appreciate the needs of the indigent and the unfortunate in our own communities in the United States, but I also suggest that international experiences are an excellent means for our residents and family practice physicians anywhere to be able to educate themselves on these issues as well as to gain an appreciation of world health (Fig. 18-1).

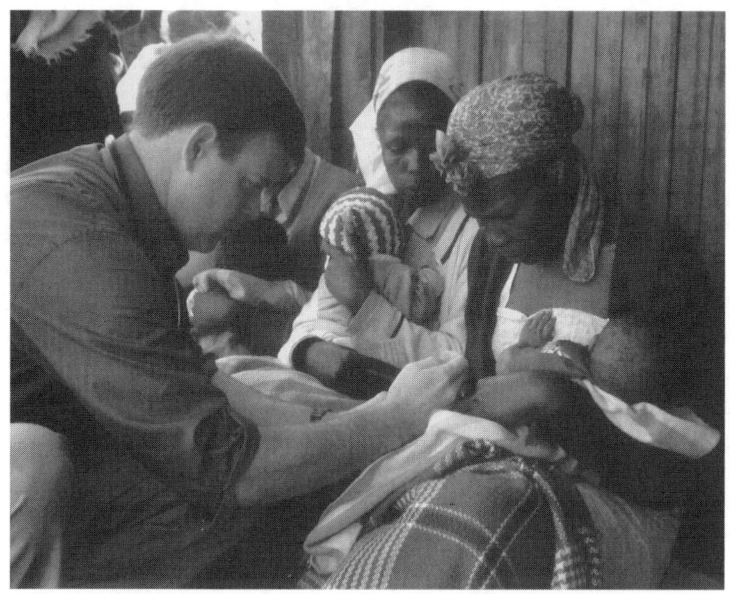

FIGURE 18-1
Some family physicians travel (often at their own expense) to Third World countries to provide care for those less fortunate.

PREPARING FOR AN INTERNATIONAL ROTATION

Mission Statement

The initial step in preparing for an international rotation is to formulate your mission statement or what you expect to gain or accomplish on an international rotation. Your mission statement does not have to be complex or keep you from being flexible, but I encourage residents to formulate a one-sentence statement that encompasses the most important goal for them. This helps you focus on what type of experience to seek.

Experience to Seek

There is nothing inappropriate about your mission statement primarily reflecting a desire to travel or to experience medicine in an exotic environment. If this is your goal, you should plan accordingly. However, if you are looking for an in-depth appreciation of medicine in developing countries or a broad experience encompassing infectious disease issues or public health concerns, then be certain as your planning progresses that you can fulfill these goals.

The greatest concern in the formulation of rotations for residents is to be certain that the international rotation has adequate precepting and teaching because many residents going on a rotation will not have had experience with many of the medical conditions or circumstances that may occur. Therefore, it is necessary continually to compare the capabilities of the site and the mission statement that has been developed for residents to be certain that the experiences will be fulfilling.

If your mission statement primarily is focused on providing humanitarian care, be certain that the site you are traveling to has the ability to help you provide this type of care. For example, if you are not bilingual, you will need interpreters for many countries and this could place a stress on an already overwhelmed medical system.

The search for an international rotation can be complex. Box 18-1 presents a synopsis of sites for prospective international rotations. Keep in mind, however, that your interest and perceived mission can change and so do the needs of these programs. The most important point is to check often and thoroughly with prospective sites to be satisfied that your mission matches your site's objective.

Administrative Preparation

This is probably the topic that many residents would least wish to deal with, but embedded in the excitement of planning an international rotation are several administrative issues that must be settled before you proceed with committing yourself to an international rotation.

From your program's perspective, do you receive appropriate credit for an international elective? Is your absence or time away from your family practice program within American Board of Family Physician guidelines for off-campus activities? Is your personal liability and professional liability insurance coverage in effect if you leave the family practice center for an off-campus or international rotation? Does your health insurance cover you during international travel?

The answers to these questions are often simple and can be handled quite easily with a few telephone calls. However, do not leave these issues to the end of your planning. For instance, if liability insurance is going to be a difficulty, you should work with the international sites, which may offer you protection, or you may need to go outside of your institution and purchase protection. Be certain to answer these questions early, and, if necessary, present your concerns to your program director or hospital administrator and have them provide a statement of understanding to send to your international host. In my experience, most international sites we have worked with do not offer liability insurance or cover any other liability for us; so be careful in looking at your personal coverage.

BOX 18-1 GETTING STARTED WITH INTERNATIONAL ROTATIONS

Eduardo Peña Dolhun, M.D. *Resident in Family Medicine, Mayo Graduate School of Medicine, Rochester, Minnesota*

There are numerous ways to create the type of experience that is right for you. Much depends on what is immediately available through your program curriculum, whether it is a formal international medicine health track or simply one person's previous experience. Even if no one in your residency program has ever worked or studied abroad, anyone can plan an international rotation with persistence, patience, and flexibility (Fig. 18-2).

Anytime one deals in an international milieu, one will encounter health care, political, and social systems that are quite different from home. These unique settings often teach much more than the immediate care of a patient. An international experience can help us understand the practical issues of treating illness within a developing country with poor health care.

WHAT IS OUT THERE?

Resources Whether you are a medical student, resident, or staff member, you may be interested in knowing that a great variety of residency programs offer international health care experiences. Roughly one-half of residency programs offer an international experience of some degree. A minority of family practice residencies have well-developed, long-standing programs.

The Directory of Family Practice Residency Programs provides a complete list of all programs and those with available international experiences. Their Web site is at: http://www.aafp.org/residencies/. Arguably the most comprehensive publication on the subject is the American Academy of Family Physician's *International Health Care Opportunities in Family Medicine—A Guide for Practicing Physicians, Resident Physicians, and Medical Students.*[1] This publication provides a list of residency programs with international health experiences, organizations sponsoring clinical and educational opportunities, professional organizations involved in international family medicine, newsletters, directories, a planning guide, and funding

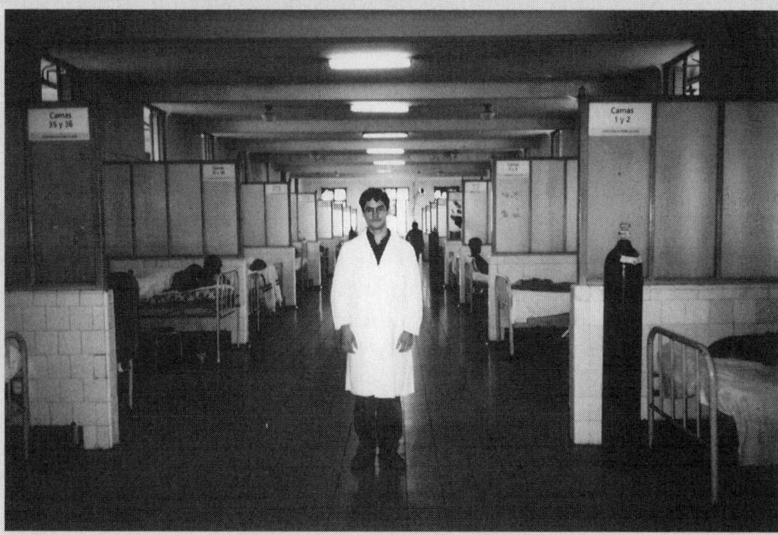

FIGURE 18-2
Dr. Peña Dolhun participated in an international rotation. At the Tuberculosis Sanitorium, Buenos Aires, Argentina, he gained knowledge of diseases he was not likely to encounter during his residency training in the United States.

BOX 18-1 Continued

sources. Copies can be requested from the Customer Service Department at (800) 944-0000. Request product #290 ($10 members, $15 nonmembers).

One other valuable source is the International Health Medical Education Consortium, an organization of faculty and program administrators interested in promoting international health and medical education in U.S. and Canadian medical schools and residency programs (Telephone [919] 962-0000; e-mail: ihmec@med.inc.edu).

Programs Listed here are several family practice programs with long-standing involvement in international medicine. This sample list is limited and intended to give the reader an idea of the level of involvement at some institutions.

MARSHALL UNIVERSITY SCHOOL OF MEDICINE, WV Believed to be the nation's first residency program featuring a 3-year International Health Track, the program offers an extensive list of foreign sites from which to choose. The experiences have been mostly clinical. Marshall receives from 75 to 100 applications for 2 to 4 slots per year. Residents have been sent to 27 countries throughout the world.

UNIVERSITY HOSPITALS OF CLEVELAND, OH Associated with Case Western University, this program offers a twice a month noon seminar series in international medicine as well as a 4-week course in the basics of tropical medicine and primary care in international health. Opportunities for research are encouraged.

BROWN UNIVERSITY, PROVIDENCE, RI The Department of Family Medicine has been involved in education in other countries. Department faculty have traveled extensively and guest faculty are regularly featured as speakers on pertinent local themes. Residents are exposed to international activities through elective opportunities and international visitors. Former sites include Zaire, South Africa, Hungary, India, Germany, Britain, Guatemala, Ecuador, Israel, Jordan, Bolivia, Nigeria, Mexico, and the Philippines.

EASTERN MAINE MEDICAL CENTER FAMILY PRACTICE RESIDENCY PROGRAM, BANGOR, ME This program offers experiences through affiliated institutions in Bolivia, Swaziland, Zimbabwe, and South Africa. Resident's clinical work has included general medicine, obstetrics, general surgery, and public health. Web site: http://www.emh.org/fprp/.

ST. ANTHONY FAMILY MEDICINE RESIDENCY PROGRAM, DENVER, CO Although there is no formal program or foreign affiliation, St. Anthony has sent one or 2 residents per year to various locations throughout the world, most recently to a banana plantation in Guatemala, through the international program of Tulane University. Former sites include Haiti, Dominican Republic, Canada, England, St. Lucia, Jamaica, the Cook Islands (South Pacific), Thailand, Nepal, and India.

SELF MEMORIAL HOSPITAL FAMILY PRACTICE, GREENWOOD, SC The strength of this program associated with international medicine is its strong association with a nonprofit organization, Volunteers in Medical Missions (VIMM), located in Seneca, SC. VIMM handles all the travel arrangements and application processing. Unlike the other programs listed, this program combines health care with ministering. The VIMM has built 6 clinics in Honduras, Ecuador, Chile, Nicaragua, and Tanzania. They have been involved in Ukraine, Vietnam, China, Russia, Bulgaria, Peru, and Belize. Web site: http://www.emeraldis.com/GreenwoodFP/.

UNIVERSITY OF CINCINNATI/PROVIDENCE HOSPITAL FPRP, OH The strength of the international experience of this program is its ongoing commitment to 2 particular communities in Latin America—one in Honduras and a newer one in Brazil. The program's strong ties to the Honduran village have gained support of the Honduran government. A series of didactic courses and relevant procedural skills workshops precede the site visits for the residents. There is Family Medicine faculty supervision with resident coordination.

SELECTING A PROSPECTIVE SITE OR HOST LOCATION

Risk Assessment

Risk assessment sounds fairly foreboding. It is important to do a risk assessment of your site and to determine if this site is in an area of political unrest or potential conflict. Be certain to check with the U.S. State Department with respect to any warnings or potential travel restrictions. Remember that in certain areas your presence may make a ''political'' statement, and you may place not only yourself but also your hosts and patients in potential danger. Admittedly, these situations are relatively infrequent, but these circumstances always must be taken into account. In general, be certain that your participation at an international site does not strongly suggest some type of political support for a cause or a certain political bias. I prefer to use the term ''medical neutrality'' and state that when one of our teams plans to work at a site we will care for any patient and provide education to anyone who wishes or needs it. This is essentially the same as your hospital's bill of rights. Be certain that your host understands that you will work only in an atmosphere of neutrality and that your basic underlying creed will be to care for any and all patients who need your medical expertise.

Your Host or Hosts

Have a precise understanding with your host with respect to your role when you are on site. For example, will you be a primary provider in a student role, are you expected to work on your own, or will you be a preceptee? Depending on your experience, these types of situations may be quite appropriate or frustrating.

Always take additional time to research the availability of local or regional physicians and how you will interact with them. Will your presence be a hindrance to regional physicians? Usually, your site host will have an excellent appreciation for anything that you need. Inquire if there is a hospital nearby where you can refer patients, if you are working in a clinical setting. Importantly, after you leave your rotation, will the patients continue to be cared for by an ongoing medical presence? If not, this does not preclude you traveling to a site, but how and possibly what you treat will require thoughtfulness. Inquire whether you will need to bring your own supplies. If you cannot speak the local language, will that be a major problem? After you have researched your site, if you are unfamiliar with something that seems to be a major part of your host practice, you will need to prepare yourself. In my experience, this typically will be in the realm of public or preventive health issues or the treatment of certain infectious diseases. This becomes the focus of your educational preparation.

EDUCATIONAL PREPARATION

Most international sites can be researched for medical geographic issues by contacting the Centers for Disease Control (http://www.cdc.gov/ or [404] 639-3311). Physicians traveling abroad should spend additional study time on common world illnesses such as malaria, parasites, enteric fevers, and malnutrition. By being familiar with the general medical problems of your intended site, you can prepare for the diseases you are likely to encounter, and if questions arise you can use local providers to help you on common and more difficult clinical presentations of diseases and conditions that they may be more comfortable treating.

Laboratory diagnostic modalities may be relatively limited at your site. Educate yourself on the clinical diagnoses of conditions you are likely to encounter, and, if time permits, learn simple laboratory methods to diagnose common infectious diseases, such as performing blood smears for malaria and parasite identification techniques. When possible, review efficacious but low-technology procedures and protocols such as tube feedings and the preparation of oral rehydration solution to substitute for intravenous hydration. Review practical approaches to clinical presentations that occur commonly in developing countries, such as fever, diarrhea, dehydration, and malnutrition.

Most second-year family practice residents have an excellent appreciation of most common primary care illnesses. However, in developing countries, the diseases seen in routine practice in the United States are often dramatically severe. For example, impetigo and fungal infections of the skin, which are familiar to every family practice resident, are often more dramatic in their clinical presentation in tropical environments and may require more aggressive treatment. Malnutrition, which can be found in the United States, may be nearly universal and severe at international sites. If you have access to faculty who have worked at international sites, be certain to tap their expertise on the typical presentations of common illnesses as well as on how to treat conditions when you do not have a great deal of diagnostic or laboratory equipment available. These paradigms will serve you well in your international rotations and as you do many of your clinical rotations in the family practice center. Mastery of these concepts allows you to be a true clinician at the bedside rather than being dependent on high-technology laboratory evaluations of your patients.

If preparation time permits, research the disease theory of the dominant culture you will be treating. For instance, in mainstream medical practice in the United States, usually both practitioner and patient subscribe to the germ theory of disease (ie, organisms can invade the body and cause clinical syndromes). In other cultures, other disease theories and explanations for illness will be widely accepted and the practitioner should be familiar with these theories to provide the best care and explanations to the patients on their conditions. Also, do you anticipate any cultural or religious practices that might interfere with your medical care. For example, in certain cultures, males and females may be completely segregated, with males often being treated first, and patients in many cultures may expect to see a clinician of the same sex. In some cultures, female professionals are not readily accepted. If these types of cross-cultural issues are germane to your rotation, research in advance how you will deal with them. Again, talking with your site host or with faculty who have done international work often helps you deal effectively with these issues.

In many situations, you will need to converse with patients through an interpreter. If you have not dealt with an interpreter before, review some proper techniques of interpreter services. If traditional healers are used at your international site, research how you should interact with them and what traditional treatments are to be expected in the area in which you will rotate. These are often excellent topics to discuss with your international host and in many cases will create unique opportunities for discussion.

Many of these issues can be covered when you arrive, but if you can ask about these issues and research them before your rotation, it will greatly enhance your experience abroad.

PERSONAL PREPARATION

You are, in most cases, taking a personal risk when traveling internationally, but with simple risk assessment and management, you will most likely complete your trip with no problems.

Personal Preventive Health Issues

Check with your immunization clinic or the Centers for Disease Control on what immunizations are needed for your international rotation. At a minimum, hepatitis B series, hepatitis A series, a tetanus booster, and typhoid vaccine should be considered. Depending on your itinerary and the standard recommendations, meningococcal and rabies vaccines may need to be added, and yellow fever vaccine may be required in a few instances. Polio may still be endemic in certain areas. Consult with your Infectious Disease consultant regarding the need for a polio booster and which type (ie, inactivated or oral-attenuated vaccine). Other vaccines may be needed for special areas. Again, planning ahead is the key, and checking with the Centers for Disease Control or with a local authority in your vicinity is essential. For many international sites, malaria prophylaxis is required. Remember, this is a prophylaxis, not guaranteed protection. Therefore, to further decrease your risk, use appropriate protection devices such as mosquito netting and insect repellents and avoid time outdoors at night. Remember that malaria prophylaxis typically needs to be started 1 week before travel and continued for 4 weeks after your return from an international site. You may need to take additional prophylactic treatment or preventive treatments with you for diarrhea, acute malaria, enteric fever, or other infectious diseases. Some countries may require proof of HIV testing. Again, be certain that you research these issues so there are no misunderstandings or delays in getting to your site.

Legal and Personal Documentation

Take several copies of your medical license, authenticated birth certificate, passport, immunization record, and a letter of support from your program director that documents your clinical responsibilities. Always carry proof of professional liability insurance.

Before your departure, ask your international host for an unequivocal letter of support and acceptance that you will be able to provide to anyone when you arrive on site in case there is a misunderstanding about your permission to practice medicine or provide care to those in need.

SAFETY AND SECURITY ISSUES

This is a topic that no one really wants to devote a lot of time to, but laxity in this realm rapidly ruins any international experience if a problem arises.

I recommend that you wear an identification tag (''dog tag'') and carry your passport and picture identification. Never travel alone if possible. If alone, always set an itinerary that you will follow, let someone else know your itinerary, and contact them to confirm your arrival when you reach your destination. When in a group, pair up and always travel with your partner wherever you go. If you are in an area of potential conflict or political unrest, always designate an emergency evacuation location in case you must leave your host country suddenly. Inform a U.S. counselor or Embassy of your presence if you are in an area of potential unrest, and let them know how to contact you in case of an emergency. If you have a medical condition that might place you at risk, make sure you have adequate supplies and information on your person at all times. Be familiar with local medical phrases that may be appropriate to your condition and research local areas for hospitals or clinics where you can seek medical care for yourself.

ADDITIONAL PREPARATIONS

If you are going to be involved in an international experience in a well-staffed and fixed facility, you may not need to bring supplies.

However, if you are going to be in an area of considerable need or a remote environment, you will have different logistical needs. It is impossible to bring everything that you might need for any particular trip. Some planning allows a reasonable approach.

Never bring medications that might cause problems after you leave if given out by well-meaning but less knowledgeable health workers. Avoid medications that might be harmful to children or pregnant women. Avoid medications that have toxic effects on renal, vestibular, or hematologic systems.

Purchase medications in stock bottles if possible, or if you use samples from pharmaceutical companies, keep the medications in their smallest original packages with a few of the package inserts available. Focus on antibiotics, dermatologic preparations, gastrointestinal tract drugs such as H_2 blockers, and respiratory tract pharmaceuticals such as bronchodilators (both inhaled and oral forms), including preparations for symptomatic treatment of upper respiratory tract illnesses. Ocular antibiotics, corticosteroids, and analgesics are also useful. Do not bring any schedule drugs. Possession of a narcotic medication can be difficult to explain to a custom agent. Take items to give to patients who do not need a medication. We typically take toothpaste, small bars of soap, and antacid tablets. Vitamins are useful, but be careful in giving out iron-containing vitamins because of the toxic reactions that can occur with these tasty, attractive vitamins when they are consumed by children. Avoid medications that require considerable mixing, preparation, or refrigeration. Instead, take chewable tablets or tablets that can be divided by a pill splitter or knife.

If your rotation is likely to involve surgery or invasive procedures, remember that medical waste disposal is relatively scarce internationally. Consider how you can dispose of medical waste safely on your rotation. Remember that medical waste may appear to be attractive toys for young patients.

Whatever supplies you bring, include an easy to follow and well-documented packing list for the custom agent. If you have considerable supplies, send a copy of your list ahead of your arrival and ask a member of your host group to ''clear'' your arrival. I typically bring a notarized letter stating that the supplies that I transport are to be given away during humanitarian care and that no money will be collected during distribution. Without such documentation, custom officials may ask you to pay tax on your supplies because they are concerned that you will be selling them for profit.

SPECIAL SUBJECTS

Organizing a Group

You may have already had considerable experience in international rotations or humanitarian medical work abroad. In this case, you may wish to establish a group that will perform international service. As mentioned previously, formulate a clear mission or goal statement and allow this to be your guide as you select a team and perhaps an organization to work with. Our team typically formulates a mission statement that emphasizes first the humanitarian approach and second education for both the community we will serve and the team members. Using this as a mission template, we contact groups with overseas sites who have a large patient care need and who will allow us to have team members encompassing various levels of medical sophistication (eg, medical students, residents, and staff physicians). We generally have predetermined sites located mostly in Central or South America, which have relatively short travel times from a major southern U.S. airport. This allows us to leave the United States, reach our destination, and be ready to work within 24 hours. Our team includes all levels of medical providers, nurses, interpreters, and community members with special talents or interests. If possible, we try to have cross-trained members of the team. For example, one of our physicians spent time with a dentist so he could perform simple dental extractions. A community member who is a journalist accompanied us on a trip and was trained to help with initial triage, height and weight measurements, and assessment of vital signs. Members of the team may also volunteer to develop special language skills or to focus on a particular medical procedure. We ask members of our teams to commit to several weeks of supply gathering and group and self-education on pertinent medical issues. We may cover basic language familiarization if time allows.

The group leader must constantly check on the details of the administrative and personnel issues for the team. We usually prepare several educational presentations for local village health workers. This provides us with a mechanism to be welcomed into many areas, with our initial contact being a presentation to village health workers. Then, we work side by side with them in a clinic.

Site Set Up

After establishing a location for service, the team must formulate plans for patient care. We typically set up our treatment areas in a public building such as a school or a church.

The first task is to determine who will provide triage and initial interview of patients. We like to select an experienced bilingual interpreter, if possible, with a good cross-cultural appreciation to have the initial contact with the patient. A single or multiple person triage area can be used. Patients are typically seen at several stations where the triage note is reviewed for the chief complaint and a brief history, if taken. Availability of interpreters is a critical factor in how many treatment stations are possible. We usually have a resident physician, medical student, and nurse at each station. This allows the resident to be the primary teacher. The staff physician or resident serves as a roaming preceptor. One resident or staff physician can function as a pharmacy supervisor. A brief medical record is kept, and diagnoses are noted and tabulated. Patients who do not require medications are always given some health-related items such as soap, vitamins, or toothpaste. Patients who require follow-up are carefully instructed by the interpreter and a written statement is given to the patient to show the triage office at the next visit. If the team is providing basic ambulatory surgery or dental extractions, we try to have this done in a separate area to provide infection control and appropriate privacy.

If the team is to function effectively, especially if large numbers of patients are likely to be seen, it is essential for village or local authorities to help triage in the most needy cases. Above all, do not allow your team to be overwhelmed. Set a definite stop time to close clinical services for the day with dignity, decorum, and safety.

Near the end of your clinical rotation, explain to village health workers what medications you are leaving behind and how they should be used. If it appears that a medication's use may be misunderstood, destroy it promptly. While providing care abroad, volunteers should be encouraged to make home visits and to travel to remote areas as necessary. These added encounters are often remembered by the team as the most poignant of the experience.

Working With Your Fellow Professionals

Imagine your reaction if a group of foreign professionals arrived at your family practice center only partially fluent in your language and announced that they have arrived to help you care for your unfortunate patients, especially if you had been doing village medical care in this location for years and did not invite anyone to present suddenly at your clinic. If this causes you discomfort, excellent. It reflects your sensitivity. With this in mind, before selecting and traveling to a site, be certain that you have contacted your local host professional and explain you wish to be a help, not a hindrance. I have found the best way to ensure a welcome is simply to ask "may we come and learn from you" and "what can we bring you to help care for your patients." Ask in plain language if your presence will cause any professional or personal hardship to local providers. Remember that many physicians serving in the poorest international areas struggle with their own livelihood. You may be providing free care to patients who ordinarily pay a meager but practice-sustaining fee to the local host professional. When in doubt, be humble, gracious, and remember that you are a visitor.

CONCLUSION

A trip abroad to provide medical care has many rewards. It often broadens the horizons of physicians and opens their eyes to the multitude of problems and illnesses that people face in developing countries. Diseases that have essentially been eradicated in developed countries continue to kill millions of people daily. But with these rewards come risks. Many diseases that we face in Third-World countries may be life threatening and put us in danger. In addition, many areas of the world are faced with political unrest and safety may not be ensured. Despite these significant risks, an educational experience abroad can ultimately make a better family physician by exposing the physician to many different cultures and customs. And it allows us to treat multitudes of needy people—a role we obviously enjoy and to which we are committed.

REFERENCE

1. American Academy of Family Physicians: International Health Care Opportunities in Family Medicine—A Guide for Practicing Physicians, Resident Physicians, and Medical Students. Second edition. Kansas City, Missouri, American Academy of Family Physicians, 1997

19

OSTEOPATHIC MEDICINE IN FAMILY PRACTICE

R. John Presutti, D.O.

Osteopathic medicine has been in existence for more than 100 years. Originally conceived by an M.D. who started the first osteopathic medical school, the popularity of the osteopathic philosophy and osteopathic physicians continues to grow and prosper during this age of primary care. Osteopathic medical schools now span America and osteopathic physicians are fully licensed in all 50 states. Osteopathy also has a growing presence in the European community, with more physicians, including M.D.s, practicing manual medicine. The concept of family medicine has always been an integral part of the training in osteopathic medicine. One of the key components in osteopathic training is the notion of wellness and the integration of a whole person approach to medical treatment.

HISTORY OF OSTEOPATHIC MEDICINE

A frontier physician from Kansas named Andrew Taylor Still, M.D., founded the osteopathic profession. After members of his own family died of meningitis in 1864, he became discouraged with the traditional medicine of that era. He believed that there must be more effective treatments for disease than the toxic remedies available at that time. In an effort to synthesize a new philosophy for medical treatment, he embarked on a detailed study of anatomy and physiology.[1] After a decade of work, he formulated the osteopathic philosophy and the practice of osteopathic medicine as it is known today.[2] He developed techniques to facilitate healing by using the body's natural reparative functions, relying, in part, on the underlying structure of the body.[1] His treatment methods met with opposition from the religious and medical community, but patients continued to seek his assistance. In 1875, Still moved to Kirksville, Missouri, to develop his practice and continue research.

BOX 19-1 STUDENTS ENROLLED IN COLLEGES OF OSTEOPATHIC MEDICINE

COLLEGE OF OSTEOPATHIC MEDICINE	STUDENTS ENROLLED, NO. (1997–1998)
Arizona	
Arizona College of Osteopathic Medicine, AZCOM	210
California	
Western University of Health Sciences College of Osteopathic Medicine of the Pacific, Western U/COMP	687
Touro University College of Osteopathic Medicine-San Francisco, TUCOM-SF	66
Florida	
Nova-Southeastern University College of Osteopathic Medicine, NSU-COM	573
Illinois	
Chicago College of Osteopathic Medicine Midwestern University, CCOM	630
Iowa	
University of Osteopathic Medicine and Health Sciences College of Osteopathic Medicine and Surgery, UOMHS/COMS	798
Kentucky	
Pikeville College School of Osteopathic Medicine, PCSOM	60
Maine	
University of New England College of Osteopathic Medicine, UNECOM	401
Michigan	
Michigan State University College of Osteopathic Medicine, MSU-COM	512

After a slow beginning, Still soon reached his capacity for treating patients and felt the need to teach his philosophy to others. He opened the first successful school of osteopathy in 1892 with a class of 21 students and 2 faculty members: Still and one of his apprentices.[1] Class size doubled the next year, and by 1897 there were enough local graduates to found the American Association for the Advancement of Osteopathy. This association was formed to develop educational standards for the profession. In 1901 this association was reorganized and renamed the American Osteopathic Association (AOA); its charge included inspection and accreditation of training programs.[3,4] Word of his success in treatment and training rapidly grew, and by 1900 there were more than 700 students in more than a dozen schools.[1] Students were granted the degree Diplomat of Osteopathy (later to be called Doctor of Osteopathy) (D.O.). They were trained in medicine and surgery and integrated their understanding of osteopathy and manipulative medicine

BOX 19-1 Continued

COLLEGE OF OSTEOPATHIC MEDICINE	STUDENTS ENROLLED, NO. (1997–1998)
Missouri	
University of Health Sciences College of Osteopathic Medicine, UHS-COM	791
Kirksville College of Osteopathic Medicine, KCOM	578
New Jersey	
University of Medicine and Dentistry of New Jersey/School of Osteopathic Medicine, UMDNJ-SOM	304
New York	
New York College of Osteopathic Medicine, New York Institute of Technology, NYCOM	940
Ohio	
Ohio University College of Osteopathic Medicine, OUCOM	420
Oklahoma	
Oklahoma State University College of Osteopathic Medicine, OSU-COM	350
Pennsylvania	
Lake Erie College of Osteopathic Medicine, LECOM	417
Philadelphia College of Osteopathic Medicine, PCOM	982
Texas	
University of North Texas Health Science Center at Fort Worth/Texas College of Osteopathic Medicine, UNTHSCFW/TCOM	454
West Virginia	
West Virginia School of Osteopathic Medicine, WVSOM	261

Modified from Kowert.[5]

into the total care of the patient.[3] There were now 2 types of accepted physicians in the United States: D.O.s or osteopaths and M.D.s or allopaths. The philosophy and charter of the osteopathic schools described general practice with an emphasis on a holistic approach and patient and physician education.[1]

OSTEOPATHIC MEDICAL SCHOOLS

As of May 1998, there were 19 Osteopathic Medical Schools (also called Colleges of Osteopathic Medicine, or COMs) with a total enrollment of 9,434 students (Box 19-1). Of the 2,648 first-year students during 1997–1998,

58.3 percent came from within the state of their COM.[5] Of the 1998 graduating class, 37 percent were women.[6] It is estimated that in the year 2000, 2,492 physicians will graduate with the D.O. degree. COMs must be evaluated for accreditation every 7 years after initial approval. The AOA continues to perform these accreditation evaluations. Sixteen of the current schools are accredited, and 3 of the newer schools are awaiting approval.[5]

The curriculum for the D.O. degree spans 4 years. The first 2 years consist of didactic and laboratory study in the basic sciences, including anatomy, biochemistry, histology, microbiology, pharmacology, and physiology. Students are introduced to osteopathic manipulation and osteopathic principles in the practice of medicine. The last 2 years consist of clerkship rotations in all major fields of medicine, with an emphasis in the field of primary care.

> *"It is worth-while to secure the happiness of the patient as well as to prolong his life."*
>
> —William J. Mayo

INTERNSHIP AND RESIDENCY

Graduates of osteopathic medical schools are encouraged to complete a 1-year rotating osteopathic internship before beginning a residency program. This allows for training in the osteopathic philosophy to continue throughout internship. During the osteopathic internship, interns apply to residency programs. Approximately 50 percent of all osteopathic graduates enter the field of primary care. Others go for additional training in any of the specialty fields of medicine. There are 114 AOA-approved family medicine residency programs in the United States, with 1,391 positions available as of the 1997-1998 academic year.[7] The duration of the family medicine residency program is 2 years. Thus, a physician will study for 3 years in postgraduate training to complete the requirements for board certification in family practice.

CERTIFICATION IN FAMILY MEDICINE

After completion of an osteopathic residency in family practice, osteopathic physicians may apply for board certification. Requirements include, but are not limited to, the following: graduating from an AOA-accredited COM, holding an unrestricted license to practice medicine in the state where the physician's practice is located, being a member in good standing of the AOA, completing an AOA-approved internship or its equivalent, and successfully passing the certification examination.[4] Osteopathic family practice board certification is valid for 8 years. Board certification cannot be granted to osteopathic physicians not completing AOA-accredited internships or residencies except with special approval from the American Osteopathic Board of Family Physicians. Mechanisms are in place for approval of allopathic training when special circumstances exist and a petition is made to the board. In 1997–1998, 132 petitions for internship approval were received, 32 of which were denied.[8]

As a Board-Certified Family Physician, osteopathic physicians must maintain a minimum amount of Continuing Medical Education activity. Continuing Medical Education hours are classified in the traditional (1-A, 1-B, 2-A, 2-B) manner. The AOA and the Family Medicine Board require a minimum of 50 category 1-A or 1-B, AOA-approved hours, with a minimum total of 150 continuing medical education hours for each 3-year cycle. Individual states may have specific requirements for licensure.

Certificates of added qualifications are also available for Geriatrics, Adolescent and Young Adult Medicine, Addiction Medicine, Sports Medicine, and Occupational Medicine. These certificates are awarded to osteopathic family physicians after passing the certification examination and either completing a fellowship or satisfying specific practice requirements in their field.[8]

OSTEOPATHIC MEDICINE TODAY

Osteopathic Medicine has come a long way from Andrew Taylor Still's original concept. Osteopathic physicians are active in all medical specialties and play a significant role providing health care in the military services and for the general public. There are now more than 41,000 osteopathic physicians in the United States (Box 19-2). More than half of these physicians are in primary care: 18,000 in family medicine.[9] The profession is active in legislative and regulatory functions throughout the country. In regard to public policy, osteopathic physicians are viewed as separate but equal. The end of the 20th century has seen a rekindled interest in manual medicine and primary care, strengthening the osteopathic profession. This, coupled with the preventive health care philosophy inherent in osteopathic medicine, ensures a strong future for osteopathic medicine in family practice.

BOX 19-2 ORGANIZATIONS AND PERIODICALS IN OSTEOPATHIC MEDICINE

Organizations

American Osteopathic Association
142 East Ontario Street
Chicago, IL 60611
Telephone: (312)202-8000
http://www.am-osteo-assn.org/

American College of Osteopathic Family Physicians
330 East Algonquin Road
Arlington Heights, IL 30005
Telephone: (847)228-9755

Periodicals

The DO
Published monthly by the American Osteopathic Association

The Journal of the American Osteopathic Association
Published monthly by the American Osteopathic Association

REFERENCES

1. Ward RC, editor: Foundations for Osteopathic Medicine. Baltimore, Williams & Wilkins, 1997
2. Greenman PE: Principles of Manual Medicine. Baltimore, Williams & Wilkins, 1989
3. Ward WD, Retz KC: History of osteopathic medical education accreditation. J Am Osteopath Assoc 98:583-584, 1998
4. American Osteopathic Association: Yearbook and Directory of Osteopathic Physicians. Chicago, American Osteopathic Association, 1998
5. Kowert C: Undergraduate osteopathic medical education. J Am Osteopath Assoc 98:589-594, 1998
6. Wallis ML: Snapshot of the profession. The DO 39:46, 1998

7. Swallow CS, Bronersky VM, Falbo PW: Osteopathic graduate medical education. J Am Osteopath Assoc 98:599-606, 1998
8. Glatz L, Dolan S: Certification of osteopathic physicians. J Am Osteopath Assoc 98:609-613, 1998
9. American Osteopathic Association: Facts About Osteopathic Physicians. American Osteopathic Association, Chicago, 1998

20

DIVERSITY IN FAMILY MEDICINE

Rhonda M. Medows, M.D.

Diversity is an issue that affects all industries including medicine and especially family medicine. Establishing some degree of knowledge of the current situation and predicted future trends as well as developing cultural competency is imperative for those who want to prosper and grow as competent professionals. In the practice of family medicine, it may seem easy to assume that the patient, physician, and staff all speak some kind of universal language—the language of medicine, with its focus on a disease state or medical problem. We may assume that all involved know and comprehend this universal language. But this is far from reality. Not everyone understands our complex medical language or interprets it in the same manner. Diversity allows us to share values and beliefs.

Remember that,

Before Anna Henderson became a patient. . .

Before David Noggin became an attending physician. . .

Before Katherine Johnson became a junior resident. . .

Before John Keeler became a nurse working the 11–3 shift. . .

each of these people is a separate individual with unique life experiences, coming from various backgrounds and cultures. Each participant brings into the patient-physician encounters individual and sometimes different expectations (Fig. 20-1).

As a family physician, part of the challenge of developing and delivering quality health care is to recognize the increasing diversity among our colleagues, staff, and patient populations and to respect these differences and

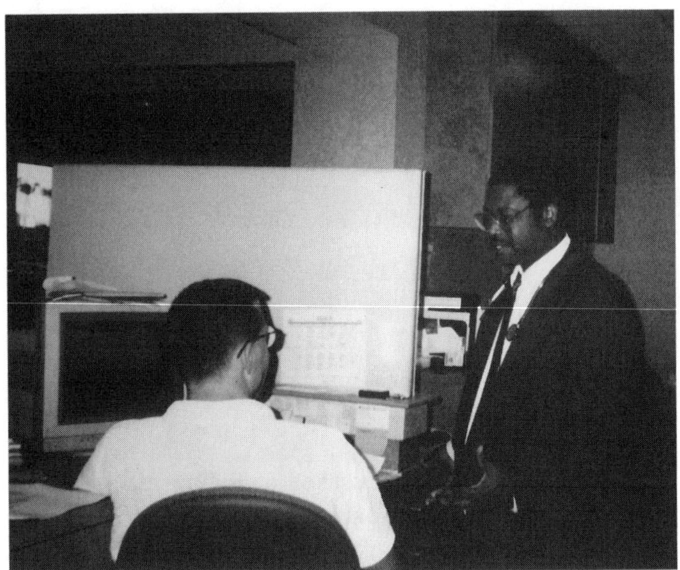

FIGURE 20-1
Racial and ethnic diversity can help make a successful practice by attracting people from many varied backgrounds.

integrate this information into our plans to achieve the best outcomes for our patients.

The following is the who, why, what, and where associated with diversity in family practice.

WHO MAKES UP A CULTURAL GROUP?

Culture is defined in the broadest definition as a group of people with a common set of beliefs, customs, and institutions and a shared set of socially accepted norms.

The more easily recognized cultural groups can be identified by race or ethnic group (eg, Hispanic and non-Hispanic). Subgroupings or microcultural groupings may include sex, linguistic background, age, and perhaps sexual orientation. It is obviously not reasonable or possible to expect to know everything about every cultural group you encounter as a physician. What is important is being aware that cultural differences exist and to be aware of changes occurring within your own evolving community.

> *''The wit of science not only expresses but actually reveals the science and art of medicine.''*
>
> —William J. Mayo

Statistics regarding the population composition of the United States with respect to the general public and specifically the physician population are readily available. The following figures are summaries of this information. In addition to information regarding racial, ethnic, and sexual demographics, consider 2 additional facts: the impact of linguistic barriers—as reported by the 1990 census, 32 million US citizens (ie, 14 percent of the population) spoke a language other than English at home. This percentage varied from state to state. States higher than the national average included New Mexico (36 percent) and California (31 percent). New York, New Jersey, Texas, and Arizona each had 20 percent (Source: *Diversity Rx*).[1] In the 1980s almost 10 million people immigrated to the United States, 80 percent of whom came from areas other than Europe. According to the US Bureau of the Census,[2] our population in 1998 changes with:

1 birth every .... 8 seconds

1 death every .... 8 seconds

1 net immigrant every .... 36 seconds

Who ''we'' are and will be, as predicted by the US Bureau of the Census, is illustrated in Tables 20-1 and 20-2. In the years to come, all races will increase in the United States except for whites. In view of this, it is obvious our society is becoming more racially diverse. Women, in the years to come, will increase in numbers and remain the majority in population statistics.

TABLE 20-1

SUMMARY OF PREDICTED POPULATION TRENDS (NUMBERS IN THOUSANDS) IN THE UNITED STATES: 1990–2005

DATE	ALL RACES	WHITE	BLACK	NATIVE AMERICAN, ESKIMO, ALEUT	ASIAN, PACIFIC ISLANDER	HISPANIC
7/1/1990	249,440 (100%)	209,185 (83.9%)	30,623 (12.3%)	2,074 (0.8%)	7,558 (3.0%)	22,575 (9.1%)
1/1/1998	268,922	222,207	34,172	2,340	10,203	29,882 (11.1%)
7/1/2000	274,633	225,532	35,454	2,402	11,245	31,366 (11.4%)
7/1/2005	285,981 (100%)	232,463 (81.3%)	37,734 (13.2%)	2,572 (0.9%)	13,212 (4.6%)	36,057 (12.6%)

From United States Bureau of the Census.[2]

TABLE 20-2
US RESIDENT POPULATION (ALL RACES AND ETHNIC GROUPS)

	CENSUS PREDICTIONS (NUMBERS IN THOUSANDS)	
DATE	**FEMALES**	**MALES**
7/1/1990	127,815	121,624
1/1/1998	137,236	131,686
7/1/2000	140,453	134,181
7/1/2005	146,196	139,785

From United States Bureau of the Census.[2]

WHY CONCERN OURSELVES WITH DIVERSITY ISSUES?

Because family physicians are a diverse group treating a diverse population, the delivery of quality health care is impacted by cultural differences brought into the clinical setting, especially in family practice (Fig. 20-2). Failure to recognize this potentiates the consequences of misunderstanding and miscommunication. More specifically, culture-based beliefs and expectations can affect each of our working relationships (physician to patient, physician to physician, and physician to staff). Culture influences the patient's interpretation and presentation of symptoms. It influences the interpretation of this presentation by the health care professional. It influences the patient's willingness to accept the medical advice given and therefore compliance with treatment plans.

Limitations in understanding owing to language barriers and poor familiarity with acceptable behavior within cultural norms add an additional level of complexity to medical care. Consider the limitations that can occur when there is a language barrier. At times physicians can be dependent on family members, sometimes children, to interpret for non-English-speaking patients instead of trained staff. The reliability of information exchanged and confidentiality of it are often diminished. With this in mind, it is evident that actively enhancing our knowledge base regarding ethnic differences and becoming cross-culturally competent improves the accuracy and efficiency in exchanging information with our patients; enhances the physician-patient and physician-staff relationships; encourages more accurate diagnosis and treatment plans; encourages patient compliance; improves our working environment and staff relationships; encourages networking and the flow of information among consultants dealing with common issues; stops the com-

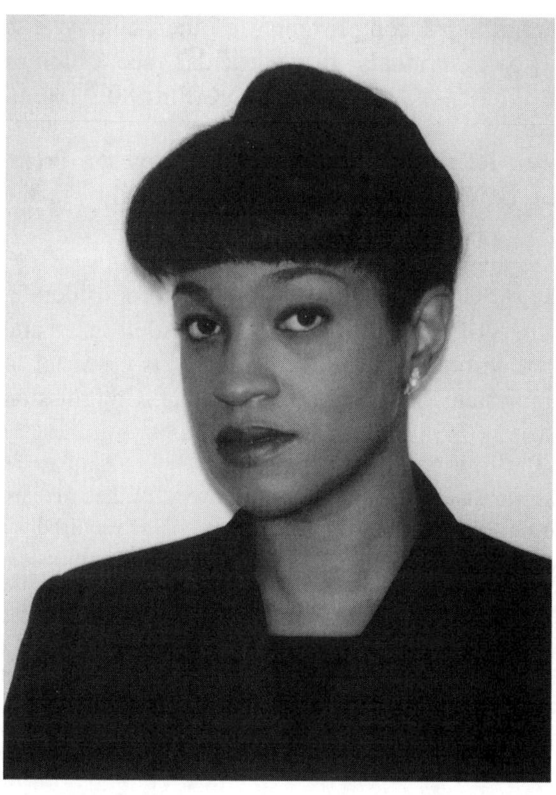

FIGURE 20-2 Sexual, racial, and ethnic barriers should not exist in the practice of medicine.

mon human responses to the familiar symptoms of anxiety, fear, and frustration; and clarifies preconceived ideas and stereotyping.

Legislation Concerning Diversity

Diversity in the workplace has legal ramifications. The following are important legislative enactments that involve diversity issues, especially the legislation regarding diversity and civil rights issues.

Title VI of the Civil Rights Act of 1964 Summary Statement: ''No person in the United States shall, on grounds of race, color, or national origin, be excluded from participation in, be denied the benefits of, or be subjected to discrimination under any program or activity receiving Federal financial assistance.'' [42 U.S.C. 2000d eq seq.][3]

(All recipients of federal funds) ''may not . . . utilize criteria or methods of administration which have the effect of subjecting individuals to discrimination because of their race, color or national origin, or have the effect of defeating or substantially impairing accomplishment of the objectives of the program [with] respect [to] individuals of a particular race, color or national origin.'' [42 C.F.R. 80.3(b)(2)][3]

Consumer Bill of Rights and Responsibilities (Proposed by the President's Advisory Commission on Consumer Protection and Quality in the Health Care Industry)

RESPECT AND NONDISCRIMINATION Consumers have the right to considerate, respectful care from all members of the health care industry at all times and under all circumstances. An environment of mutual respect is essential to maintain a quality health care system. To ensure that right, the Commission recommends the following.

> Consumers must not be discriminated against in the delivery of health care services consistent with the benefits covered in their policy, or as required by law, based on race, ethnicity, national origin, religion, sex, age, mental or physical disability, sexual orientation, genetic information, or source of payment.
>
> Consumers eligible for coverage under the terms and conditions of a health plan or program, or as required by law, must not be discriminated against in marketing and enrollment practices based on race, ethnicity, national origin, religion, sex, age, mental or physical disability, sexual orientation, genetic information, or source of payment. (Summary Statement from the Commission Fact Sheet.)[4]

The Hill-Burton Act Summary Statement: This act requires that all facilities receiving federal funds ensure services are ''available to persons residing in the facility's service area without discrimination on the basis of race, color, national origin, creed or any other ground unrelated to the individual's need for the service or the availability of the needed service in the facility.'' [42 C.F.R. 124.603(a)][5]

The Patient Protection Act of 1997 Title III: Health Plan Standards

> *§ 304 Describes the requirement that health care plans make ''reasonable efforts to address issues of cultural competence and appropriateness with respect to providers.''*[3]

These are a few of the important legislative acts that deal with discrimination related to health care. In addition, there have been efforts to address racial equality in medical schools and residency programs.

A federal study was performed from 1993 to 1994 regarding diversity in medicine entitled ''Balancing the Scales of Opportunity: Ensuring Racial and Ethnic Diversity in the Health Professions.'' It was performed by the National Academy of Sciences, Institute of Medicine, Washington, DC, and was sponsored by the Public Health Service, National Institute of Mental Health, and National Institutes of Health. The following is the summary of the study abstract.

''Although many [residency] programs over the past twenty years have tried to rectify the imbalance, minorities are still underrepresented in the health professions. In 1992, only 10.3 percent of medical school enrollees were minority students, even though the minority share of the population is 22 percent. Figures for minority faculty members are even lower.''[6] This report examined the problem of minority underrepresentation in the health professions and proposed a strategy to rectify the situation. The report found that 1) the entire educational continuum must seek to increase the number of minorities prepared for and taking part in the health professions through mentoring, an appreciation for cultural diversity, intervention programs, and educational reform; 2) a national effort is needed to track progress; 3) federal support is needed for programs which use early interventions to get minorities interested in the health professions, public and private scholarships, and faculty development and curricular revision at the university level; and 4) health care reform should recognize and promote opportunities for greater minority participation in the health professions. The report recommended that 1) the federal government, foundations, and the private sector support activities that promote minority representation and 2) a national clearinghouse and information network be developed to track these activities.[6]

The federal government is increasing legislation regarding civil rights protection and diversity. The government is concerned about discrimination and wants to support diversity not only in business but also in medicine (Box 20-1).

WHAT IS THE STATUS OF CULTURAL DIVERSITY?

The status and statistics regarding the cultural composition of the physician and medical student populations are available through agencies such as the Association of American Medical Colleges (AAMC), the U.S. Bureau of the Census, and, for specialty specific information, the American Academy of Family Practice.[7–9]

After a period of initial growth in the number of minorities in medicine from the late 1960s to the 1970s, the rate of growth slowed. This extended from approximately 1975 to 1990. From 1991 to 1995, the AAMC reports there was a 27 percent increase in the number of matriculating students

BOX 20-1 HEALTH CARE LEGISLATION

The following is a listing of 50 bills from the 105th Congress in 1997 regarding health care issues. Those with * involve human rights issues.

1. Antitrust Health Care Advancement Act of 1997 (Introduced in the House) [H.R.415.I]
2. Federal Prisoner Health Care Copayment Act (Introduced in the Senate) [S.494.IS]
3. Health Care Liability Reform Act of 1997 (Introduced in the House) [H.R.1091.I]
4. Health Fraud and Abuse Act of 1997 (Introduced in the House) [H.R.362.I]
5. Medicare Patient Choice and Access Act of 1997 (Introduced in the Senate) [S.701.IS]
6. Rural Telemedicine Demonstration Act of 1997 (Introduced in the Senate) [S.848.IS]
7. Rural Preventive Health Care Training Act of 1997 (Introduced in the Senate) [S.128.IS]
8. Federal Health Care Quality, Consumer Information and Protection Act (Introduced in the Senate) [S.795.IS]
9. Patient Right to Know Act (Introduced in the Senate) [S.449.IS]
10. Comprehensive Preventive Health and Promotion Act of 1997 (Introduced in the House) [H.R.177.I]

*11. Patient Abuse Prevention Act (Introduced in the Senate) [S.1122.IS]

12. Health Care Liability Reform and Quality Assurance Act of 1997 (Introduced in the Senate) [S.886.IS]
13. Comprehensive Telehealth Act of 1997 (Introduced in the Senate) [S.385.IS]
14. Improved Access for Telehealth Act of 1997 (Introduced in the House) [H.R.966.I]
15. Comprehensive Managed Health Care Reform Act of 1997 (Introduced in the House) [H.R.5078.I]

*16. Quality Health Care and Consumer Protection Act (Introduced in the House) [H.R.1222.I]

17. To require the Secretary of Health and Human Services to submit a report to the Congress regarding the national health care systems of certain industrialized countries (Introduced in the House) [H.R.5078.I]
18. Patient and Health Care Provider Protection Act of 1997 (Introduced in the House) [H.R.1191.I]
19. Patient Right to Know Act (Introduced in the House) [H.R.586.I]
20. To provide a Federal response to fraud in connection with the provision of or receipt of payment for health care services, and for other purposes (Introduced in the House) [H.R.2584.I]
21. Uniformed Services Retiree and Dependents Health Care Availability Act (Introduced in the House) [H.R.1456.I]
22. To amend section 552a of title V, United States Code, to provide for the maintenance of certain health information in cases where a health care facility has closed or a health benefit . . . (Introduced in the House) [H.R.2105.I]
23. Medicare Subvention Fairness Act (Introduced in the House) [H.R.1357.I]
24. To amend title 38, United States Code, to require that health care professionals of the Department of Veterans Affairs be assigned to facilities of the Department only in States in . . . (Introduced in the House) [H.R.2338.I]
25. Josephine Butler United States Health Service Act (Introduced in the House) [H.R.1374.I]
26. To amend title X, United States Code, to permit beneficiaries of the military health care system to enroll in federal employees health benefits plans; to improve health care

BOX 20-1 Continued

benefits . . . (Introduced in the House) [H.R.1356.I]

27. Primary Health Care Education Act of 1997 (Introduced in the House) [H.R.739.I]
28. Medicare Patient Choice and Access Act of 1997 (Introduced in the House) [H.R.66.I]
*29. Patient Protection Act of 1997 (Introduced in the Senate) [S.346.IS]
30. Uniformed Services Medicare Subvention Program Act (Introduced in the House) [H.R.414.IH]
31. Health Care Commitment Act (Introduced in the House) [H.R.76.IH]
32. To amend section 541 of the National Housing Act with respect to the partial payment of claims on health care facilities (Introduced in the Senate) [S.334.IS]
33. Uniformed Services Medicare Subvention Demonstration Project Act (Introduced in the House) [H.R.192.IH]
*34. Access to Medical Treatment Act (Introduced in the Senate) [S.578.IS]
35. To amend title X, United States Code, to permit covered beneficiaries under the military health care system who are also entitled to Medicare to enroll in the Federal Employees Health . . . (Introduced in the Senate) [S.224.IS]
36. Equity in Prescription Insurance and Contraceptive Coverage Act of 1997 (Introduced in the Senate) [S.743.IS]
37. Equity in Prescription Insurance and Contraceptive Coverage Act of 1997 (Introduced in the Senate) [S.766.IS]
38. Equity in Prescription Insurance and Contraceptive Coverage Act of 1997 (Introduced in the House) [H.R.2174.IH]
39. Alaskan Community Health Aide Program Expansion Act of 1997 (Introduced in the Senate) [S.1402.IS]
40. To prohibit discrimination by the States on the basis of nonresidency in the licensing of dental health care professionals, and for other purposes (Introduced in the House) [H.R.541.IH]
41. Expressing the sense of the Congress with respect to the establishment of waivers in State medical-licensing laws regarding the provision of health care to indigent individuals (Introduced in the House) [H.CON.RES.69.IH]
42. Family Planning and Choice Protection Act of 1997 (Introduced in the Senate) [S.1208.IS]
43. Family Planning and Choice Protection Act of 1997 (Introduced in the House) [H.R.2525.IH]
44. Health Care Worker Protection Act of 1997 (Introduced in the House) [H.R.2754.IH]
*45. Managed Care Bill of Rights for Consumers Act of 1997 (Introduced in the House) [H.R.2606.IH]
46. Advance Planning and Compassionate Care Act of 1997 (Introduced in the Senate) [S.1345.IS]
*47. Access to Medical Treatment Act (Introduced in the House) [H.R.746.IH]
48. Advance Planning and Compassionate Care Act of 1997 (Introduced in the House) [H.R.2999.IH]
49. Federal Employees Health Care Protection Act of 1997 (Introduced in the House) [H.R.1836.IH]
50. To amend title X, United States Code, to establish a demonstration project to evaluate the feasibility of using the Federal Employees Health Benefits Program to ensure the availability . . . (Introduced in the Senate) [S.1334.IS]

representing 4 minority groups: blacks, Native Americans, Mexican Americans, and mainland Puerto Ricans. Unfortunately, this trend did not continue. From 1995 to 1996, there was no increase in the number of matriculating minority students, raising concern that the rapid growth of the minority population in general was not being matched within the medical community.

In view of these trends, some interventions have been undertaken within the medical community to increase the proportion of underrepresented ethnic and racial minority groups in the medical profession. The AAMC created the Division of Minority Health, Education, and Prevention in 1988. This division was later renamed the Division of Community and Minority Programs in 1995. Through this program, the AAMC initiated PROJECT 3000 by 2000 in 1991, with the stated goal of increasing the number of underrepresented minority students entering medical school. The predicted minority portion of the U.S. population by the year 2000 is 19 percent based on trends predicted from the 1990 census. The intent was to match this percentage within the medical profession population (ie, 19 percent of all medical school students = 3000 students). This model for proactive change proposed and developed educational partnerships between public school systems, colleges, and medical schools that would target minority students interested in medicine. A nationwide network of educational partners, which now has more than 3000 members, was created called NESPA—National Network for Health Science Partnerships. As of the AAMC 1996 report, 66 of the nation's 125 medical schools have implemented this plan. Additional information about this program and its publications are described in the AAMC *Project 3000 by 2000: Year Three Progress Report* published by the AAMC in April 1996.[8] Despite concern for racial and ethnic equality, the representation of minorities has remained about the same for the last 10 years. Tables 20-3 and 20-4 describe important statistics for medical students based on racial and ethnic composition.

WHERE CAN YOU LOCATE REFERENCES FOR DIVERSITY ISSUES IN MEDICINE?

As a resident in training or physician in practice the following references provide important resources describing ethnic and cultural diversity related to medicine and the practice of Family Medicine:

Spector RE: Cultural Diversity in Health & Illness. Fourth edition. Stamford, CT, Appleton & Lange, 1996[10]

TABLE 20-3
NATIONAL MEDICAL SCHOOL APPLICANT POOL STATISTICS: 1991–1997

	APPLICANTS, NO. (%)		
RACE	**1991**	**1994**	**1997**
White	22,086 (59.0)	29,188 (62.6)	26,295 (61.1)
Black	2,659 (7.1)	3,659 (7.9)	3,133 (7.3)
Native American	161 (0.4)	261 (0.6)	311 (0.7)
Asian and Pacific islander	5,487 (14.7)	8,804 (18.9)	8,641 (20.1)
Hispanic	1,926 (5.1)	2,538 (5.4)	2,368 (5.5)
Total applicants*	37,410	46,591	43,020

* Includes 982, 915, and 452 in Unknown category for 1991, 1994, and 1997, respectively.
Data from Jolly and Hudley.[7]

Spector RE: Cultural Diversity in Health & Illness: Guide to Heritage Assessment and Health Traditions. Fourth edition. Stamford, CT, Appleton & Lange, 1996 (sold as a package—a book and free guide)[11]

Gropper RC: Culture and the Clinical Encounter: an Intercultural Sensitizer for the Health Professions. Yarmouth, ME, Intercultural Press, 1996[12]

Juliá MC, editor: Multicultural Awareness in the Health Care Professions. Boston, Allyn and Bacon, 1996[13]

Purnell LD, Paulanka BJ, editors: Transcultural Health Care: a Culturally Competent Approach. Philadelphia, FA Davis Company, 1998[14]

TABLE 20-4
ENROLLMENT STATISTICS FOR FIRST YEAR MEDICAL STUDENTS: 1991–1992

RACE OR ETHNICITY	**ENROLLED, NO.**	**% OF STUDENTS, 1991–1992**	**% OF STUDENTS, 1981–1982**
White	11,677	68.4	82.3
Black	1,304	7.6	6.9
Native American	93	0.5	0.4
Asian or Pacific islander	2,744	16.1	4.4
Hispanic	1,006	5.9	5.2

Data from Jolly and Hudley.[7]

BOX 20-2 REFLECTIONS ON RESIDENCY TRAINING

The following speech was given in 1998 by Kim M. Barbel-Johnson, D.O., a third-year Mayo Clinic family practice resident (Fig. 20-3) at a gathering of Mayo Clinic patrons called the ''Mayo Legacy Group.''

Legacy Speech

The late Georgia O'Keeffe once said: ''Where I was born and where and how I have lived is unimportant. It is what I have done with where I have been that should be of interest (1976).''

I have always embraced these words, for they seem to have leveled the playing field yet perpetuate and promote a principle for productivity.

You see, I have never had to look for motivation, inspiration, explanation, or substantiation of my career choice—family medicine. I grew up on a Caribbean island where I learned about poor health care and the consequences of the lack of quality care. While thousands of tourists were attracted to this vacation paradise, I saw another picture that was colored by shades of economic and political despair.

I acquired a more global understanding of health care as I pursued my college and graduate career in the continental United States. I began to appreciate that many health care problems encompass broad-based societal issues. Motivated by a desire to advocate for those who were unable to advocate for themselves, I earned a master's degree in Public Health Administration. I soon realized that life as an advocate is often isolated from the people and

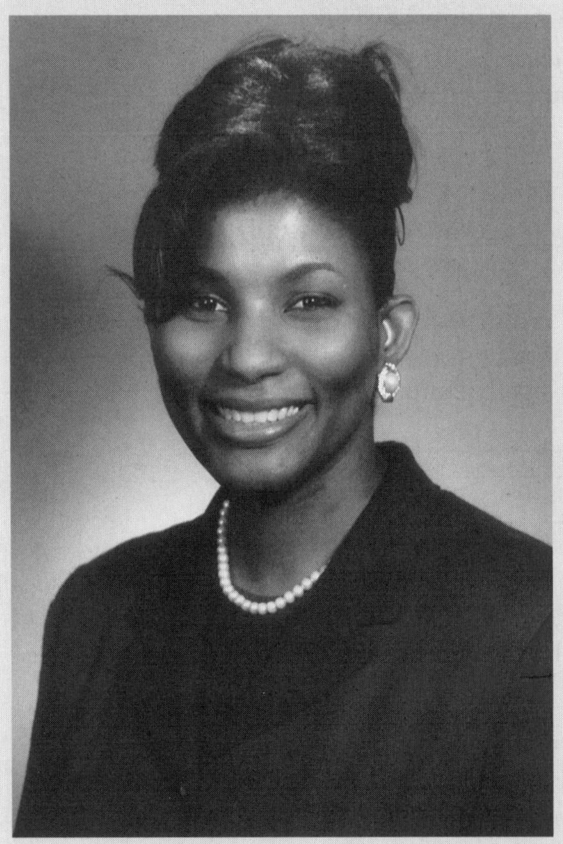

FIGURE 20-3
Kim M. Barbel-Johnson, D.O.

BOX 20-2 Continued

place one hopes to assist. As the richness of clinical medicine continued to intrigue me, I armed myself with my insatiable desire to improve the health status of the global community and attended medical school to fashion a career centered on patient care.

Later, I was successful in earning the opportunity to complete my Family Medicine Residency Program training at the Mayo Clinic Jacksonville. As a resident, my training is dominated by my desire to promote positive changes in health care and fueled by my passion to infuse competence, compassion, and commitment into the social context of health.

While developing excellent clinical skills and judgment, I am gaining exposure to ambulatory and preventive care and training at an institution where leadership in medicine means outstanding medical care and commitment to improving the quality of life of its patients.

The Mayo Clinic residency experience uniquely equips young physicians to realize our full potential as physicians. However, our experience is so much more.

Please indulge me as I return to a day in my life in 1996, during my internship year at Mayo, when I wrote in my journal:

> October 10, 1996, pre-call on a Tuesday
>
> What an incredible year this has been. Even a reflection on the last 4 months is incredible. Managing patients, delivering more than 30 babies, participating in life-reviving codes, 36 hours of sleep deprivation . . . and clinic patients who call **me** their physician. What an experience! As exasperated as I am sometimes, I am loving what I am doing . . . but then, maybe Grandma was right—that the best work in life is work worth doing.
>
> I continue writing in February 1997:
>
> I am at the Wolfson's Children's Hospital on my pediatric specialty rotations—Pediatric Hematology, Oncology, Cardiology, Endocrinology, Neurology, and Gastroenterology. I remember my anxiety as I began this month. I knew it would be overwhelming. I thought I might be underprepared, but I am surviving yet another residency challenge. I've learned so much from my patients this month. So much about their diseases: AML, ALL, SLE, VSD, IDDM, malignant melanoma, Crohn's, lupus, Cushing—but I've learned so much about life and living. I've seen honest fear and honorable bravery in children too young to pronounce my name. From the tiniest hearts with ventricular septal defects to the biggest souls with unmistakable courage, my patients—my babies—have been such a blessing to me. My prayer is that I can do all things within my power to translate the Mayo majesty into their personal miracle.

You see, the Mayo residency experience is about more than disease management and clinical acumen. It is about people—the patients and families we serve and the physicians (the staff consultants) who equip us to do this and to do it well.

We, the Mayo residents, are nurtured and fortified by staff attendings who are committed to our academic development. Their guiding principle is pride in personal commitment and performance that separates excellence from mediocrity. As residents, we embrace their vision—Mayo's vision to uphold the promise to dutifully demonstrate and develop the values of discipline, respect, and responsibility: *discipline* in an approach to the correct diagnosis, *respect* for the patient and the disease, and *responsibility* to the legacy that has made this institution great!

The Mayo residency experience is one in which diligence overcomes difficulties. It is no wonder that like staff consultants, Mayo residents and fellows are drawn to this institution from all parts of the world and bring with us our experiences with people and our diverse educations.

Once here, we are joined together by one common goal—*To advance Mayo's commitment to clinical innovation, medical research, and education.*

Once here, we too are guided by one principle, the principle of Dr. William Mayo, "The best interest of the patient is the only interest to be considered. . . ."

Quershi B: Transcultural Medicine: Dealing With Patients From Different Cultures. Second edition. Boston, Kluwer Academic Publishers, 1994[15]

Kavanagh KH, Kennedy PH: Promoting Cultural Diversity: Strategies for Health Care Professionals. Newbury Park, CA, Sage Publications, 1992[16]

Galanti G-A: Caring for Patients From Different Cultures: Case Studies From American Hospitals. Second edition.

Philadelphia, University of Pennsylvania Press, 1997[17]

Internet listings for additional diversity information include:

American Academy of Family Physicians	www.aafp.org/
Association of American Medical Colleges	www.aamc.org/
United States Bureau of Census	www.census.gov/
Health Care Financing Administration	www.hcfa.gov/
Agency for Health Care Policy and Research	www.ahcpr.gov/
Department of Health and Human Services	www.dhhs.gov/
President's Advisory Commission on Consumer Protection and Quality in Health Care	www.hcqualitycommission.gov/
Diversity Rx	www.diversityRx.org/
National Conference of State Legislatures	www.ncsl.org/

Although this is not a complete list of all resources, these references will give the family physician insight to diversity issues that affect the practice of medicine.

CONCLUSION

Cultural and ethnic diversity are important issues in all of our lives. As family physicians we will be faced increasingly with interactions involving people from all walks of life. Our colleagues and staff may represent minorities, and as medical professionals we must respect individual differences. Through understanding and knowledge we may achieve greater wisdom and in turn better serve our patients as well as the practice of family medicine (Box 20-2).

REFERENCES

1. Fortier JP, editor: Diversity Rx, who we are. Revised July 25, 1997. Available from the World Wide Web: http://www.diversityRx.org
2. United States Bureau of the Census—Population Division: Current Population Reports, Series P25–1130. Population Projections for the United States by Age, Sex, Race, and Hispanic Origin: 1995-2050. Washington, DC, Government Printing Office, 1997
3. United States Code (current Public Laws Enacted by Congress) 1997. Pittsburgh, Government Printing Office, 1997
4. (Fact sheet) President's Advisory Commission on Consumer Protection and Quality in the Health Care Industry. Retrieved November 20, 1997 from the World Wide Web: http://www.hcqualitycommission.gov
5. Code of Federal Regulations. Office of the Federal Register. Government Printing Office, Washington, DC, 1997
6. Lewin ME, Rice B, editors: Balancing the Scales of Opportunity: Ensuring Racial and Ethnic Diversity in the Health Professions. Washington, DC, National Academy Press, 1994
7. Jolly P, Hudley DM, editors: AAMC Data Book: Statistical Information Related to Medical Education. Washington, DC, Association of American Medical Colleges, 1998
8. Association of American Medical Colleges. Division of Minority Health Education and Prevention: Progress to Date: Project 3000 by 2000: Year Three Progress Report. Washington, DC, Association of American Medical Colleges, 1996
9. American Academy of Family Physicians: Facts About Family Practice. Kansas City, MO, American Academy of Family Physicians, 1995, pp 222–223; 224–225
10. Spector RE: Cultural Diversity in Health & Illness. Fourth edition. Stamford, CT, Appleton & Lange, 1996
11. Spector RE: Cultural Diversity in Health & Illness: Guide to Heritage Assessment and Health Traditions. Fourth edition. Stamford, CT, Appleton & Lange, 1996 (sold as a package—a book and free guide)
12. Gropper RC: Culture and the Clinical Encounter: an Intercultural Sensitizer for the Health Professions. Yarmouth, ME, Intercultural Press, 1996
13. Juliá MC, editor: Multicultural Awareness in the Health Care Professions. Boston, Allyn and Bacon, 1996

14. Purnell LD, Paulanka BJ, editors: Transcultural Health Care: a Culturally Competent Approach. Philadelphia, FA Davis Company, 1998
15. Quershi B: Transcultural Medicine: Dealing With Patients From Different Cultures. Second edition. Boston, Kluwer Academic Publishers, 1994
16. Kavanagh KH, Kennedy PH: Promoting Cultural Diversity: Strategies for Health Care Professionals. Newbury Park, CA, Sage Publications, 1992
17. Galanti G-A: Caring for Patients From Different Cultures: Case Studies From American Hospitals. Second edition. Philadelphia, University of Pennsylvania Press, 1997

SUGGESTED READING

Essed P: Diversity: Gender, Color, and Culture. (Translated by R Gircour.) Amherst, MA, University of Massachusetts Press, 1996

Gardenswartz L, Rowe A: The Managing Diversity Survival Guide: a Complete Collection of Checklists, Activities, and Tips. Burr Ridge, IL, Irwin Professional Publishing, 1994

Carr-Ruffino N: Managing Diversity: People Skills for a Multicultural Workplace. Cincinnati, OH, Thomson Executive Press, 1996

21 PLANNING FOR THE FUTURE AND SELECTING THE RIGHT JOB

Frederick D. Edwards, M.D.

The task of selecting a site for practice after residency training is important and, at times, intimidating. Unfortunately, many residency programs do not teach the basics involved in such a difficult process. In most cases, the resident physicians are left to find their way through the multiple interviews and practice opportunities until they select their first practice site. The purpose of this chapter is to add some insight and organization to this often chaotic process.

WHAT ARE YOU LOOKING FOR?

Completing residency training and beginning the search for your first practice is one of the most exciting times of your medical career. For those in family practice the options are almost limitless. For the first time, you are not limited by the location of major academic medical centers or residency training programs. Primary care opportunities are not constrained by location, population density, or demographics. Although this wide range of possibilities means that your perfect practice setting is almost certainly out there somewhere, it can make finding it a daunting task.

DEFINING YOUR VALUES AND GOALS

The most important first step in finding the perfect practice setting is deciding what you want. In doing so, you must first define your values and goals. Finding a job requires a specific definition of who you are and what is important to you. Introspection is key. *Random House Webster's College Dictionary* defines *values* as "the abstract concepts of what is right, worthwhile, or desirable; principles or standards," whereas a *goal* is the "the result or achievement toward which effort is directed; aim; end."[1] Any practice setting that does not fulfill your individual goals and reflect your values will surely not become a long-term commitment. Even if your purpose after completing residency training is in attaining short-term goals (fulfillment of a Public Health Service commitment, travel, or maximization of income to pay off loans), the eventual desire for a career and the need for stability make the defining of values and goals necessary.

Often the struggles of getting through medical school or a rigorous residency program can cause you to lose touch with your core values. Whereas the definition of values can be difficult for some, others may have maintained a set of values that are honed by years of religious or philosophical commitment. Beginning a job search is a good time to write down the values that guide your life so they can be taken into account during the process.

Once your values have been outlined, it is time to become more concrete in defining the specific goals for your future practice situation. Career choices for a well-trained family physician are almost unlimited. It is up to you and the other significant people in your life (spouse or partner, children, parents, and friends) to decide whether you become a cruise ship physician or work in an urgent care center, open a solo practice or work for a health maintenance organization (HMO), live in rural Kentucky or lower Manhattan, and work full time or part time. Defining your goals will go a long way in identifying the sort of practice situation that is right for you. Things to consider are your desired scope of practice (obstetrics, intensive care, a focus on pediatrics, or geriatrics), practice location (rural, urban, near family or far away), procedures (flexible sigmoidoscopies, vasectomies, cesarean sections, endoscopies), and opportunities for research or teaching. Although some of these decisions will be made by you individually, others are best made together with the significant people in your life.

HOW TO FIND WHAT YOU WANT

When to Start Looking

There are no rules regarding when to start looking for a practice opportunity. Some will have completed their job search before or during medical school, because they plan to return to a hometown or the practice of a mentor, friend, or relative. For most, however, the search for the first job is something that takes place during the final year of postgraduate medical education. In general, it is best to begin the search as soon as possible. It can take several months to obtain credentials such as a state medical license, hospital privileges, insurance billing numbers, and managed care plan provider numbers. Late summer or early fall of the final year is probably the best time to begin the search. Even though some programs allow extra time away for interviews, it may be best to reserve several vacation days in the final year of training to be used for job interview trips. If possible, it can be helpful to arrange an elective educational experience at the practice setting that seems most promising.

Where to Look

There are several ways to locate potential practice opportunities. The resource that might be most helpful depends on the factors that are most important in directing the search. For instance, if geographic area or locale is the most important factor, contacting the state or county medical societies in the desired area might be best. If a career in academic medicine is sought, the Society of Teachers of Family Medicine might be the best resource. In general, the following resources can be helpful.

Journal Ads Nearly every medical journal features several pages of classified advertisements. These can be primarily directed to all specialties and a national audience (as in the *New England Journal of Medicine* or the *Journal of the American Medical Association*), all specialties and a more regional audience (as in the *Western Journal of Medicine*), or specialty specific (as in the *American Family Physician* or the *Journal of Family Practice*).

Medical Societies If you have decided to limit your search to a specific state or county, the medical society for that area is often an excellent resource. State and county medical societies, as well as a state's chapter of the American Academy of Family Practice, often have their own physician placement services or maintain a list of practice opportunities available in their areas. Addresses and telephone numbers for these resources usually can be found in the local telephone directory.

Specific Employers Or Local Resources If you are able to narrow your search to a specific community or metropolitan area, it is often helpful to contact specific employers in that area. This might include hospitals, managed care plans, or physician groups. Hospitals often have fairly complete information about opportunities in their service areas or may be recruiting primary care physicians for their own physician networks.

Government Agencies These resources are most often dedicated to placing physicians in underserved areas. Many state governments maintain physician recruiting offices or use an Office of Rural Health to recruit physicians.

The Internet The electronic superhighway is rapidly becoming an excellent resource for finding employment opportunities. Most residency programs now have computers available with Internet access that allow you to browse the Web without the need for your own computer. Many large medical employers and recruitment firms have their own Web sites where employment opportunities are listed.

Recruitment Firms In the past several years, many firms have emerged that specialize in finding suitable applicants for particular positions. This phenomenon is not unique to medicine; companies in a wide array of industries use recruitment firms or headhunters to identify suitable applicants. A good recruiter can be helpful in locating a position that suits your specific needs and will work with you to screen out opportunities that are not appropriate. It can be helpful to remember, however, that recruiters usually charge large fees (often tens of thousands of dollars for each successful physician recruitment), and these fees are paid by the employer. The situation is somewhat analogous to that of a real estate agent. The agent will make every effort to satisfy the needs of the homebuyer, but the commission is paid by the seller only after the deal is closed. Recruitment firms are sometimes asked to fill positions that are difficult to fill through other means, but some employers find it more economical to hire a recruitment firm when needed rather than maintaining an in-house physician recruitment department. Professional physician recruiters can often perform much of the legwork of finding the best job for you. They should be treated with honesty and respect for their efforts but always remember they are in the job of selling a practice opportunity—whether good or bad.

Networking Finding the best practice setting is often not so much what you know, but *who* you know. Some of the best positions will be filled by word of mouth before there is ever a need to advertise them. Physicians already in the practice call people they know when the need for additional physicians arises. By maintaining contacts with medical school classmates, former graduates from your residency program and your residency director or attendings, you may keep yourself in a position to learn of job opportunities before they are advertised publicly. Networking with physicians who have similar goals also can take place at national conferences or continuing medical education activities that are geared to areas of your particular interest.

EVALUATING A PRACTICE OPPORTUNITY: WHAT MIGHT IT LOOK LIKE WHEN YOU FIND IT?

Once you have decided what sort of position and practice location will best suit your personal values and goals and have started a search using the methods outlined above, you need to begin evaluating various opportunities. To understand which opportunities best suit your needs, it is important to have a basic understanding of the various practice models, legal structures, and types of health care organizations that exist in modern medical practice. Although the potential combinations of these elements are almost unlimited, a review of the following points may be of some value.

PRACTICE MODELS

Solo Practice

Even though solo practice has been made more difficult by the competitiveness of most urban health care markets, the complexities of modern medical practice, and the development of large integrated health care organizations, it is still possible to hang out a shingle and begin a new practice. Whereas solo practice was once the preferred method of practice for the majority of primary care physicians, the number of new physicians entering solo practice has decreased dramatically in recent years. Despite this trend, there may always be a place for solo practitioners in rural areas because of the isolated nature of the practice setting. In urban and suburban areas, solo practices will survive because they are better able to provide specialized services. They also can lend a more personalized touch to the provision of care, for which many patients are willing to pay extra. Special services such as weight loss, alternative therapies, travel medicine, and health and fitness can often provide a competitive edge to a solo practice.

The greatest advantages of solo practice are the independence and autonomy that come with running your own office and the potential for a higher income than physicians working in groups. Solo physicians have complete control over their office settings, including the hours worked, the office staff hired, and the patients seen. The price paid for such independence and control can be high because the solo practitioner must take responsibility for running a business as well as for practicing medicine. Navigating the complexities of the legal requirements and insurance billing procedures of modern medical practice while maintaining a compatible, competent, and trustworthy office staff can take several hours a week. There is also the burden imposed by the reality that your office staff rely solely on you for their livelihoods. It can be difficult to arrange coverage for days out of the office for vacation or continuing medical education. The amount of time spent on call tends to be much higher, but the difficulty of call is less because you are covering a smaller number of patients with whom you are much more familiar.

Before opening a solo practice or purchasing a practice from a colleague, it is important to research the local medical community to assess the degree of managed care penetration, how care is paid for in the community, and whether or not the contracts of any existing practice are transferable to a new physician (many are not). For the independent, entrepreneurial physician who values autonomy and the potential for greater income more than security and free time, solo practice may be the best practice model.

Single Specialty Groups

The increase in the number of young physicians joining groups is an indicator of how complex modern medical practice has become. College, medical school, and residency training prepare you for the practice of medicine but not for running a business. Joining a group of other family practitioners allows you to be a part of a practice that can run more efficiently than a solo practice, with less duplication of administrative services, a more structured environment for dealing with office personnel, and increased bargaining power or market clout when dealing with insurance contracts. Joining an established group usually also allows you to achieve a guaranteed income instantly without the need to go through the process of building up a patient base, because the group will most often subsidize a new physician's income while the new physician builds a practice. Being a member of a group also makes it much easier to have a life outside of medicine, because other members of the group are available to cover call and vacations. Many physicians also prefer the collegiality of working in a group setting where other physicians are present to discuss difficult cases or new therapies. Physician income tends to be more dependable in group practices because the group can develop capital reserves to be used to even out the month-to-month or seasonal variability present in many practice settings.

When joining a group of any sort, the individual physician sacrifices a certain degree of autonomy. The effective management of a group mandates that the individual's interests and priorities be superseded by those of the group. In many groups, the governance may favor the more established, vested partners. Most groups definitely develop a group culture that ultimately controls the group's actions. The advantage of joining a single specialty group is that the physicians in the group tend to maintain a commonality of purpose, and group decisions are more likely to reflect the goals and values of the individual.

Multispecialty Groups

The advantages of single specialty groups are increased by multispecialty groups, but so are the disadvantages. Because of their ability to care for more of a patient's total health care needs, larger multispecialty groups usually gain even more market clout than single specialty groups and are in a better position to negotiate managed care contracts. The size of most multispecialty groups allows for the development of a more well-defined infrastructure of business services for such things as marketing, human resource management, risk management, and regulatory compliance. In general, multispecialty groups can provide more steady physician income and better benefit packages. The collegiality between specialties can facilitate patient care and create a satisfying work environment, with good follow-up of patients and communication between specialties (Fig. 21-1).

Multispecialty groups bring with them their own set of problems, however. The disparities in income between specialties can be a source of group divisiveness unless there is agreement among specialties regarding an equitable income distribution scheme that rewards the efforts of both primary care and specialty physicians. The group culture becomes even more important because there is often not the commonality of purpose enjoyed by single specialty groups. The patient demographics, managed care contract provisions, administrative structure, and governance that are best suited for specialty medicine may not be the best for primary care and vice-versa. Before joining any group, but especially a multispecialty group, a physician must be willing to contribute to the group process by spending time in meetings to help ensure that all viewpoints and needs are fairly represented in the decision-making process. On the other hand, it is important to be sure that the group culture allows for fair representation of various opinions and viewpoints during the process of governance.

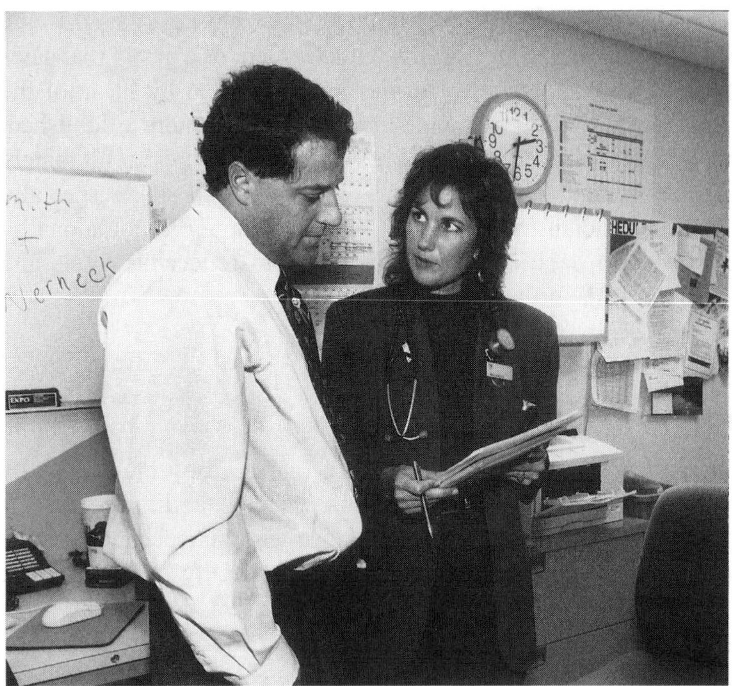

FIGURE 21-1
Group practice settings allow physicians to share knowledge and expertise.

LEGAL STRUCTURES

There are several legal structures possible within the practice of medicine. The choice of which structure is appropriate for any given practice depends on several factors, including state law, goals of the organization, and pension planning requirements. The choice of structure can affect an individual physician's income, tax liability, malpractice exposure, retirement planning, and professional autonomy. The most common legal structures are summarized in the following discussion.

Sole Proprietorships

This is the simplest organizational structure and the most common for solo practices and small groups. In this structure, one person (the proprietor) controls everything, owns everything, and is responsible for everything. Sole proprietors can hire other professionals to work in the business, so there is no true limit on the size of the proprietorship, but for practical purposes medical sole proprietorships remain relatively small. Sole proprietors can band together to form groups for the purposes of sharing expenses, but they must remain as separate entities within the group, because they cannot share profits. If profits are shared, the entity becomes a partnership.

Partnerships

The key difference between a group of sole proprietors and a partnership is that the partners agree to share all profits as well as expenses and liabilities. The partners act as co-owners of the business. In general partnerships, the partners share all risks, including malpractice. There is no limit to a partner's exposure to malpractice liability for his or her own acts or the acts of a partner, so personal assets are also at risk. Income is not necessarily equally distributed, but most partnerships have a well-defined income distribution formula as a component of the partnership agreement.

Limited partnerships were created to limit the obligations and risks of certain partners to encourage investment. In this entity, the limited partners enjoy some protection from the risks of investing in the business (with the amount of liability limited to the amount invested and the assets of the partnership), but in exchange they have little say in the day-to-day running of the business, which is left to general or managing partners. Limited partnerships are used most often in medicine to generate capital for the acquisition of land, buildings, or equipment.

Another type of partnership created for a specific purpose is the joint venture, but various state and federal laws, such as Medicare antikickback regulations, may limit a physician's participation in such entities.

> *''Commercialism in medicine never leads to true satisfaction, and to maintain our self-respect is more precious than gold.''*
>
> —William J. Mayo

Corporations

A corporation is an entity that is distinct from its individual shareholders (owners), employees, and directors. It is governed by corporate bylaws that define such things as who can vote, how decisions are made, the duties of the corporate officers, and what happens to the corporate assets on dissolution. Corporations are managed by a board of directors elected by the shareholders. The primary difference between a corporation and partnership is that the owners of the corporation are generally protected from individual liability for corporate obligations and liabilities.

Corporations are regulated by state laws, and the specific structure varies from state to state. Many states also have laws that prohibit the corporate practice of medicine. A for-profit corporation can generate a profit that is paid to the shareholders of the corporation. On the other hand, a nonprofit corporation cannot distribute any profits (or excess revenues) to its owners, directors, or officers. The profits must be reinvested in the institution. Nonprofit status does not automatically confer tax-exempt status. Such status must be applied for through the Internal Revenue Service and comes with a strict set of regulations. Professional corporations are business corporations that can be formed only by shareholders who are licensed to practice the same profession as that practiced by the corporation.

Physicians practice in a highly regulated professional environment. The laws regulating physician organizations often differ greatly from those governing nonmedical entities. Legal counsel should be employed with specific knowledge of the state and federal regulations as well as partnership and corporate law when defining a legal structure for the practice of medicine.

HEALTH CARE ORGANIZATIONS

In general, practice models tend to be selected based on an individual physician's desire for such things as autonomy, security, and flexibility. Legal structures tend to be selected based on legal and regulatory issues as well as the balancing of issues such as control and liability. The selection of the best organizational structure for an individual physician or a group of physicians tends to be driven by the desire to be competitive in the managed care marketplace. Often the organizational structure becomes a vehicle through which a physician gains access to contracts from a managed care organization that would not be available to an individual practitioner. In general, the following organizational structures involve large groups of physicians.

Preferred Provider Organizations

A preferred provider organization (PPO) is a group of providers (that may include physicians, hospitals, pharmacies, and other providers) that has agreed to provide services at a discounted rate in exchange for preferential treatment from an insurance carrier. The providers may or may not have any other formal affiliation, either legally or financially. They have, in effect, offered to provide an insurance carrier a volume discount. Patients enrolled in the PPO have financial incentives to see preferred physicians rather than nonparticipating providers. They therefore tend to favor the preferred providers, thus increasing business for the participating physicians. The method of payment to the providers is most often a discounted fee-for-service, so the providers don't assume any risk other than that of receiving less reimbursement for each unit of service.

Independent Practice Associations

To increase their bargaining power, individual physicians or separate groups often band together to form an independent practice association (IPA). In doing so, they do not forfeit their autonomy to run their practices individually, but they form a larger unit, much like a consortium or cooperative, that is better able to bargain more aggressively for specific managed care contracts. Often, the IPA is large enough to assume enough risk to be able to take on capitated contracts. With such contracts, the IPA receives a set amount of money to provide a set amount of health care services for a defined patient population for a predetermined time. This capitated amount of money is usually a set amount per member per month for each person covered by the plan (covered lives). The IPA can then distribute this income to the participating independent practitioners by a formula determined in advance by the member physicians.

Management Services Organizations

A management services organization (MSO) is an entity formed when individual physicians or groups of physicians enter into an agreement with a larger entity (usually a hospital or insurance carrier) for the provision of certain management functions. The agreement can be for a limited array of services (such as billing or payroll), or it can include all of the services necessary to provide patient care (such as office space, marketing, contract negotiations, personnel management, and recruitment). Presumably, the larger entity is able to provide such services more efficiently and at a lower cost, thereby benefiting the individual physicians. For each service that is turned over to the MSO, however, there is a concomitant reduction in physician autonomy and control.

Health Maintenance Organizations

HMOs are essentially insurance companies that have shifted from the traditional insurance role of collecting premiums from patients and using that money to pay for care rendered by individual physicians (indemnity insurance) to a role of actually providing the care. HMOs developed as an effort to control health care costs by better managing how the care is provided and eliminating unnecessary services, duplication, and waste. They are generally organized into either staff model (closed panel) HMOs or group model (open panel) HMOs. Staff model HMOs employ physicians to provide care exclusively to their patients. The physicians are usually salaried and work in facilities that are owned by the HMO. Group model HMOs, on the other hand, contract with other medical groups to provide care for their members. The contracted groups may actually be best described as PPOs or IPAs.

SALARIES AND CALL

Many will argue that we have entered the renaissance of generalism, or the golden age of primary care. It is true that managed care and cost consciousness have placed a premium on well-trained family physicians capable of managing and appropriately referring a wide variety of patient problems. The income of family physicians is beginning to reflect this new reality. Between 1990 and 1994, the median compensation for family physicians overall increased 20%, and for those in practice only 1 to 2 years, it increased 33%. Data from the Medical Group Management Association for 1996 (collected from physician groups) indicates that the median income for all family physicians increased to $134,500 for those who do obstetrics and to $132,400 for those who do not. There are variations in income depending on the size of the group, geographic location, practice setting, and physician sex (Table 21-1).

When evaluating a new practice opportunity, it is important to understand how your compensation will be calculated and how the costs of starting your new practice will be covered. Few would argue that to earn $130,000 by working 40 hours a week is a better rate of compensation than to earn $150,000 by working 60 hours a week. Some basic questions to consider before signing on the dotted line are the following.

How is the compensation calculated? This question has a fairly straightforward answer if you will be paid a straight salary or hourly wage. More often than not, however, there are subtleties that are best dealt with if understood before beginning work. If compensation is based on production, what is

TABLE 21-1
1997 FAMILY PRACTICE COMPENSATION IN DOLLARS (BASED ON 1996 DATA)

	WITH OB	WITHOUT OB
Overall		
Mean	141,800	142,500
25th Percentile	113,900	111,900
Median	134,500	132,400
75th Percentile	160,400	162,700
90th Percentile	193,600	197,025
Median by group type		
Single specialty	125,000	129,000
Multispecialty	135,600	132,600
Median by geographic section		
Single specialty		
Eastern	118,300	127,000
Midwest	136,400	120,000
Southern	160,200	150,000
Western	109,600	125,327
Multispecialty		
Eastern	127,200	120,000
Midwest	136,000	129,500
Southern	149,900	148,300
Western	130,900	133,000
Median by geographic class		
Urban/central city	132,500	136,900
Suburban	141,200	132,200
Small city	137,500	128,000
Rural	128,300	123,700
Median by sex		
Male	137,100	134,400
Female	112,500	116,100

OB, obstetrics.

Data from Medical Group Management Association: Physician Compensation and Production Survey: 1997 Report Based on 1996 Data. Englewood, CO, Medical Group Management Association, 1997.

the formula? Are all physicians dealt with equally, or are there "special circumstances" that influence compensation for some individuals but not for others? If overhead costs are a part of the formula, how are they calculated and monitored? Are there periodic bonuses? If so, how are they calculated? Do the current compensation formulas violate any antikickback principles (such as the prohibition against receiving direct compensation for ordering laboratory tests or generating referrals)? Does the compensation system reward cost-effective care? This is especially important in managed care settings that use a capitated payment mechanism, in which traditional production-based compensation formulas tend to reward overutilization and, therefore, the wrong behavior. Are non-patient care activities (especially administrative or committee activities that benefit the entire group) fairly compensated? If not compensated, are they fairly distributed among physicians in the group?

Are opportunities available to increase your income, such as after-hours clinics or Urgent Care/Emergency Department shifts? If such opportunities exist, are they purely optional or required?

How is call distributed? Are newer physicians required to take extra call? Is there extra compensation for extra call? If some members of the call panel do obstetrics and others do not, is the resulting inequality of call load dealt with fairly?

How long is the work week? Is there flexibility in how many days a week or how many hours a day must be worked? Is flexible scheduling of hours allowed? Is part-time practice allowed?

What are the provisions for Continuing Medical Education and vacation? Are Continuing Medical Education expenses covered in addition to the basic compensation, or must they be absorbed by the individual physician? Are vacations paid time off, or does any time away from patient care result in lower compensation?

In addition to the above questions and considerations, it is important to recognize that it usually takes a new physician a certain amount of time to develop a busy, financially rewarding practice. Depending on the extent of the unmet patient demand, this can take weeks to years. A young physician moving into a practice from which previously established physicians have recently left or retired will be working at full capacity much sooner than the physician who is opening a brand new practice, either in an established group or at an entirely new practice setting. During the time required to reach full productivity, the practice will almost certainly operate at a net financial loss. It is important to understand how this initial loss (and your compensation during this period) will be dealt with. Will a larger organization (hospital system, multispecialty group, or HMO) absorb this cost as a normal cost of business growth, or will you be required to repay it in some form, either by paying it back as a loan, accepting a lower level of compensation initially, or being prohibited from sharing in certain bonuses or profit sharing for a time?

Before signing on to a new practice situation, understand what will happen if either you or your new associates decide that the association is not working. Is there a restrictive covenant or noncompete clause? This is usually a clause in the contract stating that if you leave the practice for any reason, you cannot practice within the same geographic area for a certain time. It is important to understand the implications of this clause, because it might prohibit you from staying in the community that was the focus of your job search to begin with. It is sometimes possible to pay a financial penalty instead of suffering a geographic restriction on your practice. This not only discourages you from leaving but also allows the group to recoup some of the expenses incurred in the development of your practice.

WHAT NEXT?

The first practice situation for a new physician is often the culmination of years of sacrifice, dedication, and hard work. Regardless of when the decision is made to become a physician, it is inevitably followed by years of moving from one stage to the next, with the transition to the next stage becoming the immediate goal. Years are spent performing specific goal-oriented tasks that make the achievement of the next level or stage possible. Medical school and residency demand extremely long hours and extraordinarily hard work. Many essential elements of who you are must be put on hold while you study for one more examination, work up one more admission, or recover from one more long night on call.

As you search for your first practice setting on completing training, it is worthwhile to reflect on who you are and what you want to become. Without this reflection it is sometimes difficult for young physicians to achieve the inner balance required to develop a long, satisfying career in medicine. New goals need to be set and challenges defined without an admissions committee or residency director defining for you what constitutes success. It is important to define your new goals (family, community, or profession) in a way that allows you to work toward them in a positive manner while avoiding a pattern of hard work and long hours at the office that can be destructive to ultimate personal fulfillment. Physicians often become so work centered that they lose the balance necessary to live a healthy life. This is promoted by the first new job, where the allure of an income substantially greater than any you have ever received, the need to pay off educational loans, and the demands of others (including colleagues, administrators, and patients) promote the tendency to ignore your values and long-term goals. By defining your goals as clearly as possible and working toward those goals, you can avoid many of the pitfalls of modern medical practice. Happy hunting!

REFERENCE

1. Random House Webster's College Dictionary. New York, Random House, 1996

SUGGESTED READING

American Academy of Family Physicians: From Residency to Reality: Practice Management Teaching Tools. Kansas City, MO, American Academy of Family Physicians, 1997

Medical Group Management Association: Physician Compensation and Production Survey: 1997 Report Based on 1996 Data. Englewood, CO, Medical Group Management Association, 1997

Ross A, Williams SJ, Pavlock EJ: Ambulatory Care Management. Third edition. Albany, NY, Delmar Publishers, 1998

22 FAMILY PRACTICE BOARD CERTIFICATION, RECERTIFICATION, AND IN-TRAINING EXAMINATIONS

Robert F. Avant, M.D.

Each year the American Board of Family Practice (ABFP) administers certification, recertification, and in-training examinations to physicians in practice and physicians in training. Founded in 1969, the ABFP was the 20th specialty board within the American Board of Medical Specialties (ABMS). The first Family Practice Certification Examination was administered in 1970. A pioneer in ensuring the highest standard of medical care, the ABFP was the first board to require recertification, and as of 1998, all 24 boards of ABMS have recertification plans or procedures in place. Diplomates of ABFP are certified for 7 years and must complete a Recertification Process, which includes passing a proctored, written examination (just as in certification) to become recertified. This requirement ensures that physicians in practice maintain an appropriate level of cognitive skills to be recognized as specialists in family practice (Fig. 22-1). The In-Training Examination serves as a measure of cognitive knowledge for residents in training that can be used to assess the resident's progress compared with residents both in their program and nationally.

DESCRIPTION OF EXAMINATIONS

Certification Examination

Physicians may take the ABFP Certification Examination after successful completion of a family practice residency training program approved by the Accreditation Council for Graduate Medical Education (ACGME). If successful in passing this examination, the physician will obtain Diplomate

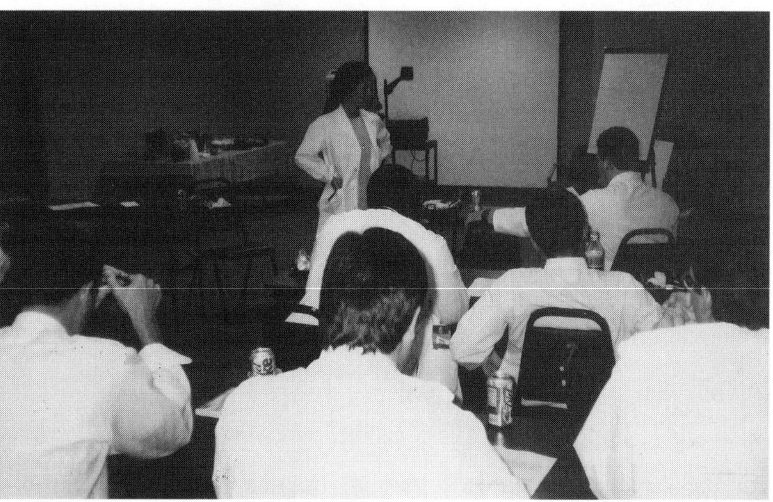

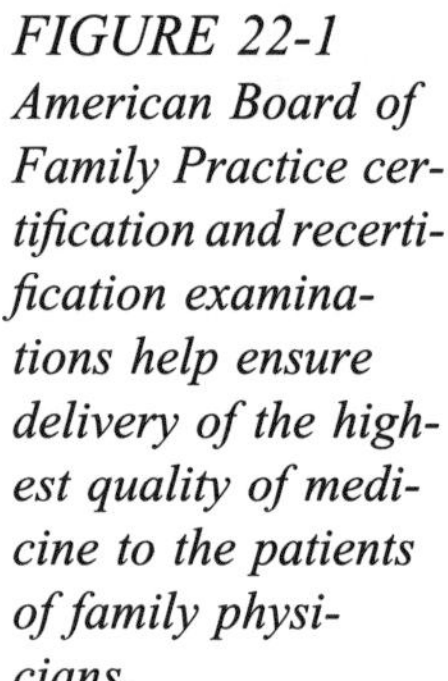

FIGURE 22-1 American Board of Family Practice certification and recertification examinations help ensure delivery of the highest quality of medicine to the patients of family physicians.

status, which is valid for 7 years, at which time the physician will be required to recertify by successful completion of the Recertification Examination. Although certification is a voluntary process, gaining Diplomate status may be essential to receiving hospital privileges at many institutions, and in some cases, to obtaining jobs and providing care for Health Maintenance Organizations (HMOs). This is a phenomenon created by managed care organizations and has changed the perceived value of certification during the past several years. In many cases, if physicians do not have board certification or fail to keep their certification status, it can have significant impact on their ability to maintain practice opportunities and privileges. Because of these factors, the majority of family practice residents completing training do seek certification by ABFP.

The ABFP Certification Examination is given on the second Friday in July after residents have completed their family practice residency programs. Materials for registration are sent to residents in December and must be returned completed to ABFP by February 1. Late applications are accepted until May 1, but significant late fees are applied. The registration information includes a list of testing sites. Test sites are assigned on a first-come, first-served basis; therefore, candidates should return their applications promptly to ensure their first choices. The following is a list of test sites for 1999.

Anchorage, AK
Atlanta, GA
Houston, TX
Kansas City, MO

Bellevue/Seattle, WA
Boston, MA
Chicago, IL - Downtown
Chicago, IL - O'Hare Airport
Cincinnati, OH
Dallas, TX
Denver, CO
East Brunswick, NJ
Honolulu, HI
Lexington, KY
Los Angeles, CA
Minneapolis, MN
Orlando, FL
Philadelphia, PA
Sacramento, CA
San Juan, PR
Washington, DC

Registration requires 2 recent passport-type photographs, demographic information, proper examination fee, and confirmation by the program director of successful completion of an ACGME-approved residency training program. Importantly, all candidates must hold a currently valid, full and unrestricted license to practice medicine in the United States or Canada and must provide a copy of that license with the submitted application materials. After completion of registration, the materials should be mailed to the ABFP. On approval of the application, candidates will be notified of their assigned testing locations, given information concerning registration procedures, and provided their admission tickets.

". . . it is better to think and sometimes think wrong than not to think at all."

—William J. Mayo

The Certification Examination consists of a full day of testing that begins about 7:45 AM and ends at 5:00 PM. One test booklet, containing 2 sections, is given during the morning session. The questions in the first section are multiple-choice (one-best answer) questions and true-false questions. Below is a sample question.

Which one of the following is true regarding medical therapy for chronic congestive heart failure (CHF)?

A) Angiotensin-converting enzyme (ACE) inhibitors often improve the symptoms of CHF.
B) Vasodilators other than ACE inhibitors should be first-line therapy.
C) Digoxin is most likely to be useful in patients with mild symptoms.
D) Diuretics are more effective for treating symptoms related to low output than for treating symptoms of fluid overload.
E) Antiarrhythmia agents should be used routinely for all patients.

The second section consists of clinical set problems which are designed to assess certain aspects of clinical problem solving. Each problem consists of a clinical framework in which information is given about a patient. The candidate is asked to make choices regarding diagnosis and management in a series of true-false options. Below is a sample question.

A 45-year-old business executive is found to be mildly hypertensive, with blood pressure measurements of about 145/100 mm Hg on 3 successive visits to your office. The patient is approximately 20 lb overweight; otherwise, the physical examination is unremarkable. The family history is negative.

Minimum baseline laboratory tests which should be done before starting therapy include

A) serum potassium
B) serum cortisol
C) fasting and 2-hour postprandial blood glucose
D) urinalysis
E) 24-hour urine for metanephrines
F) rapid sequence intravenous pyelogram

Reasonable management for this patient includes which of the following?

G) weight reduction diet
H) restricting daily protein intake to 40 g
I) advising the patient to avoid caffeine
J) advising the patient to avoid alcohol

During the examination, there are no scheduled breaks. Examinees are permitted to leave the examination room for a break but are asked to remain in the general area. No additional testing time is given for the time spent on break.

Following the morning session, examinees are given a lunch break of approximately 1 1/4 hours. After lunch, the registration process is repeated. Candidates are allotted 3 hours for the afternoon session, which consists of one test booklet containing 180 multiple-choice (one-best answer) and true-false questions. There is also a pictorial insert consisting of approximately 30 items (eg, electrocardiograms, radiographs, photographs of skin conditions) about which the examinee will be asked.

All answers for the examination are recorded on a standardized grid sheet, which contains alphabetized ovals that must be filled in with a standard number 2 pencil.

The cost of the Certification Examination for 1999 is $725.00. Late fees are assessed if the application is received after the published deadline.

Recertification Examination

The Recertification Examination is given annually on the same day and at the same locations as the Certification Examination (Fig. 22-2). Although Diplomate certificates are valid for 7 years, candidates are given the option of taking the examination to renew their certificates in either the sixth or seventh year. This opportunity is offered in the event that the Diplomate is either unable to sit for the examination in the seventh year or is unsuccessful in the sixth year. It allows an additional chance to take the examination before the expiration of the certificate and loss of Diplomate status.

The application for the Recertification Examination requires the candidate to provide evidence of a valid and unrestricted license to practice medicine in the United States or Canada and to affirm that all licenses held are valid and unrestricted. In addition, candidates must show evidence of 300 hours of continuing medical education in the last 6 years, provide demographic

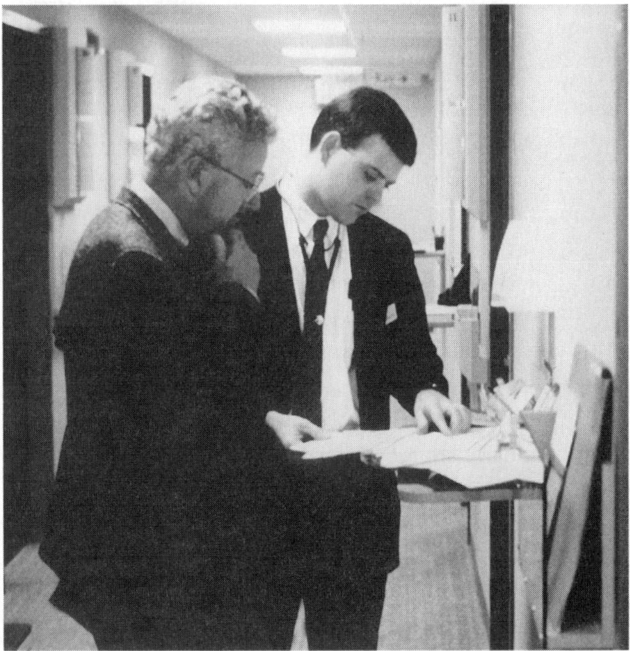

FIGURE 22-2 Although clinical expertise is important, the successful family physician must participate in continuing medical education and successfully pass certification and recertification examinations.

TABLE 22-1
OFFICE RECORD REVIEW

The following is a list of clinical problems that may be used in the Office Record Review for the ABFP Recertification Examination. The examinee must choose one office progress note from Group I and one from Group II that outlines the care you have provided recently for that clinical problem. The office record is sent to the ABFP for grading purposes. Following successful completion of the Office Record Review, the candidate may sit for the Recertification Examination.

COMPUTERIZED OFFICE RECORD REVIEW DEFINITIONAL CRITERIA	
GROUP I	**GROUP II**
CORONARY ARTERY DISEASE: A patient with angina, or a history of myocardial infarction as the primary diagnosis. You need not have made the initial diagnosis, but you should have provided care for this condition for at least one year. **HYPERTENSION:** An adult patient with confirmed primary hypertension for which you initiated management or initiated a significant change in regimen and which you have managed for at least six months. **URINARY TRACT INFECTION:** An adult, nonpregnant **female** patient with acute microbial lower urinary tract infection, which you diagnosed, and a history of at least one previous episode. (Note: "UTI" refers to lower urinary tract inflammatory nonvenereal disease only and does not include gonococcal disease or acute or chronic renal disease. Acceptable diagnoses are cystitis and urethritis.)	**CARCINOMA OF THE BREAST:** A patient whom you have diagnosed or referred for a definitive diagnosis of carcinoma of the breast. Information regarding the management of the patient should be reflected in the record even though management is provided by a consultant. At least one chart should be for a patient for whom you have provided follow-up care for a period of at least three years. **DEPRESSIVE DISORDERS:** An adult patient whom you have diagnosed as having a Depressive Disorder and who has been under management for at least three months since the diagnosis. **MENSTRUAL DISORDERS:** A patient who is at least three years postmenarchal, is premenopausal, and whose presenting complaint is either abnormal vaginal bleeding (if any menses) or lack of menses. **WELL CHILD CARE:** A patient who is now at least three years old but not more than eighteen, and who has been seen for at least three well child visits. You should have provided care for a minimum of three years, and both of the charts must be for patients who have been under your care since birth.

Continued

TABLE 22-1
OFFICE RECORD REVIEW (Continued)

COMPUTERIZED OFFICE RECORD REVIEW DEFINITIONAL CRITERIA

GROUP I

DUODENAL ULCER:
An adult patient with confirmed duodenal ulcer which you have diagnosed and managed medically.

DIABETES MELLITUS:
A patient with adult onset, non-insulin dependent (Type 2) diabetes mellitus which you have diagnosed. You should have followed the patient for at least one year.

CHRONIC HEART FAILURE:
An adult patient with chronic heart failure which you diagnosed. You should have managed the patient for at least six months.

OSTEOARTHRITIS:
An adult patient with osteoarthritis. You should have made the initial diagnosis and seen this patient for at least three visits for this condition.

URETHRAL DISCHARGE:
A male patient who is 15 years old or older, with an initial complaint of urethral discharge which you have diagnosed and managed, and whom you have seen at least twice for this problem.

COPD (Chronic Obstructive Pulmonary Disease)
An adult patient with chronic generalized airway obstruction in whom the diagnosis has been established and who has been under your care for at least three years. Acceptable diagnoses include chronic bronchitis or chronic emphysema. This category excludes asthma.

GROUP II

IRRITABLE BOWEL SYNDROME:
An adult patient whose complaints may include chronic abdominal discomfort and/or alterations in bowel function. Acceptable diagnoses include any functional bowel disorder or syndromes, e.g., spastic colitis, mucous colitis, irritable colon, etc. This category does not include infectious hepatitis.

GERIATRIC PATIENT:
A patient who is at least 70 years old, who is not institutionalized in a long-term care facility, who has been under your care for at least three years, who is usually ambulatory, and who comes to the physician's office for a major portion of his/her medical care. At least one of the charts must be for a patient who is 75 or older.

ALCOHOLISM & ALCOHOL ABUSE:
A patient in whom alcoholism or alcohol abuse has been identified as a problem and who has been under your care for this problem for at least one year.

ACUTE APPENDICITIS:
A child or adult patient for whom you have made the diagnosis of acute appendicitis.

LOW BACK PAIN:
An adult patient with an initial complaint of low back pain for whom the final diagnosis was lumbosacral strain, lumbar disc disease, or osteoarthritis. You should have seen the patient at least three times for this problem for a minimum of six weeks.

NORMAL PREGNANCY (Delivered):
A patient, aged 17-35, who has had an uncomplicated pregnancy. You need not have delivered the baby.

From the 1999 Recertification Examination application. By permission of the American Board of Family Practice.

information, submit the proper examination fee, and provide 2 recent passport-type photographs.

"Once you start studying medicine you never get through with it."

—Charles H. Mayo

Candidates are also required to participate in the Office Record Review process. From 19 categories, the candidate selects 2 patient charts from 2 of these categories (Acute Appendicitis, Alcoholism and Alcohol Abuse, Carcinoma of the Breast, Chronic Heart Failure, Chronic Obstructive Pulmonary Disease, Coronary Artery Disease, Depressive Disorders, Diabetes Mellitus, Duodenal Ulcer, Geriatric Patient, Hypertension, Irritable Bowel Syndrome, Low Back Pain, Menstrual Disorders, Normal Pregnancy, Osteoarthritis, Urethral Discharge, Urinary Tract Infection, and Well Child Care) and completes questionnaires using information from the charts (Table 22-1). These forms are returned to ABFP for scoring. On successful completion of the Office Record Review and the formal application, the candidate is approved to sit for the written examination.

The Recertification Examination is identical to the initial certifying examination in the morning session; however, the afternoon session consists of 3 preselected modular examinations that are chosen by the candidate at the time of application. The choices for the modules are internal medicine, surgery, obstetrics, pediatrics, geriatrics, gynecology, and emergent/urgent care. Each of the modules contains 50 multiple-choice (one-best answer) questions and 10 true-false questions. The candidate has 3 hours to complete the 3 modules chosen. On successful completion of the Recertification Examination, the candidate is recertified for 7 years. The cost of the Recertification Examination in 1999 is $725.00, and as with the Certification Examination, late fees are assessed for applications submitted after the published deadline.

In-Training Examination

Each year the ABFP offers the In-Training Examination to family practice residents. The test is given on the first Friday in November and 5 hours is allowed to complete the examination. Residency directors are responsible for registering residents with the ABFP, receiving the test, and providing an appropriate site to administer the test. This test consists of 2 booklets. The first booklet contains 180 multiple-choice (one-best answer) and true-false questions. Residents have 3 hours to answer these questions. After the completion of the first booklet, residents are allowed a 10- to 15-minute break, which is followed by a second booklet consisting of clinical set problems, similar to those in the Certification and Recertification Examinations (Fig. 22-3). Residency programs pay $30/resident for the In-Training Examination; there is no cost to the resident.

EXAMINATION SCORING

Scoring for all ABFP written examinations is accomplished by computer analysis performed on standardized answer grids. There is no penalty for guessing; thus, it is advantageous for the examinee to answer *all* questions.

Passing scores for the Certification and Recertification Examinations are determined by committees of the American Board of Family Practice, using accepted psychometric procedures. Scores for the In-Training Examination are determined by national averages and reported to the residency director approximately 6 weeks after the examination.

SUGGESTIONS FOR STUDY AND TEST TAKING FROM ABFP

The key to preparing for the ABFP examinations is to remain active in practice, learning from each patient encounter and each consultation. Regular attendance at hospital conferences, attendance at continuing medical education programs, and regular reading of current literature for family physicians

(*Continues on page 279*)

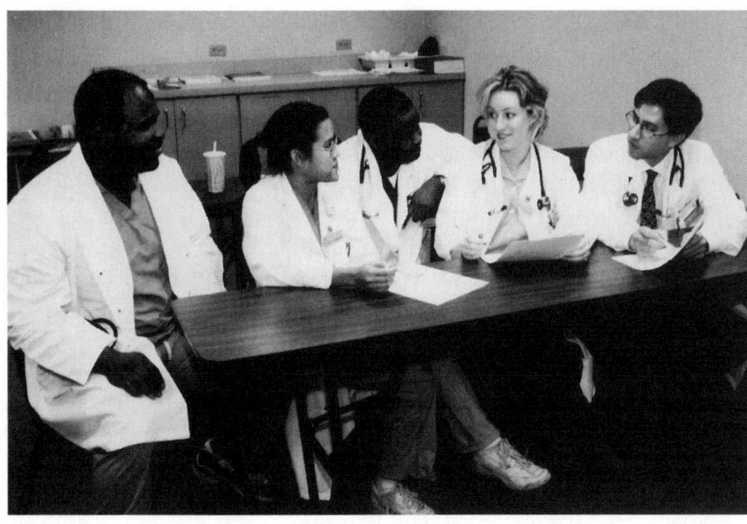

FIGURE 22-3
Review of the results of in-training examinations with other residents is an excellent way to prepare for the actual ABFP certification examination.

BOX 22-2 SPECIFIC STUDY TIPS FROM ROBERT L. BRATTON, M.D.

The following are tips from the editor, not from the American Board of Family Practice or Dr. Avant.

Each one of us has taken hundreds of tests on the journey to becoming a licensed physician. It is a rite of passage that every physician must endure. Although all of us are successful at completing and passing tests, we continue to dread these experiences. As we have learned, the secret to passing tests and reducing the anxiety associated with them is to prepare adequately for examinations. The following are tips for studying and taking ABFP Certification, Recertification, and In-Training Examinations.

1. Prepare yourself

Although by most standards ABFP examinations are not exceedingly difficult, they should not be taken for granted. A poor score could result in not becoming board certified or losing board certification status (thus prohibiting hospital privileges in many areas). In addition, for residents who perform poorly on their In-Training Examination, their efforts may give attending physicians concern and perhaps a different attitude toward their overall performance as they progress through their residency training.

A typical study schedule might include a structured study program that you begin 6 weeks before the examination. Some individuals may need longer; however, if the review process takes too long, you may forget some of the material before the test. Each night during the week (reserving the weekends for rest), I suggest reviewing for 2 to 3 hours with frequent breaks. During the 3 days before the test, I suggest a brief cramming period that covers the topics you have reviewed in the last 6 weeks, to refresh and fine tune your memory just before the test.

2. Review the structure of the test

Although your knowledge of the topics covered is the most important aspect of the test, it is also important to be familiar with the structure of the test, including the types of questions and sections as well as the time allotted for each section. All tests are graded from a computer-readable answer sheet that requires the participant to fill in a circle for the answer to a question. Make sure each answer circle is appropriately filled in.

3. Familiarize yourself with the test site

In-Training Examination Each residency program provides the In-Training Examination at their institution. To adequately prepare, it is a good idea to find out where the test is going to take place and locate the room and nearby restrooms before the day of the test. It may be important to listen for any noises, such as nearby construction or loud traffic, which may be distracting during the test. In these situations, earplugs may be helpful. If you live far from the test site and the weather is bad, it may be wise to make arrangements for an alternative place to stay the night before the test. Other suggestions include arranging call schedules so that you are not on call the night before the test. On many rotations, there are residents in other fields who are not taking the test and could take call the night before the test. Think ahead and discuss this with your chief resident or supervising staff well in advance of the rotation. In most cases, your residency director will help arrange this for you.

Certification and Recertification Examinations These tests are given at specific locations across the United States and may require a significant amount of travel to reach the location. You will receive an updated list of locations with your registration material. Remember, it is important to register early to improve your chance of getting your first choice of location. Because of the travel that may be involved, it is extremely important to arrive at your destination in plenty of time

BOX 22-2 SPECIFIC STUDY TIPS *(Continued)*

to locate the test site. In many cases, the Certification and Recertification Examinations are given in hotel meeting or convention rooms; therefore, it is usually most convenient to stay at the hotel hosting the examination. Always inform the hotel reservation agent that you are there for the test; you may be given a discounted room rate. In addition, make sure you try to reserve a quiet room. Also, if possible, arrange your call schedule with your partners to allow you to get plenty of sleep the week before the test.

4. Prepare for comfort

The In-Training, Certification, and Recertification Examinations require you to sit for extended periods—often at a hard and uncomfortable desk. Prepare yourself. You may want to consider a soft pillow to sit on, a light jacket in case it gets cold, and loose-fitting clothing with comfortable shoes. If you wear glasses, don't forget them.

5. Food and exercise

As we all know, food and exercise are important. A regular exercise program during the weeks of preparation can help you to retain the information you have studied and put you in a better frame of mind for the test. A good diet can help fuel the brain with high-octane energy that helps those brain cells retain information. Think of the test as a marathon, and avoid high-fat meals. Choose high-carbohydrate foods, especially the night before the test. Also avoid alcohol and its deleterious effect on sleep during your preparation. The morning of the test, I suggest a light meal and perhaps a snack to take with you to the test if you get hungry. I also suggest that you take your lunch for the Certification and Recertification Examination; this is not necessary for the In-Training Examination because you are usually through with the test at about 1 PM.

6. Sleep

Adequate sleep is imperative as you prepare for any test, and this test is no exception. The mind works better when it is rested.

Unfortunately, adequate sleep is not always possible for residents in training and physicians in practice. If at all possible, try to arrange your schedule so that it allows for maximal sleep during your preparation and, as mentioned above, make sure you are not on call the night before the test. Try to maintain a regular schedule of going to bed and rising at the same times during the weeks before your test.

7. Miscellaneous items to bring

Bring aspirin, ibuprofen, or acetaminophen in case of a headache during the test. Cough drops and allergy medication (preferably nonsedating) should be brought. Chewing gum or mints should be packed to help break the monotony of the long test sessions. Remember that calculators or watches with calculators are not allowed, and beeping electronic devices should be left at home for the courtesy of others. Earplugs may help to block unwanted noises.

8. Relax

Anxiety is a natural response when faced with a test situation. The important thing is to not let anxiety affect your performance deleteriously. In most cases, simple relaxation techniques, such as exercising, deep breathing, meditation, or biofeeback can be used. Remember, a little anxiety is usually good for you and in most cases helps improve performance.

9. Listen and read the instructions

Before each section, the proctors usually explain the instructions. Also, an explanation and sample

BOX 22-2 SPECIFIC STUDY TIPS *(Continued)*

question usually are given for each section. Listen carefully to the instructions and ask questions if you do not understand something. In addition, take a minute to read the instructions and sample questions before starting. Make sure you adequately fill in the response area on the answer sheet with a number 2 pencil and make sure there are no stray marks on the answer sheet when you have completed it.

Another precaution is to make sure that at the end of each booklet you note that there is a statement that the section has ended.

10. Answer the easiest questions first
Start with the first question of the section and answer all the questions you can with reasonable certainty. If there is a difficult question whose answer you are unsure of, skip it and return to it when you have finished the section. Don't spend an excessive amount of time on one question and risk not being able to answer easy questions at the end of the test because you ran out of time. Circle the numbers of the questions you skip, and be careful on the answer sheet that you skip the numbers of the answers you have omitted. It is an empty feeling when you get to the end of the answer sheet and realize you have answered in the wrong boxes for the last 50 questions. To help prevent this, check that the number of the question in the test book corresponds to the number of the answer on the answer sheet each time you turn a page of the test booklet.

11. Check your pace
Throughout the test, you will receive a reminder of the time remaining. Pay attention to these reminders and adjust your pace as necessary. Having your own watch is helpful. In some situations, there may not be a clock available but only announcements of how much time is left.

12. Guess if you do not know the answer
You are penalized only for an incorrect answer or an unanswered question; therefore, all questions should be answered, even if they require a guess. Remember any answer is better than no answer. If you are unsure of an answer, try to narrow the options down to 2 or 3 selections and choose from them. If you have no clue to the answer, be sure you make a guess. Also, remember that if the question uses absolute terminology such as ''always,'' ''never,'' ''all,'' or ''none,'' it is usually false. Little in the world of medicine is absolute.

13. Review your answers
If time allows during the multiple-choice question section, review your work. There is an old saying, ''you should always stick with your first impression.'' For a multiple-choice test, this is not always the case. If after further consideration, you feel you need to change the answer—go ahead. For true-false questions, it is usually better to stick with your first answer.

14. Try to anticipate the answers
Before looking at the choices available for the answers, try to answer the question. Then see if your answer matches one of the alternatives given. This will allow more certain responses for questions and help to save time.

15. Do not read extra meaning into the questions
The ABFP is not interested in structuring questions to try to outwit the test taker. Questions are designed to be fair and do not have hidden agendas. Above all, the most important thing to remember is to remain confident that you can perform well on the test. The mind can work miracles, and a positive

BOX 22-2 SPECIFIC STUDY TIPS *(Continued)*

attitude with confidence can be achieved by adequate preparation. Remember, a test gives you the opportunity to show what you know. Do not think of it as a test of what you do not know. Study and prepare yourself, and these tests will be nothing more than time away from your practice. Once the test has been completed, take some time to reward yourself for the hard work you've done in preparation. After all, you deserve it.

and primary care help to prepare for the examination. Board review courses offered by the American Academy of Family Physicians and other educational institutions have helped many, especially those preparing for recertification. Those just completing family practice training should be well prepared for the examination through their learning experiences in residency programs.

In taking the examination, the candidate should be prepared, relaxed, and approach the questions as a patient in the office (Box 22-1). The questions are written by practicing family physicians and precautions are taken to ensure that the questions are not trick questions. All questions are referenced either to standard texts or to current journal literature. Although test taking is naturally a stressful experience, coming to the examination rested, prepared, and focused enhances the examinee's experience.

23

OBSTETRICS IN FAMILY MEDICINE

Michele A. Hanson, M.D.

The phone rings. You open one eye to see the digital clock glaring 3:02 AM. You answer the phone. Mrs. Jones is at the birthing center and dilated to 8 cm—and it's her third baby! You jump out of bed, throw on some clothes, run a comb through your hair, and run downstairs. You glance at the thermometer outside the window: −10°F, brrrr! You grab your keys and hospital keycard and jump into a cold car. As you drive through the snowy streets, you start to wake up and sort through the details of Mrs. Jones' history: third pregnancy—uncomplicated. You've already delivered 2 healthy boys to her. She didn't ask at her ultrasound examination about the sex of the baby. Maybe it's a baby girl! You arrive at the hospital and race in. The nurse remarks "Just in time, doc!" You scrub quickly, throw on a gown, and call out "push!" Three pushes later a 7 lb 5 oz baby girl is born. There are tears of joy from mom and dad—and a tear in your eye, too. You shake dad's hand, give mom a hug, and head back home hoping to get a couple hours of sleep before your alarm goes off, signaling the time to do your morning workout before you go to the office.

That's real life obstetrics (OB) in family medicine.

FAMILY MEDICINE AND OBSTETRICS

The basic philosophy of family physicians is to care for the everyday medical needs of their patients, with an emphasis on the psychosocial interactions of the family in health and disease. Family physicians, with their deep understanding and comprehensive approach to patients and their families, are ideally suited to provide care and support to women and their families throughout pregnancy, labor, delivery, and child rearing.

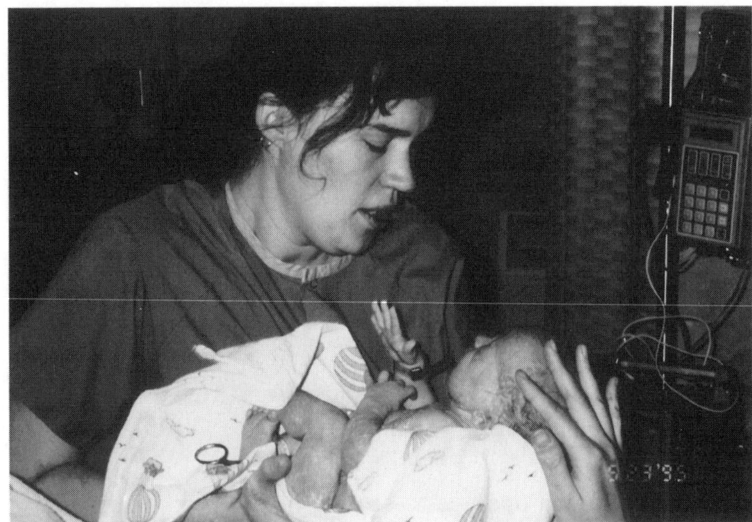

FIGURE 23-1
Approximately one-third of family physicians are involved in obstetric care.

Since the beginning of the specialty, OB care has been an important part of the training of family medicine residents. Yet, not all family physicians choose to provide OB services once they enter practice. A 1991 survey of the American Academy of Family Physicians indicated that about one-third of the members who responded provided OB care in their practices (Fig. 23-1).

Why do some family physicians choose OB and others do not? There are many personal and professional reasons surrounding this decision. Let's try to sort through these areas.

PERSONAL SATISFACTION AND LIFESTYLE ISSUES

Providing OB care to your patients and committing to be there for their deliveries has obvious implications for your personal and family life. You may suddenly be called away from your daughter's birthday party. You may not see the end of that movie. You may miss your son's Little League pitching debut. Do you have a spouse who can support you in your efforts? Who else is available to cover your family's needs or perhaps to cover the delivery if needed? These are real issues that must be faced when making the decision to include OB services in your practice.

Your needs and personal situations may change, and thus your ability to provide OB care may change throughout your career. Many feel after residency that they need to do it all so they don't lose their skills. This may not be necessary and may contribute to early burnout.

For example, my first practice position allowed me to provide prenatal services until 36 weeks, at which time I turned the mother's care over to my obstetrician colleagues. My husband (also a physician) was still in training, and I was uncertain how long I would be in that position. My malpractice coverage would be considerably more expensive if I chose to do deliveries, so the group and I decided on this compromise. It actually worked well for my patients, too. I was in a branch office in a small town, so the availability of local prenatal care until 36 weeks saved patients travel time and distance to an OB's office. Plus, they had an automatic follow-up in my office for well-child care.

After my husband finished medical training, we needed to find a clinic that would have positions for both of us. The clinic that seemed to suit both our needs most closely wouldn't allow me to provide OB services. The family medicine group there had decided not to provide OB care. (Ironically, I would have full cardiac- and intensive-care unit privileges.) At this point in my life, I had a 1-year-old child and another child on the way, and this clinic seemed like the best choice for my family. I thought I might be able to negotiate for OB privileges at a future date if I desired.

> *''Knowledge is static; wisdom is active and moves knowledge, making it effective.''*
>
> —William J. Mayo

This was satisfactory at the time, but when I moved to my next position I had to make more decisions. I would be a family physician but have a concentrated experience in an Urgent Care Center accounting for 50% of my clinical time. OB care would not be required but could be considered. I still had a young family, so initially I chose not to provide OB care. However, as my practice matured, I found it more and more difficult to diagnose pregnancy and then send patients away. I asked the practice committee if I could resume OB, and permission was granted. I also had to discuss this with my husband who agreed to support me in this practice and lifestyle change.

I now provide prenatal care and delivery for my patients, with excellent backup from our OB department. Although this story involves me personally, there are many family physicians who I'm sure have experienced similar circumstances. The important thing to remember is to pursue your goals if you wish to practice OB. Often, there may be obstacles, but in almost all cases these can be overcome.

LIABILITY ISSUES AND RISK MANAGEMENT

Everyone wants a perfect baby. This wish looms over all who have an OB practice. Having good backup is essential to providing OB care as a family physician, unless the family physician has enough advanced training to be able to do cesarean sections. An important part of residency training is helping each individual decide on a level of comfort and at what level to transfer patients to obstetricians if the need arises. This can help residents decide if, how, and where they would feel comfortable delivering OB care (Fig. 23-2). Ultimately, risk management needs to be assessed carefully to decrease liability.

Malpractice insurance is more expensive for family physicians who provide OB care than for those who choose not to provide OB care. However, in most states, reasonably priced malpractice insurance coverage is available for family physicians who provide OB services. Typically, the rates are low in the first years of practice and increase over 6 to 7 years to a level premium.

Good prenatal care, complete documentation, and timely OB consultation reduce malpractice exposure. Most family physicians delivering 25 to 50 babies per year feel they have an adequate volume to be able to respond to OB management problems. Also, this volume seems to provide professional satisfaction without being too disruptive for personal or professional life.

FINANCIAL AND PRACTICE MANAGEMENT CONSIDERATIONS

Whether or not there is a financial incentive to provide OB care is a confusing and controversial subject. Family physicians who provide OB care pay a higher malpractice premium—as much as $8,000 more in California—than family physicians who choose not to provide OB care. If a physician sees an adequate number of OB patients, this can be made up through income generated for delivery services. An additional benefit is that a practice that includes OB can enhance income, not only in fees for maternity services but also in spin-offs such as newborn care, circumcisions, colposcopies, intrauterine device insertions, or dilatation and curettage procedures. This can be significant not only in respect to financial rewards but also in physician satisfaction.

The studies that have reviewed net pay of family physicians based on whether or not they provide OB care have yielded some confusing results. In 1989, Bredfeldt et al.[1] reported the highest annual income accumulated in practices that provided a full range of OB services, including cesarean

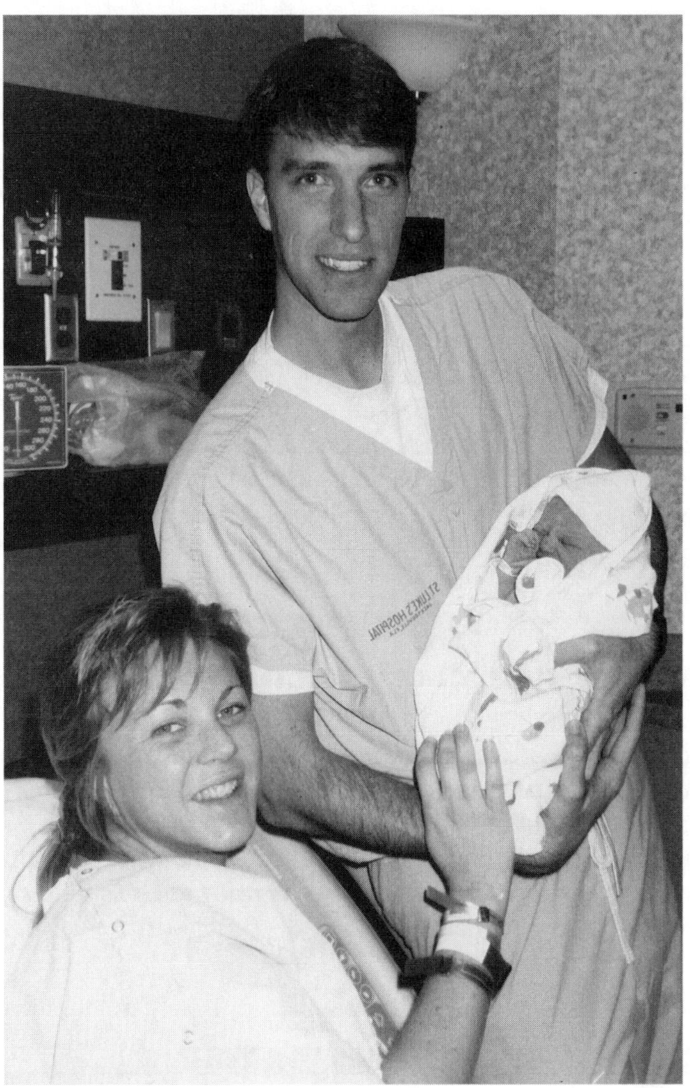

FIGURE 23-2
Residents in training are assigned obstetric patients. They are followed in the Family Practice Clinic for prenatal care and delivered by the resident, with supervising staff physicians in attendance.

section. This was followed by those who never provided OB care. The next group was those who provided OB care, excluding cesarean sections, and the lowest income was in practices that provided prenatal care but no delivery care.

In addition to financial issues, there are practice management issues that need to be considered. For new physicians in practice, delivering babies provides a steady infusion of pediatric patients and young families. Some studies have shown that family physicians who do not provide OB services eventually have a practice composed of adult medicine and geriatrics. Therefore, if a family physician wants to ensure a broad base of young patients, OB should be considered.

THE PRACTICE SETTING

Family physicians have the opportunity to work in almost any practice setting. Location is often the first variable decided when choosing a practice. OB can be a part of nearly any practice setting in nearly every location (Table 23-1). Some areas are known to be more receptive to family physicians providing OB care, such as the midwest. Other areas may be less receptive, but OB care by family physicians may be found in less traditional sites such as residency teaching centers (Fig. 23-2) or extremely rural areas where OB care is limited.

WORKING WITH OBSTETRICAL CONSULTANTS

Part of providing quality OB care is timely referral. Thus, a good working relationship with OB consultants and local referral centers is essential. Contacting OB consultants should be done even before the decision is made on a practice location if you plan on practicing OB. A good working relationship with family physicians provides OB consultants with ready referrals for both OB and gynecologic surgery services.

MAKING THE CHOICE—IS OBSTETRICS FOR YOU?

Providing OB care can be a satisfying part of your practice (Fig. 23-3). It may help your patient population to be more diverse and well rounded. Providing OB care requires a personal commitment and a full understanding of how this will affect your personal and professional life. Given the sleepless nights and long hours spent in the hospital or on call, the desire to practice OB is special and OB practice is not meant for everyone. Having committed myself to this type of practice, I can truly say that the joy of delivering babies, watching them grow into adults, and then delivering their children is a special opportunity that only a family physician can fully appreciate.

TABLE 23-1

BABIES DELIVERED BY FAMILY PHYSICIANS IN 1997* BY CENSUS DIVISION AND PRACTICE LOCATION,† MAY

CENSUS DIVISION/ PRACTICE LOCATION	RESPONDENTS	PERCENT OF PHYSICIANS REPORTING THEY DELIVERED ONE OR MORE BABIES	MEAN NUMBER OF BABIES DELIVERED‡
Total	2,200	27.4	30.2
Urban	869	19.5	30.6
Rural	428	38.4	36.3
New England	207	29.0	26.0
Urban	85	20.0	26.7
Rural	37	18.9	36.4
Middle Atlantic	253	16.6	27.0
Urban	137	10.9	25.7
Rural	25	20.0	35.0
East North Central	273	31.1	30.3
Urban	113	23.9	30.4
Rural	47	53.2	33.2
West North Central	270	50.7	30.5
Urban	85	44.7	34.2
Rural	83	61.4	36.0
South Atlantic	237	15.2	26.5
Urban	80	10.0	18.9
Rural	35	11.4	37.5
East South Central	213	16.9	37.9
Urban	65	7.7	30.4
Rural	64	15.6	33.6
West South Central	230	21.3	39.6
Urban	93	14.0	42.5
Rural	52	32.7	46.5
Mountain	276	36.2	28.6
Urban	95	20.0	26.2
Rural	63	57.1	31.9
Pacific	241	32.4	28.5
Urban	116	24.1	31.4
Rural	22	45.5	39.9

* Includes only active member respondents of the American Academy of Family Physicians. Number of respondents in an urban or rural practice location may not add to the total number of respondents in the census division because some respondents in the census division did not report urban/rural practice location. Estimated percentages were adjusted by the sampling fraction and the response percentage for each division.

† Respondents were asked to indicate city and county of practice. ''Urban'' and ''Rural'' were determined based upon federal definition of counties as either metropolitan or non-metropolitan, except in New England and other selected cities where township or city determines a metropolitan area.

‡ By those physicians reporting that they delivered one or more babies.

From American Academy of Family Physicians: Facts About Family Practice. Kansas City, Missouri, American Academy of Family Physicians, 1998. By permission of the Academy.

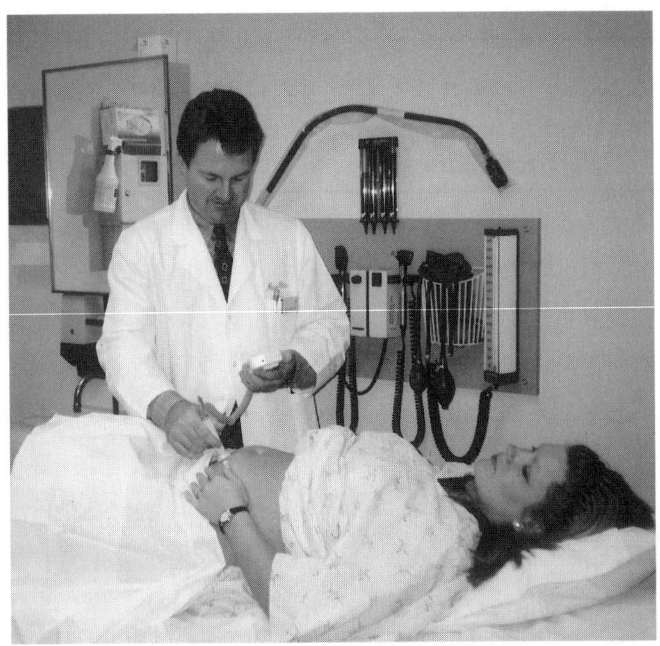

FIGURE 23-3
Family physicians find obstetric care rewarding because they develop lasting relationships with families.

REFERENCES

1. Bredfeldt RC, Sutherland JE, Wesley RM: Obstetrics in family medicine: effects on physician work load, income, and age of practice population. Fam Med 21:279, 1989

SUGGESTED READING

Mehl LE, Bruce C, Renner JH: Importance of obstetrics in a comprehensive family practice. J Fam Pract 3:385, 1976

Scherger JE: The family physician delivering babies: an endangered species. Fam Med 19:95, 1987

Smith MA, Howard KP: Choosing to do obstetrics in practice: factors affecting the decisions of third-year family practice residents. Fam Med 19:191, 1987

24

SPORTS MEDICINE IN FAMILY MEDICINE

Walter C. Taylor III, M.D.

Sports medicine can be integrated easily into the practice of family medicine. One must first acquire the necessary skills, as with any area of family medicine, to feel comfortable in evaluating and treating athletes. Depending on the physician's level of interest and needs, these skills can be developed during residency training, by fellowship training in sports medicine, or by continuing medical education courses after postgraduate training. One does not need to have completed a fellowship or to have obtained a certificate of added qualifications to achieve some level of sports medicine competency.

The practice of sports medicine within family medicine can vary from evaluating and treating athletes in a family practice office setting to evaluating these patients in a formal sports medicine clinic or facility. The latter usually requires a fellowship in sports medicine. The practice of sports medicine can involve athletes ranging from children involved in youth or scholastic sports to older persons trying to exercise for health reasons. Physicians may want to become team physicians, which can range from high school sports to collegiate or occasionally professional sports.

> *"Education must concern itself with the aspirations and needs of the common man."*
>
> —William J. Mayo

RESPONSIBILITIES OF SPORTS MEDICINE PHYSICIANS

Team physician duties vary with the needs of the school or organization and the amount of time the physician can spend in this role. Frequently, they are called on to perform preparticipation sports physicals as well as to provide medical coverage for various athletic events. In some cases, particularly on the collegiate and professional levels, the team physician is asked to provide one or several injury-related clinics per week. These services are often provided in the training room at the team's practice facility.

Compensation for these services varies from region to region, and some areas may be so competitive that the physician may have to volunteer time to be involved with a team. In some cases, physicians caring for professional teams pay large sums of money to have the opportunity to care for professional athletes and have their names associated with these teams. As they see it, it is an opportunity to add prestige and to publicize their practice. There are some colleges and universities (primarily National Collegiate Athletic Association Division I schools) that have salaried positions for full-time team physicians. Acting as a team physician can be an excellent way to build your family medicine practice, because you not only come in contact with student athletes but also with their families. Unfortunately, in most cases caring for athletes and their teams can be more or less a donation of time and effort for those who truly enjoy taking care of athletes.

Emergencies Facing Team Physicians

When providing sports event coverage, the physician must be comfortable in dealing with various emergencies: cardiac arrest, closed-head injuries (sometimes severe), neck injuries (with possible neurologic compromise), heat illness, and anaphylaxis (often to bee stings). In addition, the qualified team physician must deal with minor musculoskeletal injuries such as ankle sprains, shoulder dislocations, and various overuse injuries. Physicians are asked to determine whether or not the athlete can return to play after injury. Various people may place pressure on the injured athlete or physician for a premature return to play. These pressures may come from coaches, parents, or other players. Unfortunately, in some cases the athlete may be concerned about losing a scholarship opportunity if not able to play that particular game. The team physician must look out for the best interest of the athlete, so that a safe return to sports does not risk further injury.

Working with Trainers

Team physicians are responsible for coordinating the on-the-field care of the athlete. They may be the only medical provider on site. In many cases the physician works with an athletic trainer. These individuals have a college degree in athletic training and are certified by a national examination through the National Athletic Trainers Association. They are proficient in evaluation of on-the-field injuries and emergencies. The physician who is involved in sports medicine should come to understand the training and background of athletic trainers. The combined care from trainer and team physician can enhance the medical care provided to team-related sports. Adequate communication and appropriate delegation of duties between the two are qualities that best serve the athlete and team.

Emergencies in Sports Medicine

Despite adequate preparation and training, injuries are bound to occur. In a true emergency, the medical team including trainer and team physician must coordinate efforts to ensure the best outcome possible for a particular medical condition. It is important to know each individual's role in these unfortunate situations and to have discussed multiple scenarios before any actual event. The medical staff should know how to summon ambulance transport. For instance, where is the nearest telephone within the athletic venue and who will be responsible to make the 911 call while the medical team is attending the athlete. Other examples may include staff responsible for back and neck braces, staff responsible for taping ankles and wrists before competition, and staff specifically trained in the delivery of cardiopulmonary resuscitation and advanced cardiac life support. The American College of Sports Medicine's *ACSM's Guidelines for the Team Physician*[1] is a good reference, which gives some of the basics in this area.

Office-Based Sports Medicine

The office-based practice of sports medicine most often deals with athletes with simple musculoskeletal complaints but can also encompass exercise prescription, medical conditions affecting athletes, and exercise physiology. Examples of medical conditions affecting the athlete are exercise-induced asthma or anaphylaxis, exercise in people with diabetes, concussions, or exercise during pregnancy. The sports physician needs to become familiar with eating disorders, which can become a problem for some female athletes and rarely male athletes. It is important for the physician who deals with athletes to understand the athlete's sport as well as the physical and emotional demands required by that sport. This promotes better rapport between the athlete and the physician. Examples of physical demands of a sport involve the biomechanics of a certain activity, such as the tennis serve or golf swing;

BOX 24-1 SPORTS MEDICINE FELLOWSHIP PROGRAMS (FAMILY PRACTICE)*

Ball Memorial Hospital	Muncie, IN
Bayfront Medical Center Program	St. Petersburg, FL
Christiana Care Health Services Program	Newark, DE
Crozer-Keystone Health System Program	Springfield, PA
DeWitt Army Community Hospital Program	Bethesda, MD
Fairview Health System Program	Cleveland, OH
Franciscan Medical Center (Dayton) Program	Dayton, OH
Halifax Medical Center Program	Daytona Beach, FL
Hennepin County Medical Center Program	Minneapolis, MN
Indiana University School of Medicine Program	Indianapolis, IN
Kalamazoo Center for Medical Studies/Michigan State University Program	Kalamazoo, MI
Lutheran General Hospital Program	Park Ridge, IL
MacNeal Memorial Hospital Program	Berwyn, IL
Maine Medical Center Program	Portland, ME
Medical College of Wisconsin (St. Mary's) Program	Milwaukee, WI
Memorial Hospital of South Bend Program	South Bend, IN
Mercy Health System Program	Janesville, WI
Moses H. Cone Memorial Hospital Program	Greensboro, NC
Ohio State University Program	Columbus, OH
Palmetto Health Alliance-University of South Carolina School of Medicine Program	Columbia, SC
Providence Hospital and Medical Centers Program	Farmington Hills, MI
San Jose Medical Center Program	San Jose, CA
Shadyside Hospital/UPMC Program	Pittsburgh, PA

the strength and flexibility of a football or basketball player; or the endurance of a track star. Speaking in the vocabulary associated with their sport grabs the athletes' attention and increases their confidence in the treating physician.

EDUCATION IN SPORTS MEDICINE

Medical students interested in receiving training in sports medicine during residency should look for programs that have both office-based sports medicine and on-the-field team physician-based experiences, preferably under the direction of a family physician or primary care physician with significant experience in this field.

BOX 24-1 (CONTINUED)

Sharp HealthCare (La Mesa) Program	La Mesa, CA
Southern California Kaiser Permanente Medical Care (Fontana) Program	Fontana, CA
Sparrow Hospital Program	East Lansing, MI
St. Joseph's Medical Center of South Bend Program	South Bend, IN
Thomas Jefferson University Program	Philadelphia, PA
Toledo Hospital Program	Toledo, OH
UCLA Medical Center Program	Los Angeles, CA
UMDNJ-Robert Wood Johnson Medical School Program	New Brunswick, NJ
University of Alabama Medical Center (Huntsville) Program	Huntsville, AL
University of California (San Diego) Program	San Diego, CA
University of Maryland Program	Baltimore, MD
University of Michigan Program	Ann Arbor, MI
University of Oklahoma College of Medicine-Tulsa Program	Tulsa, OK
University of Oklahoma Health Sciences Center Program	Oklahoma City, OK
University of Pittsburgh Medical Center, St. Margaret Program	Pittsburgh, PA
University of Tennessee Medical Center at Knoxville Program	Knoxville, TN
University of Texas Health Science Center at San Antonio Program	San Antonio, TX
University of Texas Southwestern Medical Center (Methodist) Program	Dallas, TX
University of Washington Program	Seattle, WA
Wake Forest University School of Medicine	Winston-Salem, NC

*An up-to-date list can be accessed at the American Medical Association Web site (http://www.ama-assn.org), American Academy of Family Physicians (http://www.aafp.org/fellowships/), or Accreditation Council for Graduate Medical Education (http://www.acgme.org/).

Fellowships in Sports Medicine

Those who may want to consider fellowship training in sports medicine are individuals who are considering postgraduate positions in an academic family medicine or sports medicine practice or a university or collegiate full-time team physician position or those with a particular interest in this field (Box 24-1). It is wise to have significant sports medicine experience during medical school and residency when applying for these fellowships, because they have become competitive. It may help to have published on a sports medicine topic. One can obtain a listing of sports medicine fellowships, which go through a matching process similar to residency, from The American Medical Society for Sports Medicine, 11639 Earnshaw, Overland Park, KS 66210. The general application form for the sports medicine fellowship match can be obtained via this society. Another source for fellowship information is *The Physician in Sportsmedicine,*[2] which publishes a list of fellowships annually.

Fellowship training involves 1 and in some cases 2 years of training after residency. The structure of the programs varies somewhat, but most include primarily office-based sports medicine rotations with primary care and orthopedic sports medicine specialists. The fellow may rotate with other orthopedic specialists such as hand, foot, spine, and pediatric orthopedists. On the orthopedic rotations, the sports medicine fellow may be requested to make rounds and assist in surgery. Significant time is spent with the Primary Care Sports Medicine faculty during clinic and some sporting event coverage. There are usually rotations in cardiac stress testing and exercise physiology and some exposure to drug testing. There are many team physician or related opportunities at various levels. Some programs require a research project. A Certificate of Added Qualifications (CAQ) in Sports Medicine is available through the American Board of Family Practice. After 1999, one must have completed an accredited fellowship to sit for the CAQ examination (Box 24-2).

Sports Medicine Conferences

Another option for those family physicians who want to gain more knowledge and expertise in sports medicine is to attend continuing medical education courses related to the field. There are numerous courses on the topic of sports medicine in every region of the country. The American College of Sports Medicine sponsors ''The Team Physician'' course in 2 parts and an ''Advanced Team Physician'' course, which are excellent sources of information. In addition, the American Academy of Family Physicians and many regional and some local sports medicine clinics offer continuing medical education courses in sports medicine.

Sports Medicine Organizations

There are several professional organizations which those interested in sports medicine might want to consider joining. As a student, resident, or physician in practice, one can join the American College of Sports Medicine, P. O. Box 1440, Indianapolis, IN 46206-1440. This society is represented by exercise scientists, athletic trainers, physical therapists, physicians, and other health professionals involved in Sports Medicine. The American Medical Society for Sports Medicine (AMSSM) is composed of physicians, mostly those in primary care. To join the AMSSM, certain criteria must be met.

BOX 24-2 AMERICAN BOARD OF FAMILY PRACTICE REQUIREMENTS FOR CERTIFICATE OF ADDED QUALIFICATIONS IN SPORTS MEDICINE

SPORTS MEDICINE

The American Board of Family Practice participates in a joint program for certification in sports medicine. This Certificate of Added Qualifications (CAQ) in Sports Medicine examination is offered biennially in odd-numbered years in conjunction with programs sponsored by the American Board of Emergency Medicine, the American Board of Internal Medicine, and the American Board of Pediatrics.

REQUIREMENTS

1. Family physicians must be certified by the American Board of Family Practice and must be Diplomates in good standing at the time of the examination. The Diplomate must hold a valid and unrestricted license to practice medicine in the United States or Canada.
2. Family physicians must qualify through one of the following plans.

Plan I (Fellowship Pathway) A candidate must have completed a minimum of 1 year in a sports medicine fellowship program associated with an Accreditation Council for Graduate Medical Education-accredited residency in Emergency Medicine, Family Practice, Internal Medicine, or Pediatrics.

Plan II (Practice Pathway)* A candidate must have 5 years of practice experience consisting of at least 20% professional time devoted to sports medicine, defined as one or more of the following: 1) field supervision of athletes; 2) emergency assessment and care of acutely injured athletes; 3) diagnosis, treatment, management, and disposition of common sports injuries and illness; 4) management of medical problems in the athlete; 5) rehabilitation of ill and injured athletes; and 6) exercise as treatment. In addition, all candidates must show evidence of participation in 30 hours of sports medicine-related American Medical Association Category I (or its equivalent) continuing medical education during the past 5 years.

3. Diplomates must achieve a satisfactory score on a half-day written examination.

RECOGNITION OF SUCCESSFUL CANDIDATES

Successful CAQ candidates will be awarded the American Board of Family Practice CAQ. The certificate is valid for 10 years, at which time completion of a recertification process is required for renewal of the certificate.

LOSS OR EXPIRATION, REINSTATEMENT

Loss or expiration of primary certification in Family Practice automatically results in simultaneous loss of the CAQ. In cases in which a CAQ is lost as a result of loss of the primary certificate and later the primary certificate is reinstated, the CAQ will be reinstated for the remaining period, if any, as stated on the CAQ certificate.

American Board of Family Practice 1996 Directory of Diplomates, American Board of Family Practice, Lexington, KY 1996.

*This pathway will be available through the 1999 examination. After 1999, completion of a 1-year sports medicine fellowship will be required for eligibility.

Sports medicine fellows usually meet those criteria. Physicians who have not completed a fellowship may join but must have significant experience in sports medicine.

CONCLUSION

Sports medicine can be a rewarding aspect of family medicine. Some family physicians may choose sports medicine fellowships to further their educational endeavors, whereas others may be satisfied with serving as the local high school's team physician. The level of involvement varies. One of the most refreshing aspects of the practice of sports medicine is that athletic patients are usually highly motivated in their desire to get better. This can be a ray of sunshine to family physicians who see patients day in and day out who are sedentary, possess harmful habits, and lack motivation to improve their health. Family physicians involved in sports medicine can enhance their enjoyment of the practice of medicine while at the same time serving as role models for young athletes and providing much needed care.

REFERENCES

1. Cantu RC, Micheli LJ, editors: ACSM's Guidelines for the Team Physician. Philadelphia, Lea & Febiger, 1991
2. Anonymous: Sports medicine fellowships for physicians. Phys Sportsmed 25:118, Mar 1997

25

GERIATRICS IN FAMILY MEDICINE

Joseph W. Furst, M.D.

The field of geriatrics offers both great challenges and great rewards. Our population is aging. In light of this trend, the phrase ''squaring of the pyramid'' accurately defines this phenomenon. The phrase refers to the fact that there will be fewer younger people in the population and more older people in the years to come. In 1989, there were 31 million people older than age 65 years in the United States, and it is anticipated that by the year 2030, there will be 65.6 million[1] (Table 25-1).

As older Americans become more populous, demand for health care services will increase as well. Older Americans already account for more than one-third of health care expenses in this country. Forty-nine percent of noninstitutionalized persons age 65 years and older have arthritis, 37 percent have hypertension, 30 percent have some form of heart disease, and 9 percent have diabetes.[1]

The challenges offered by the field of geriatrics are obvious. There is a higher incidence of chronic illness, and many patients are affected by multiple medical problems. Further, the symptoms and signs of acute illness are often more subtle and difficult to detect in the elderly population. In addition, complicating social issues often compound the delivery of health care to the elderly. Truly, in treating the geriatric patient, one must use all of the honed skills of a family physician.

> *''The old should remember that they represent the past, and that the young represent the future.''*
>
> —William J. Mayo

TABLE 25-1
THE ELDERLY POPULATION OF THE UNITED STATES: TRENDS 1900-2050

	PERCENT OF THE TOTAL POPULATION						
AGE, YR	**1900**	**1940**	**1960**	**1990**	**2010**	**2030**	**2050**
65–74	2.9	4.8	6.1	7.3	7.4	12	10.5
75–84	1	1.7	2.6	4	4.3	7.1	7.2
85+	0.2	0.3	0.5	1.3	2.2	2.7	5.1
65+	4	6.8	9.2	12.6	13.9	21.8	22.9

From Kane RL, Ouslander JG, Abrass IB: Essentials of Clinical Geriatrics. Third edition. New York, McGraw-Hill, 1994, p.19–43, as adapted from US Senate, 1991.

REWARDS OF GERIATRIC CARE

Geriatric care can be very satisfying. I have debated with colleagues regarding what aspect of medicine provides the physician the greatest reward. Some say delivering a newborn child provides the greatest bond between physician and patient and, therefore, the greatest reward. Others say nurturing the growing child and educating new parents. Still others find interactions with patients of their own age most rewarding. No matter what our role becomes as family physicians, the feeling is universal: what we find most rewarding is simply being there for patients in need, whatever stage of life they are in, and whatever problem they bring to us. Geriatric patients, with a greater frequency of chronic illnesses, are seen more often, and their needs are substantially greater. The rewards, therefore, are greater as well.

CERTIFICATE OF ADDED QUALIFICATIONS IN GERIATRIC MEDICINE

In the 1970s and 1980s, most family practice programs had no formal geriatric rotations. As time passed and our patient demographics changed to a more elderly population, so has our focus in training family physicians. At Mayo Clinic Rochester, we are presently constructing a formal rotation in geriatric family medicine. This will include didactic lectures, hospital experience with geriatric patients, nursing home care, and an outpatient geriatric experience. The structure of the geriatric rotation is similar to the structure of a geriatric fellowship. Such fellowships have been established throughout the country

BOX 25-1 GERIATRIC MEDICINE FELLOWSHIP PROGRAMS (FAMILY PRACTICE)*

Ball Memorial Hospital Program	Muncie, IN
Case Western Reserve University (MetroHealth) Program	Cleveland, OH
East Carolina University Program	Greenville, NC
Florida Hospital Program	Orlando, FL
Georgetown University/Providence Hospital Program	Washington, DC
San Bernardino County Medical Center Program	San Bernardino, CA
Southern California Kaiser Permanente Medical Care (Los Angeles) Program	Los Angeles, CA
St. Joseph's Hospital and Medical Center Program	Phoenix, AZ
St. Lawrence Hospital and Health Care Services/Michigan State University Program	Lansing, MI
Thomas Jefferson University Program	Philadelphia, PA
UMDNJ-Robert Wood Johnson Medical School Program	Piscataway, NJ
University Hospital/University of Cincinnati College of Medicine Program	Cincinnati, OH
University of Minnesota Program	Minneapolis, MN
University of Missouri-Columbia Program	Columbia, MO
University of Missouri at Kansas City Program	Kansas City, MO
University of Pittsburgh Medical Center, St. Margaret Program	Pittsburgh, PA
University of Puerto Rico Program	Caguas, PR

*An up-to-date list can be accessed at the American Medical Association Web site at http://www.ama-assn.org.

and vary from institution to institution in duration and curriculum (Box 25-1). Rules set by the American Board of Family Practice (ABFP) require that one complete a 1-year geriatric fellowship before taking the ABFP-sanctioned examination for the Certificate of Added Qualifications (CAQ) in Geriatric Medicine.

The ABFP has offered a CAQ in geriatrics since 1988. As with other new certifications, grandfathering, which allowed those interested in receiving certification to sit for the examination without successfully completing a geriatric fellowship, was allowed for several years but ended in the early 1990s. The current examination is offered jointly by the ABFP and the American Board of Internal Medicine on a yearly basis. To date, there are 2,848 diplomates who have received CAQs in geriatric medicine.

Certification requirements for the geriatric CAQ include the following.

1. Family physicians must be certified by the ABFP and must be diplomates in good standing at the time of the examination.

2. The diplomate must hold a valid and unrestricted license to practice medicine in the United States or Canada.
3. Diplomates may qualify by satisfactorily completing a 2-year fellowship training program in Geriatric Medicine accredited by the Accreditation Council for Graduate Medical Education. Pending formal accreditation procedures by the Residency Review Committee, candidates completing a 1-year clinical Geriatric Fellowship Program may be accepted for examination on approval from the ABFP.
4. Diplomates must achieve a satisfactory score on a 1-day written examination.

(From The American Board of Family Practice Booklet of Information. Lexington, Kentucky, American Board of Family Practice, September, 1996. By permission of the publisher.)

The geriatric certification examination covers the following topics.

1. Biology of aging. The examination covers the biology of aging and longevity, including changes in drug metabolism, immunology, and nutritional requirements of the elderly. Epidemiology and research methodologies related to geriatric medicine are included.
2. Geriatric care issues. Issues specific to the care of the elderly are covered, including geriatric assessment; preventive medicine; management of patients in long-term care settings; and psychosocial, ethical, legal, and economic issues important to geriatric patients.
3. Medical diseases. Diagnosis and treatment of diseases that require a modified approach to management in the elderly are included. Situations of special concern are covered: falls and incontinence, preoperative assessment, and preoperative and postoperative management of geriatric patients. The examination encompasses all of the relevant organ systems and includes other specialty areas relevant to the practice of geriatric medicine such as otorhinolaryngology, ophthalmology, gynecology, and dermatology.
4. Neuropsychiatry. The examination covers relevant topics in neurology and psychiatry, including the diagnosis and management of cerebrovascular diseases, dementia, sensory impairment, and other cognitive and affective changes that occur with aging.
5. Clinical situations involving diagnosis, treatment, prognosis, etiology, and natural history of a disease are stressed. Interpretations of physiologic data, electrocardiograms, and imaging studies used in caring for a geriatric patient may be required.

The examination fee is $750.00. Successfully completing the examination results in a CAQ in Geriatric Medicine that is valid for 10 years. The examination schedule may be found on the Internet at the ABFP Web site: www.abfp.org or by contacting the American Board of Family Practice at 2228 Young Drive, Lexington, Kentucky 40505-4294 or by telephone at (888) 995-5700 extension 250.

Recertification Requirements

The recertification process for the Geriatric Medicine certificate is completed over a 2-year period and may begin in the 8th year of the certificate. Requirements include:

1. current primary certification in family practice at the time of the examination
2. completion of a geriatric recertification preapplication form and submission of an application fee
3. successful completion of 3 Self-Evaluation Process (SEP) modules (see below)
4. completion of a formal geriatric examination application form with an accompanying examination fee
5. verification that all licenses held in the United States and Canada are currently valid, full, and unrestricted
6. successful completion of a half-day cognitive examination.

The Self-Evaluation Process modules are at-home open-book examinations of 60 questions each. All candidates must successfully complete 3 modules to be eligible to sit for the examination. The SEP modules will be scored and feedback will be provided on the incorrect answers. No references to the literature will be given with the feedback. Should a candidate be unsuccessful on any of the SEP modules, the candidate will be required to repeat the particular module until successful.
(From The American Board of Family Practice Booklet of Information. Lexington, Kentucky, American Board of Family Practice, September, 1996. By permission of the publisher.)

Geriatric Rotations

In the late 1980s and early 1990s when family physicians were grandfathered for the CAQ in geriatric medicine, it was suggested in the application process to ''immerse'' oneself in the geriatric literature to prepare for the examination. Now, there are many educational opportunities to participate in that are relevant to geriatric medicine. At the Mayo Clinic, we are structuring a resident's experience to include a formal rotation in geriatrics, but we plan to provide a longitudinal experience as well, mostly centered around the care of elderly patients in nursing homes. There is some didactic interactive experience which takes place over 3 years, but primarily, the longitudinal experience is in the nursing home setting. We believe that longitudinal experience is paramount. Residents who see nursing home patients on an itinerant basis spend most of their time in the interaction gathering information, rather than learning from the interaction. We believe that a resident's nursing home responsibilities must include: assigning patients earlier in the residency experience so that the resident will be responsible for patients' care over the entire 3 years of residency training. Given the schedules associated with residents' rotations, it is imperative that there is a team approach to the care of nursing home patients in case the individual resident is unavailable for monthly rounds from time to time. This helps ensure quality of care when continuity is lacking.

"At the close of a man's life, to estimate his worth it is wise to see him in relation to his life surroundings, to know not only the part he played as an individual, but also as a component part of the great events to which he contributed in the betterment of mankind."

—William J. Mayo

NURSING HOME ROUNDS

Many family practice residency programs have nursing home rounds, which usually are held once monthly (Fig. 25-1). This educational experience is centered around residents doing their geriatric rotations. The patients seen on these rounds have other primary physicians who follow them over time, but they would be seen on monthly rounds by the resident physician during the 1-month geriatric rotation. The geriatric resident and accompanying family medicine staff member meet these patients for an itinerant but prolonged interaction and make recommendations as to what further might be done to solve the problems at hand. The process amounts to getting a consult from colleagues in family medicine. Although there is some lack of continuity, the patient's care is often improved by having essentially a second opinion on the treatment and management of the patient. This interaction provides an excellent learning opportunity for the resident on the geriatric rotation.

"Long ago I learned from my father to put old people to bed only for

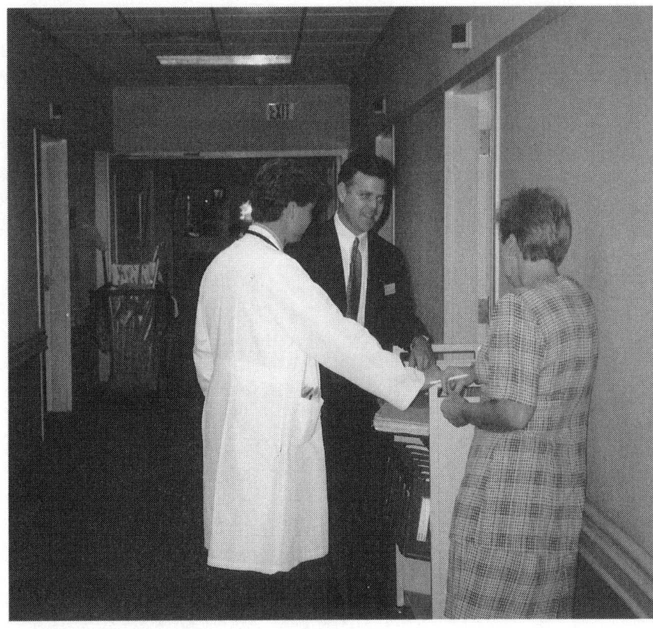

FIGURE 25-1
Family physicians often take care of nursing home patients. Patients are scheduled to be seen once a month or more often if they have complications or concerns.

as short a time as was absolutely necessary, for they were like a foundered horse, if they got down it was difficult for them to get up, and their strength ebbed away very rapidly while in bed.''

—Charles H. Mayo

On monthly rounds day, it is expected that the resident on the geriatric rotation provides an in-service presentation related to nursing home care to the nursing home staff. Requests are taken regarding what topics the nursing home staff would like covered, and there is an effort to produce a program of use to them.

ADDITIONAL GERIATRIC ISSUES

Other issues pertinent to the care of geriatric patients include living wills and the right to die. As family physicians, we are called on to address these important aspects of medical care with our patients. In most cases, the family physician has provided the most comprehensive care to the patient and the family, and it is important to discuss and plan for death. In addition, the family physician may be called on to make decisions regarding an elderly

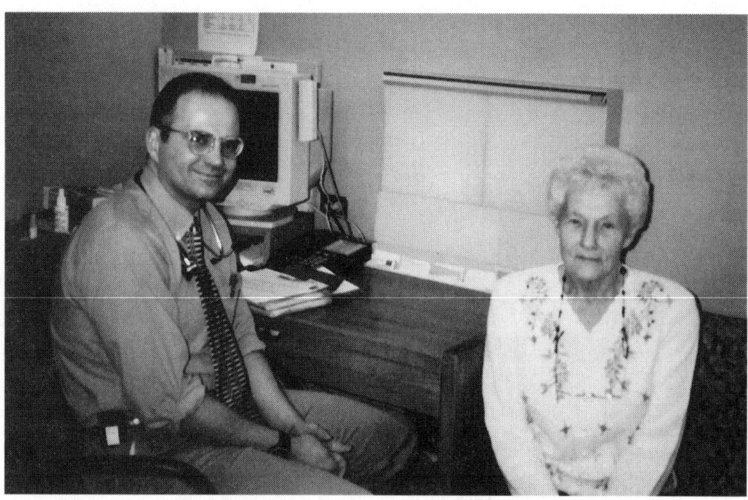

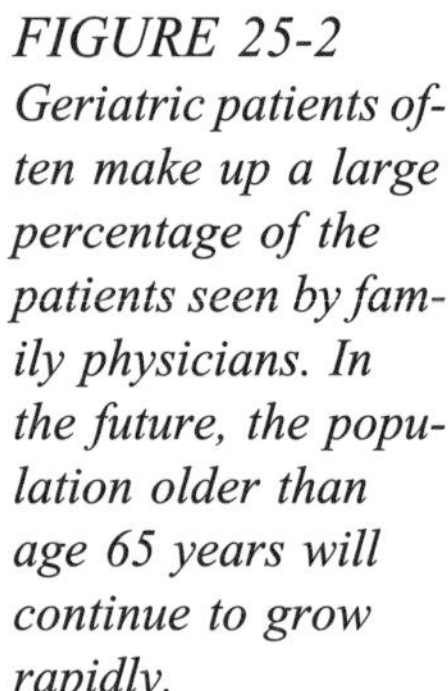

FIGURE 25-2
Geriatric patients often make up a large percentage of the patients seen by family physicians. In the future, the population older than age 65 years will continue to grow rapidly.

patient's mental competence and abilities for self-care at home. In these difficult situations the family physician must remain impartial but proactive in doing what is best for the patient. Providing education and resources to families in need may also be asked of a family physician, and it is important to remain knowledgeable of social service assistance programs, group counseling, and other assistance programs that may help patients or families.

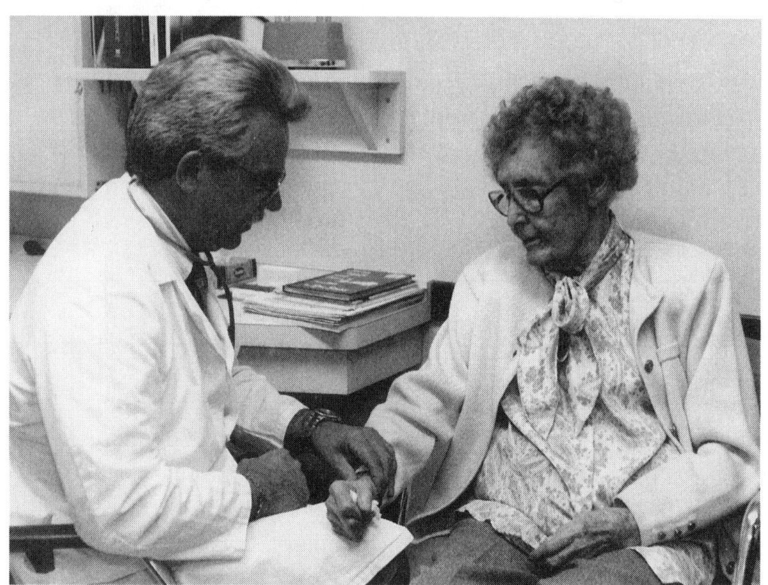

FIGURE 25-3
Family physicians often provide comfort and companionship to their older patients.

Armed with this type of knowledge, the family physician can provide superior care to the elderly population.

CONCLUSION

Geriatrics is going to become a larger part of all of our practices in the coming years (Fig. 25-2). The elderly have specific issues that need to be addressed, and the well-trained family physician is in a position to address their concerns and provide their comprehensive medical care. The challenges are substantial, but the rewards are commensurate (Fig. 25-3). Plan ahead for the demographic changes that are about to take place and remain abreast of pertinent geriatric issues. In the long run, it will make you a better family physician and an advocate for superior health care in our ever-changing medical environment.

REFERENCE

1. Fowles DG: Profile of Older Americans: 1990. Washington, DC, American Association of Retired Persons, 1990

26

MANAGED CARE

Robert E. Nesse, M.D.

In the 1990s, medical providers, including family physicians, have seen tumultuous and often chaotic change in health care systems as purchasers, payers, providers, and government work to adapt to the new demands of a troubled health care system. The accelerating pace of change and the sense of unease and foreboding among virtually all participants in health care suggest that current systems have not adequately aligned incentives and rewards with a professional obligation to provide high quality care that meets the best interests of the patient.

Health care reform must evolve to support the medical mission and provide an adequate market support for medical practice. Crawshaw et al.[1] defined medicine as "at its center, a moral enterprise grounded in a covenant of trust." This fundamental grounding of the medical profession is, in some circumstances, threatened by reimbursement systems that reward decreased use of health care services without accountability for quality, move patients between caregivers as a block, and then dehumanize the system by applying business standards and terminology to the patient-physician interaction.[2]

The medical care delivery system has failed to make a timely transition to effective practice patterns that meet society's needs for cost efficiency, service, and accountability. Health care delivery systems promoting cost discounting with only vague references to patient satisfaction and quality are opposed by systems that continue high system utilization with excessive cost and questionable interventions and provide only vague references to patient satisfaction and quality.

Health care providers often have limited their potential for influence in the managed care environment owing to a lack of understanding of the issues that led to the development of managed care systems. In addition, they fail to recognize that the change is incomplete and there is still a significant opportunity to influence the new changes that are developing.

The terms "managed care" and "health maintenance organization" (HMO) are not synonymous. HMOs are a diverse assembly of health care finance or delivery groups (or both) that have various models for payment and cost control. The development of these new systems and the other diverse support systems for managed care delivery has been accompanied by a new vocabulary that frustrates and baffles even the most knowledgeable physicians. (A glossary of common managed care terms is included in Box 26-1.) However, for most providers it is far more important to understand the forces of reform and to use this information to formulate a response that is best for the combination of forces present in the local and regional market than to spend time working to become familiar with all of the arcane details of health care finance.

This chapter explores the major players responsible for changes in the health care system and examines the essentials of success for managed care provider activities.

"Health has come to be generally recognized as an economic principle."

—Charles H. Mayo

MAJOR PLAYERS RESPONSIBLE FOR CHANGES IN HEALTH CARE

In recent years, the rapid change in the health care system has made it difficult to focus on the organizations and groups that have had a lasting involvement in the transformation of health care. However, there are some groups that are fundamentally involved, including government, health care insurance industry and HMOs, business payers, patients, and providers. The following is a review of these important players and the influence they have had in health care reform.

Government

In the early 1990s, the Clinton administration's plans for a central government-managed health care system failed to gain the approval of Congress and the American people. In spite of this failure of government-dictated reforms, the interest of federal and state government in health care is unabated. By its nature, government's interest is usually expressed through

BOX 26-1 GLOSSARY OF TERMS

Any Willing Provider—any provider who is willing to accept a health plan's terms and conditions. Any Willing Provider Laws mandate health plans to accept all such providers in the health plan.

Benefits Design—the specific set of services members are entitled to use in their health plan.

Capitation—a payment system in which a provider is given an amount of money per person usually per month to provide specific services for health plan members, regardless of the number of services provided.

Case Management—a plan developed for patients with special needs to help coordinate and manage their care.

Carve-Out—specific services that are paid separately from those covered under a capitation agreement. These services are usually paid on a fee schedule or discounted fee-for-service basis.

Case Mix—the range of sex, age, health status and illness severity of patients for which a health plan or health care organization is responsible.

Coinsurance—usually a significant portion of an HMO bill (*20–50 percent for example*) that is paid by the health plan subscriber to obtain certain medical services. Usually these services are considered by the HMO to be optional. The coinsurance is usually much greater than a copayment.

Copayment—the portion of the patient's bill paid to the provider at the time of service (*$10 per specialty visit, for example*).

Community Rating—a method of calculating the health care premiums of a defined community, or group of people, based on the anticipated utilization of health care services. Currently, most health insurance companies do not use community rating to establish health care premiums.

Concurrent Utilization Review—a review of the medical necessity of a service to determine if a patient's needs justify continued inpatient care. Named concurrent review because the review occurs at the time of service.

Deductible—the amount of individual or family out-of-pocket expense which must be incurred before the activation of insurance coverage. Typically, a higher deductible amount results in a lower monthly premium amount.

Discharge Planning—the process of establishing a plan to meet a patient's needs after discharge from a hospital or nursing facility. The discharge plan typically defines both medical and nonmedical services patients will benefit from after discharge from an inpatient facility.

Disease Management—a program in which groups of patients with specific disease processes are involved with direct interventions and educational programs aimed at improving medical and functional outcomes.

Drug Formulary—the specific list of drugs that a health plan will cover as part of the benefits package.

Experience Rating—a method of calculating the health care premium for a defined group of individuals (*employees*) based on the sex, age and health status of the employees as well as the specific company and nature of the company's business. The expected ''experience'' of the group establishes their anticipated use of medical services and the resulting premium level required to cover that use.

Gatekeeper—typically a primary care physician or case manager who controls a patient's access to other health care services.

BOX 26-1 (Continued)

Generic Medication—drugs that have the same chemical equivalents as a brand name drug. Generic medications are typically prescribed as a less costly alternative for patients because they are generally cheaper than the brand name medications.

Health Risk Assessments—written or telephonic surveys used by health plans to prospectively identify patients with special medical or other needs.

HEDIS (*Health Plan Employer Data and Information Set*)—a core set of performance measures designed to help employers understand the value of their health care dollar and to hold health plans accountable for performance. HEDIS is sponsored by the National Committee for Quality Assurance (NCQA).

Home Health Care—health care services provided to people in their homes. Coverage for home health care services varies from insurer to insurer. Typically services justified by medical necessity are covered, whereas those with no medical justification (eg, bathing, dressing, cooking, etc.) are not covered.

Hospice Services—services for terminally ill patients, including counseling and health care services that give the dying patient and patient's family comfort. Hospice services focus on assisting the patient and family through the end of life process rather than on sustaining life through continued medical care.

Independent Practice Association (*IPA*)—independent physicians or physician offices linked for purposes of contracting, quality, or other interests of mutual benefit.

Lock-In—a term used when a member in an HMO must use only those physicians, hospitals, or other health care facilities in the health plan. Services received outside of the HMO providers listing are generally not covered by the plan except in the case of an emergency.

Mandated Benefits—services required by the state legislature to operate a health plan in the state.

Out-of-Pocket—the portion of health care services patients pay for with personal funds. Insurers often define out-of-pocket limits that govern the maximum amount of money patients would be responsible to cover for deductibles, copayments, or other expenses over a certain period.

Per Member Per Month (*PMPM*)—the amount of money a health plan or provider receives per covered person per month.

Physician Hospital Organization (*PHO*)—a linkage of physician or physician offices and a hospital for purposes of contracting, quality, or other interests of mutual benefit.

Physician Profile—a summary of a physician's or group of physicians' prescribing and utilization patterns usually derived from claims paid on patients cared for by the physician or physician group.

Point Of Service Option (*POS*)—affords HMO members the option of utilizing out of plan providers and facilities. POS options usually cost more and were created to offer people more flexibility in their managed care plans.

Preadmission Review—a review before hospital admission to verify that the admission is medically necessary and appropriate.

Preferred Provider Organization (*PPO*)—health plan which gives patients lower rates for health care services if they utilize the physicians in the PPO network. Patients may still use providers outside of the preferred group, but usually they pay more for the health care services if they do.

BOX 26-1 (Continued)

Premium—the money a company or person pays a health plan every month for health insurance coverage. Premiums are adjusted based on sex, age, health status, number of family members, and other related factors.

Prior Authorization (*Precertification*)—a cost-control procedure that requires certain services or medications be approved in advance by the insurer. If prior authorization is not obtained, the health plan generally will refuse payment for the service or medication.

Provider Incentives—financial rewards built into the health care system to encourage providers to perform a certain way.

Provider Network—a group of providers who work together under contract to provide services to a group of patients.

Quality Assurance—a review process to determine if patients have received care within preestablished standards. Quality assurance also reviews and corrects problems in other parts of the health plan or health care system.

Referral—a process of transferring patient care from one provider to another based on the patient's specific condition and the provider's expertise.

Retrospective Utilization Review—a review of the medical necessity of a service to determine if a patient's needs justified the services provided. A retrospective review takes place after the services have occurred.

Risk Analysis—an examination of the expected health care utilization by a particular group or employer to define the appropriate benefits package and associated rate for the group.

Risk Sharing—a term used when hospitals and other health care providers share in the financial risk of providing services by receiving a set amount for providing specific services to a population.

Service Ratio (*Loss Ratio*)—the difference between the money received in premiums and the money spent on claims and administrative and other expenses.

UCR (*Usual & Customary Rates*)—the standard health care fees in a community or area. Fees for health care services vary by state, within state, and even within communities. The UCR establishes payment for services based on the standard fees within the community.

Utilization Management—the process health plans use to determine the appropriateness of the treatment a patient is receiving.

24-Hour Nurseline—a telephone service staffed by registered nurses designed to provide advice and direction on medical conditions phoned in by health plan members.

Modified from Gorman RS, editor: Managed Care Primer. Rochester, Minnesota, Mayo Foundation for Medical Education and Research, 1998, pp 45–48.

regulatory actions, and it is clear that government policy will continue to stimulate the growth of managed care and mandate measurement of care effectiveness and cost. In addition, it will intervene with regulations when the public's interest is not being served.

The 1998 Balanced Budget Act imposed sweeping change in the federal program for Medicare and Medicaid. Average annual patient cost calculations

(AAPCC) will be modified to decrease the inequity in calculation between counties. This will be done through a blending of local and national expenses when the AAPCC is calculated and will impose a new nationwide base rate for the AAPCC of approximately $370. The increase in money available for Medicare managed care reimbursement surely will stimulate growth in this area. At the end of 1996, several states had Medicaid experimental projects in which large percentages of the Medicaid population of the state were moved into managed care delivery systems. The population was introduced to these managed care plans by offering a new plan as a choice to improve services and reimbursement or through the direct method of mandating participation for Medicaid coverage. In 1997, 12 percent of the Medicare population and 40 percent of the Medicaid population was involved in some form of managed care.[3]

In view of this, it is obvious that the federal government continues to hold tight reigns over our health care system and may eventually provide additional regulations for the delivery of health care.

Medical Insurance Companies and Health Maintenance Organizations

A cursory look at the financial status of the health insurance and HMO industry in the early 1990s could easily have led to the impression that this industry was poised to drive health system change without major interference. In 1992, HMO assets were at record high levels and capital reserves approached record levels as well. Americans in the 1990s continued to join HMOs in record numbers (Fig. 26-1).

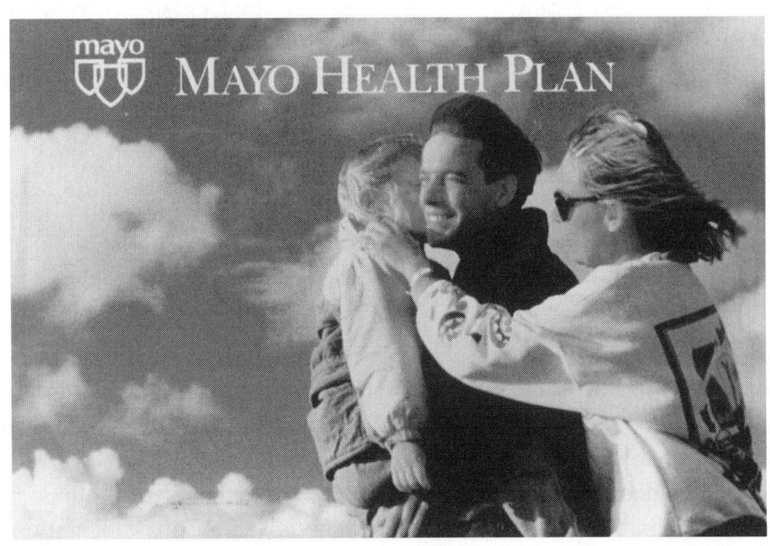

FIGURE 26-1 Mayo Clinic, realizing the importance of managed care, has formed its own health maintenance organization. Typically, members of HMOs are younger and actively working. (By permission of SuperStock Images.)

However, in the late 1990s, it is apparent that this segment of the health care industry is challenged and struggling to adapt. The Minneapolis/St. Paul, Minnesota, market has been considered an advanced HMO market on the basis of the percentage of population covered in the metropolitan area. The system is now consolidated so just 3 major insurance and delivery systems (Medica, HealthPartners, and Blue Plus) are in control of 92 percent of the HMO market, with a combined operating revenue of more than 2 billion dollars. However, in spite of this market maturity, there was significant instability and financial chaos. From 1995 to 1996, Medica lost 51.8 million dollars on clinical operations. HealthPartners and Blue Plus lost 29.6 and 5.2 million dollars, respectively. In addition, in 1997 several national managed care companies such as Oxford Health Care, PacifiCare, and Aetna lost money on clinical operations. These losses were the result of inaccurate predictions of how many services the covered population would need (the medical loss ratio).[4]

Recent HMO growth overwhelmingly favored independent practice associations (IPAs) over the more controlled staff and group model HMOs. The IPA model has burdened HMO organizations with the challenge of cost control. This system, without any direct control over the clinical care process, reinforced a growing public perception that HMO incentives for return on investment and decreased use of services outweighed the patient's best interest for quality care. HMOs are responding with a renewed emphasis on outcomes reporting and plan accountability. Whether reports of health care plan data can, in and of themselves, improve and distinguish provider performance when there is as much as 80 percent provider overlap between HMO plans remains to be seen.

Patients

The financial woes of the medical insurance industry are expanded into a larger issue by the restiveness of patients unsure of who to trust with their health. Jane Bryant Quinn addressed this problem in an opinion/editorial piece in *Newsweek* titled, ''Is Your HMO Ok—or Not?''[5] She wrote ''HMOs' own happy-patient surveys are almost entirely self-serving. The medical data that exist don't measure what we most want to know—namely, which plan delivers better results. . . .'' Dr. Regina Herzlinger spoke about the fundamental problems in many health care systems when she wrote, ''the creators of these new organizations were so blinded by the vision of the dazzling new world they hoped to forge that they neglected the details of management that would breathe life into their vision.''[6]

Despite these revelations, patients have joined managed care organizations in record numbers, and there are presently more than 75 million Americans in managed care organizations. Yet they are demanding provider choice and service delivery much as they did in more open and traditional systems. In Minnesota, 32 percent of the patients in HMOs reported they believed the health care delivery system was worse off because of the presence of managed care in the state.[7]

Business Payers

In the United States, health care expense for most employees is considered to be a work benefit and is paid by the business employer. In the 1980s, employers saw their percentage of income devoted to health care costs increase dramatically. In the face of mounting liability, the business employer has evolved from a largely passive purchaser of health care benefits from an insurance vendor to an active and aggressive managed care advocate.

The 1990s have seen a remarkable increase in big business and business coalition's direct involvement in health care reform. The Advisory Board Group of Washington, DC, has done research suggesting that, by the year 2000, 30 percent of the nation's employees will have their health care choices defined for them by a business health care coalition.

In Minneapolis/St. Paul, Minnesota, a large employer group (Buyers Health Care Action Group) has worked to change the current system and return competition to the providers. Through the use of a modified voucher system, the business group has begun to allow patients to choose from several care systems which, among them, include the vast majority of physicians in the metropolitan area. The HMO and insurance industry serves as a third-party administrator. These employers recognized that HMO channeling of patients was moving the system to consolidation of provider systems and generic care. They thought that competition at a provider level served their employees better.

This managed competition model for care delivery ultimately depends on a defined contribution toward a health care premium and on the employees and their families choosing from an approved list of care providers that can accept the patients. The patients are expected to choose the provider based on their perceptions of the value of the care offered and may pay more or less out-of-pocket money depending on the difference between the contribution from the insurance plan and the provider charges. In other words, the insurance company pays only so much money for a diagnosis and the patient has the choice of selecting a provider from an approved list of physicians.

The patient is then responsible for payment above what is contributed by the insurance company if the fee for service surpasses the insurance company's contribution.

The interests of employer groups in care value and new systems development have been stated clearly. Although still viewed with skepticism by some, the demands for integrated accountable health care have been expressed by business groups throughout the country. The full impact has yet to be realized.

Providers

The response of providers to the acceleration of health care reform has been fragmented and chaotic. This reflects the diversity of provider systems and the characteristic independence of professional organizations. However, it is fundamentally wrong to assume that the slow and disorganized approach to health care system reform by some providers represents an ignorance of the need to develop new systems or an active sabotage of current systems. Provider groups have a common professional bond but disparate financial and cultural models, which may impede rapid fundamental change.

In addition to group differences, the nation's health care markets vary widely. Market penetration by managed care is highest on the West Coast, with significant market shares owned by for-profit HMOs. On the other hand, in the Upper Midwest, Minnesota represents an advanced market, with for-profit HMOs prohibited by law. Therefore, health care markets are diverse and complicated—often by government regulation.

The size of medical groups also varies widely, and the primary care-specialist relationship varies by region of the country. In addition, whether groups are single specialty or multispecialty group models and whether they have professional administration or close relationships with insurers also varies by region of the country.

To allow for any coordinated action by providers without the specter of antitrust regulation requires that the providers examine the fundamental forces of health care markets, the essence of patient needs, and rekindle their personal involvement and resolve to provide care in the best interests of the patients, recognizing that this must include public accounting of both the quality and cost of the care.

THE FOCUS AND PRINCIPLES OF HEALTH CARE REFORM

Underlying trends driving and shaping health care reform include increased consumer concern about health care and health care service quality; increased

TABLE 26-1
DIMENSIONS OF CARE THAT INFLUENCE PATIENT EXPERIENCE

Respect for personal needs
Coordination and integration of care
Communication
Physical care and comfort
Emotional support

Adapted from Gerteis M: What patients really want. Health Manage Q 15 no. 3:2–6, 1993.

competition among providers for adequate market share; and increased demands for specific patient and system information on care, revenue, quality, and cost effectiveness.

It is essential that all of the health care industry work to integrate systems and respond to these market demands in a coordinated, coherent fashion. Within the system, it is essential that patients be arbiters of their own care; their expectations and what they consider high quality have been studied. The 5 dimensions of caregiving that most affect patients are listed in Table 26-1.

Providers deal with significant challenges in meeting expectations, and their investment and work to improve the system are essential. Many managed care systems impose demands on providers that physicians believe threaten the physician-patient relationship or impose numbing and mindless regulation on the system. Table 26-2 lists the top 10 managed care hassles dealt with daily by many physicians. It is essential to address these challenges to satisfy both patients and providers in the system. Alignment of incentives is necessary for any system to flourish long term.

New health care systems need to evolve to a point of collaboration among business, providers, patients, payers, and government. To accomplish this, it is necessary to address the need for change at a fundamentally different level. Current systems of health care have clearly recognized the inefficiencies of caregivers and the clumsiness of HMOs as they try to influence provider-patient interactions. Duplication of services, inefficient use of pharmaceuticals and formulary products, needless referrals and other care delivery foibles increase health care costs. However, it has never been clear that increasing regulation of caregivers and insurers will ever lead to the cost breakthroughs needed for our future. Indeed, it seems apparent that the fundamental reason

TABLE 26-2
MANAGED CARE HASSLES FOR PROVIDERS

Authorization and referrals
Utilization review
Termination from plan
No pay, slow pay, low pay
Repeated requests for information
Professional credentialing
Formularies
Data collection and paperwork
Records review
Difficulty getting tests done in a timely manner

Modified from Keister LW: Managed care hassles—a fact of life? Managed Care 6:55–58, June 1997. By permission of Stezzi Communications.

for the generation of costs in the first place is patient care or interventions to prevent a disease. To approach this level of system understanding requires that all interested parties unite against a common foe (disease) and work to manage caregiving with documented quality and efficiency while allowing caregivers to operate in an innovative and effective manner.

The essentials for success in managed care delivery are listed in Table 26-3. They include, first and foremost, a provider commitment to patient service and accountability for the cost and quality of services delivered. Current health care systems do not yet fully support new incentives, and providers must work to improve and evaluate their practice as a routine activity.

> *"We have never been allowed to lose sight of the fact that the main purpose to be served by the Clinic is the care of the sick."*
>
> —William J. Mayo

TABLE 26-3
ESSENTIALS FOR SUCCESS IN MANAGED CARE

Provide superior patient service, courtesy, and access
Support and document practice quality and cost; develop value (quality/cost) equation for your practice
Use principles of managed care for the entire practice
Support practice innovation every day
Develop data resource for practice evaluation

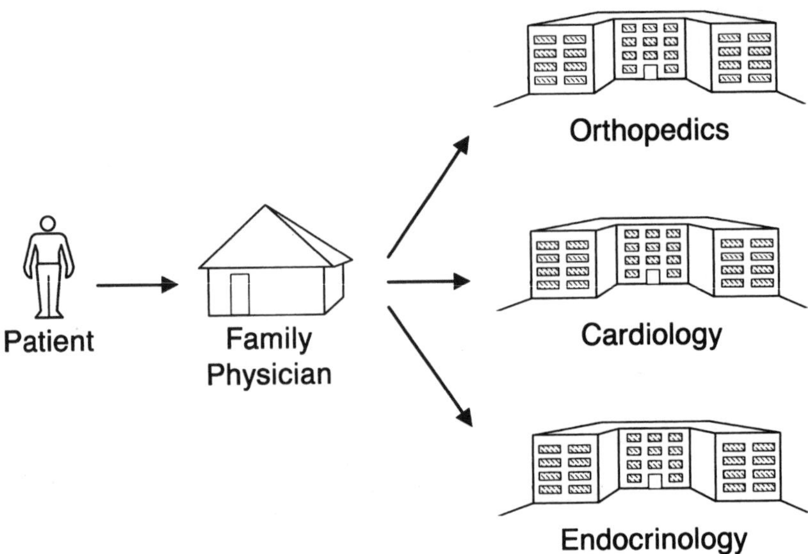

FIGURE 26-2
Gatekeeper model. This type of health care delivery requires the patient to seek the care of a family physician before any referral is allowed to a specialist. Often criticized, this type of model limits open access to care and potentially creates an adversarial relationship with the patient.

Family physicians have a primary care focus and continuing involvement in their patients' lives. They are often asked by the patient to serve as the manager for health system access and are trusted as honest brokers for the delivery of health care. This has led to the gatekeeper model in which the primary care provider is entrusted with the decision of when or when not to refer patients to specialists (Fig. 26-2). Any referral must be approved by the patient's primary physician. As expected, this often criticized system has not developed as fully as planned owing to the patient demands for open access and choice which have imposed an adversarial aspect on the physician-patient relationship and have raised the concerns of both parties. In the future, it is likely that sophisticated health care-based research will help to define the best medical and economic outcomes and relate them to the provider and the type of health care system used. Now, however, the data are not conclusive and turf wars emerge as medical-related political organizations promote their constituents. In view of these controversies, it is prudent for the family physicians in these circumstances to remember that their interests are the best interests of their patients and to err on the side of patient service and avoid financial relationships that openly threaten their values and mission.

CONCLUSION

The end of the 20th century may provide an opportunity for the health care provider and especially family physicians to respond proactively and creatively to meet patients' expectation for high-quality, cost-effective care. Patients who select a physician do so with a basic trust that the physician's overriding concern is for their health and well-being. The ultimate judges of the success of managed care will not be on Wall Street—rather they will be on Main Street in our own cities and towns, where we as family physicians provide care to the patients we know. Our patients and those who assist them with the financing of their care expect from family physicians and other primary care providers that we respect their concerns and meet their interests for cost-effective and quality health care. As family physicians dedicated to the practice of medicine, we owe them no less.

REFERENCES

1. Crawshaw R, Rogers DE, Pellegrino ED, Bulger RJ, Lundberg GD, Bristow LR, Cassel CK, Barondess JA: Patient-physician covenant. JAMA 273:1553, 1995
2. Pellegrino ED: First annual Nicholas J. Pisacano Lecture. Words can hurt you: some reflections on the metaphors of managed care. J Am Board Fam Pract 7:505, 1994
3. Managed Care Digest Series 1997. Kansas City, Missouri, Hoechst Marion Roussel, 1997
4. Solberg C: Managed carnage. Corporate Report Minnesota 28:33–34, 1997
5. Quinn JB: Is your HMO Ok—or not? Newsweek p 52, Feb 10, 1997
6. Herzlinger RE: The failed revolution in health care—the role of management. Harvard Business Rev 67 no. 2:95, 1989
7. Minnesota poll: plan members and doctors rate health care organizations. Star Tribune (Minneapolis, MN) p 20, Dec 7, 1997

27

POLITICS IN FAMILY MEDICINE

Benjamin W. Chaska, M.D.

Family physicians have always been involved in politics. Evidence to support the involvement of physicians in the political process can be traced back for millennia. Family practice as currently formulated resulted from a coordinated, well-organized political process. Much of what family physicians do in their daily practice is the result of a political process. The fact that we call ourselves family physicians rather than general practitioners is because of politics. Much of what we often believe to be science-based medical practice is really a product of a political process. Even those situations which are apparently scientific are usually the consequence of a political process of one kind or another. Who you work with, your own job, how you perform in your workplace, what kind of opportunities you receive, how much you are paid, where you work, who your patients are—in short, everything you do—is the result of some sort of political process. Whether you realize it or not you are actively involved in the political process. There are two kinds of people: those who are consciously involved (those who develop policy) and those who are not consciously involved (those who are affected by policy). The remainder of this chapter discusses ways in which you can become consciously involved in the political process.

TYPES OF POLITICS

So how do you become active in politics? As you can see, you really already are. What follows is a discussion of how you can become conscious of the political world around you and how you can become involved in politics. To begin with, there are many kinds and levels of politics. There are interpersonal politics, organizational politics, local politics, regional politics, and national and international politics. And there is medical politics. For those of us in the medical profession, there is influence from each arena that ultimately affects our lives.

Interpersonal Politics

Examples include relationships with colleagues and acquaintances in daily life. A conscious awareness and participation in interpersonal politics can bring you personal rewards and allow you to fulfill your dreams. Communication skills and dependability are keys for success. Lack of participation can result in professional and personal isolation, stagnation, and frustration as you pursue your goals. Others more involved will achieve what you had hoped to do.

Organizational Politics

Examples include hospital or institutional departments. Organizational politics can help you personally and can benefit your immediate working environment. If you do not participate in this game, it is unlikely that your personal and group goals will be achieved.

Local Politics

Examples include your local medical society, local political party, and perhaps city government. Local politics involve participation with people beyond your personal group. Your active participation with local politics helps to position your group within the community. Failure to recognize this dimension and actively be involved can lead to organizational frustration and failure. Active participation, when done well, can help you and your organization achieve your goals.

Regional Politics

Examples include your state or regional medical society and state government. Regional politics involves participation with people beyond your community. The region may be as few as a couple of cities or may include one or more states. Participation at this level can help your community and organization succeed. It also allows you to network with others like you and can offer opportunities to you that you did not anticipate.

National and International Politics

Examples include national medical organizations such as the American Medical Association or the American Academy of Family Physicians and national government. National and international political involvement directly helps your region, state, community, and organization. At this level, you determine general standards for large groups. This is where the decisions are made about who does what, where, when, how, and how much is paid for what you do. Failure to participate effectively at this level results in loss of autonomy, prestige, income, and opportunity for you, your organization, your city, state, and region.

GENERAL VS. SPECIAL INTEREST GROUPS

Many political organizations have structures at each of these levels. You can become involved in one or more types of political organization at one or more levels (Fig. 27-1). From the broadest viewpoint, there are 2 types of political organizations: those that include the general public and those limited to a special interest group. Examples of general public organizations include the Democratic, Republican, Libertarian, and other political parties. Examples of special interest groups include groups related to such professions as medicine, law, and teaching.

Within medicine there are many types of political organizations. They include your local practice or institutional organizations as well as larger organizations, which may include health maintenance organizations or other insurance organizations. Often there is a formal political structure such as an organized medical staff and there is always an informal political structure where most of the important decisions are made. In many cases, it is hard to tell the different structures apart. Also, within medicine there are formal organizations of physicians and other interested parties. These include your local, regional, state, national, and international medical societies and specialty societies.

Almost all family physicians participate in the American Academy of Family Physicians and perhaps their local or state medical society and the American Medical Association. There are a large number of smaller, mostly

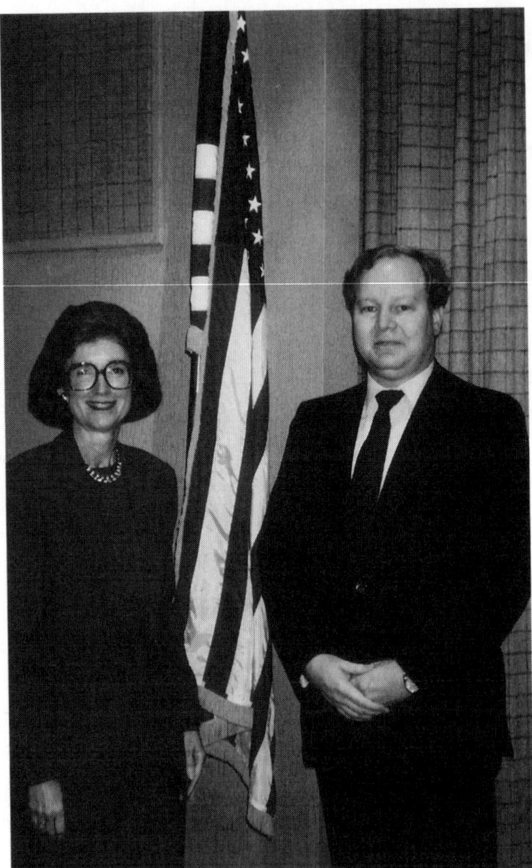

FIGURE 27-1
Family physicians often work closely with legislators both locally and at a national level on health-related issues.

national medical societies that different subgroups have formed. Many of these may be of interest to the family physician.

HOW TO BECOME INVOLVED IN POLITICS

Get Involved

The most important step in becoming involved in politics is to decide that you want to become involved. Having made this crucial decision, you need to decide what is important to you. The field of medicine is a demanding profession, which does not leave you an unlimited amount of time to do other things. Because of this, you need to decide what you are interested in achieving. For example, if your goal is to develop a new Department of

Family Medicine in your institution, you need to become deeply involved with the informal political structure and the organized medical staff structure of the institution. Involvement at the ground level is the first step in the development of new ideas.

Whether you're a resident in training or a physician in practice, the best way to become involved in politics is to explore every political opportunity and find the best one for you. The surest way to pass up an opportunity is to refuse to become involved. If you do not get involved, you cannot experience your dreams. The next step is more difficult. Once you become involved, you need to set goals and work diligently toward them. You need to fulfill your commitments in a timely manner with your best effort—in other words, always give 110 percent. Those who deliver the goods and continue to explore new opportunities will make many satisfying contributions. Consistency over time is also important. Others need to know that they can count on you, even when the going gets tough.

> *"All who are benefited by community life, especially the physician, owe something to the community."*
>
> —Charles H. Mayo

Run for Office

After gathering experience in voluntary activities, you may want to run for an elected position in a political organization. The important point to remember is to start small. Some outstanding individuals with little experience run for high offices initially. Unfortunately, that doesn't work for most organizations. In fact, many potential leaders, who in reality are not fully qualified for the position they are running for, become disinterested in political organizations if they lose an election in the early stages of their political involvement. Therefore, look for opportunities that you are qualified for and interested in. Most medically related organizations have a resident physician section that allows residents in training the opportunity to become involved early in their careers. It is no accident that those residents who hold offices in these training organizations go on to run the parent organization later in their careers once they have developed knowledge and experience. This is equally applicable in your multispecialty group practice or even in your community. One important point to remember: if you do run for an elected office, physicians and the general public generally are hesitant to make a decision about who to vote for, but once they have committed they almost always vote the way they said they would initially. Therefore, it is important to start early and let as many voters as possible get to know you and hopefully commit to you in your quest for an elected position. Remember, the first impression is often the most important.

Political Participation

Some physicians find that they are attracted to general politics. Basically, there are 2 ways to participate: personally or by contributing resources (eg, money). Participating in both ways is the most valuable. If you choose only to contribute money, there are a few key factors you should remember. Avoid giving money anonymously, and try to make a generous contribution that will be acknowledged. It is best to reserve your contributions for when it really counts and when it has the most personal impact for you. A personal request from a politician should always be addressed personally either with an offer to help or with a contribution to their campaign. People remember responses to personal requests.

An example of political influence through donations is a story about a physician who knew a politician when the politician was in high school. He had not seen the politician for 20 years; however, the politician was running for office and had goals similar to those of the physician. The physician had certain political goals he wanted to achieve and therefore was in full support of his candidacy. The physician took more than $1,000 of his personal funds, invited his 4 children to join him, and arrived unannounced on the politician's doorstep. He had his children give their college money to the politician because it was so important that the politician work on behalf of their issue. It was definitely a statement of full support. Both got what they wanted. After a successful election, the physician was appointed to a leading position in the politician's political organization. A somewhat extreme example of how to influence a politician, this type of scenario is reenacted every day in the political world. Using your child's college fund is a little dramatic and most likely a foolish move, but nevertheless the story makes a point. People are often willing to make great sacrifices in return for political influence, and politicians are usually willing to accept.

If you choose to become actively involved yourself, begin by identifying a local candidate who is running for office for the first time. Ask where you can help. Offer to run the telephone bank or to go door to door for the candidate. In other words, start with the grass roots movement to elect a candidate—often it's the most rewarding. For physicians, a good place to start is to attend the American Medical Association's campaign school to learn the nuts and bolts of the political process. You will always be remembered by the politician and the door will always be open to you if you show an interest and work for a grass roots organization. Better yet, set up a fund-raiser for the politician and then personally deliver a significant contribution to help elect the politician. You will be well received. Money talks.

TIPS FOR POLITICIANS

The ultimate example of becoming involved is running for office, within the medical profession or in general politics. For those interested in general politics, don't get trapped by getting too closely allied with organized medicine. The public won't elect you unless you are seen as representing them rather than a special interest. Be prepared for dirty politics. As a physician involved in politics, you become vulnerable to criticism and controversy. The political environment is vastly different from the highly respected daily practice of clinical medicine. It is always possible to find a disgruntled constituent who may criticize you to the media. True or not, you need to be able to deal with these issues in a diplomatic and professional manner. Also, many groups have a philosophical bias against physicians in public office. It is common and real to have such groups conduct smear campaigns against you in which innuendo and outright lies are whispered about you in and out of the public eye. This can be disconcerting to physicians who are used to a collegial environment in which your word and your character are most important.

BENEFITS AND DRAWBACKS OF POLITICS

What are the benefits of becoming active in politics during your medical career? There are many kinds of benefits. Personal influence, a wide and growing network of friends and colleagues, improved health and welfare of your patients and your community, and even professional success can derive from active involvement in politics. At a minimum, you will come to understand the forces that shape your life, your profession, and your community.

However, there are some drawbacks. The most frequent and significant is time. No one expects you to neglect your family or medical career. But as a traveling, politically involved physician, you don't get much sleep, you eat irregularly, you may not have time to exercise, and your patients and colleagues may complain about your inaccessibility. And most of all, your family can suffer. I have heard stories of physicians who end up divorced and estranged from their wives and children because they became too involved. For those involved in politics, the most important point is to set your priorities and keep a sense of balance in your life. After all, you become active in politics to improve your life and career and the life of your community or specialty, not to destroy your life or the lives of those around you.

CONCLUSIONS

Being politically involved is important for physicians. Had we done a better job in the past, we wouldn't be reading articles in our journals entitled ''Will Physicians Take Back Medicine?'' Political involvement as a physician can help you to reach your own personal and professional goals as well as goals for the practice of medicine. Medical or general community politics is seductive and rewarding in its own right. It can become a career. Be cautious; you may get what you ask for and find that it's more than you expected.

28

FAMILY MEDICINE IN THE MILITARY*

Susan S. Wilder, M.D.

Lori Heim, M.D., LTC. USAF

Ted Epperly, M.D., Col. USA

Family medicine is essential to the mission of all military services and therefore receives a high degree of respect. Regardless of one's long-term career plans, the military is an excellent venue for family practice training. It also provides economic advantages during residency and practice as well as a wide spectrum of practice opportunities and challenges. The military functions effectively as the largest health maintenance organization in the world. As such, providers in the military are well versed in the concepts of managed care and cost-effective care. Quality of care, preventive medicine, and access are emphasized. Military-trained physicians are coveted in the civilian setting because of their efficiency, high-quality training, leadership, and managerial experience. Although military medicine is not immune to the dramatic change occurring throughout the medical field, careers in military medicine can be tremendously rewarding and challenging.

INROADS TO MILITARY FAMILY MEDICINE

Medical school opportunities for a military-based education include the Uniformed Services University of the Health Sciences (USUHS) in Bethesda, Maryland, or a scholarship to a civilian school. USUHS students are commissioned as officers on matriculation and follow the customs and regulations of the parent service during training. Advantages include the school's reputation for excellent education plus the enticement of a salary during medical school in lieu of tuition. USUHS traditionally has a substantial number of

*The opinions in this manuscript are the private views of the authors and are not to be construed as official or as reflecting the views of the United States Air Force or United States Army.

graduates apply for family medicine residency positions and a strong Family Medicine Interest Group. USUHS graduates incur a 7-year active duty commitment and then 3 years as a Reserve officer (able to be recalled and obligated to periodic duty with a reserve unit). They request service affiliation on acceptance into school (Army, Navy, Air Force, or Public Health Service, although the last does not accept students in some years). USUHS graduates generally proceed to train in military residencies, although this is not always the case.

Students accepted to a civilian medical school can apply to the Health Professions Scholarship Program (HPSP) through any of the services. This pays full tuition, a living stipend, and reimbursement for insurance, text, and equipment purchases. HPSP students are commissioned as reserve officers during medical school and have 1 month of active duty required during each year of medical school. This time generally includes Officer Indoctrination training the first year, clinical rotations at military sites, and other service-specific requirements. HPSP students can apply to military residency programs or request deferment for civilian training. HPSP students pay back 1 year for every year sponsored (minimum of 3). They also incur 1 to 2 years of inactive reserve commitment after their payback period unless they have completed 5 years of active duty, excluding residency.

Residents in training in civilian programs also can apply for sponsorship by one of the services. Sponsorship results in payment of a salary during residency and potential loan-forgiveness options. The resident then incurs a payback period based on the number of years sponsored.

> *"Medicine gives only to those who give, but her reward for those who serve is 'finer than much fine gold.'"*
>
> —Charles H. Mayo

TRAINING IN MILITARY FAMILY MEDICINE RESIDENCY PROGRAMS

Overview

The 6 Army, 5 Air Force, and 4 Navy military family medicine residency programs include some of the best in the country. At this writing, all are fully accredited by the Residency Review Committee for Family Practice. All also have impressive board certification rates of graduates. The programs aim to prepare physicians to practice in a multitude of unique environments, often without the luxury of specialty support. The combination of academically competitive students and faculty with excellent leadership and teaching abilities culminates in outstanding training programs. Many residency faculty have fellowship training or Certificates of Added Qualifications in such areas as Obstetrics and Gynecology, Sports Medicine, and Geriatrics.

The mission of training physicians for remote overseas assignments includes a strong procedural skills emphasis, complete Advanced Life Support training (advanced cardiac life support, advanced trauma life support, advanced pediatric life support, neonatal advanced life support, and often advanced life support in obstetrics) required by most military programs, and strong management and leadership training. Graduates from military family medicine residency programs must be well versed in emergency medicine, orthopedics and sports medicine, disaster management and triage, public health, and epidemiology. Special requirements aside, the military residency curricula adhere to the Residency Review Committee requirements, with the same basic core elements as civilian programs. This ensures a high-quality, well-trained family physician who can step into any environment and provide the full spectrum of care.

Family medicine training programs in the military are located throughout the country. On the other hand, subspecialty programs tend to be limited to large cities and include the following locations: Washington, DC; San Diego, CA; San Antonio, TX; near Sacramento, CA; and Honolulu, HI. Many training programs are integrated among all 3 military services, meaning that a resident may rotate in Army, Navy, and Air Force facilities during training, depending on the proximity of the facilities and experiences available. There is a growing trend toward tri-service initiatives. In addition, some programs successfully integrate civilian institutions into their curricula.

> *''Civilization and intellectual growth depend largely on preventive medicine.''*
>
> —William J. Mayo

The majority of military family medicine programs are in community hospitals with limited subspecialty residencies. There are exceptions in each service. The Air Force has 5 residency programs in the following locations: California, Illinois, Maryland, Florida, and Nebraska. The 6 Army sites are in Virginia, Georgia (2 sites), Hawaii, Washington, and North Carolina. The 4 Navy programs are in Florida (2 sites), Washington, and California. Each training program has unique strengths, such as emphasis on procedures, obstetrics, or sports medicine. Applicants are encouraged to contact the programs or to visit their Web sites to evaluate these specifics. At least 2 military programs arrange experiences for residents and staff to provide medical care for underserved populations in areas such as Haiti and South America.

Service-Specific Nuances

Army Family Practice residents also receive detailed training and experience in chemical and biological warfare agents, disaster medicine, tropical medicine, travel medicine, field sanitation and hygiene, preventive medicine, field medical skills, evaluation and evacuation, military occupational health, disability determination, and managed care. In addition, military survival training, map reading, weapons qualifications, and military clinic administration skills are taught through each of the services. Air Force Family Practice residents may have exposure to aerospace medicine. Field hospital setup, disaster, and mock-wartime exercises are an ongoing part of military medicine during and after residency.

Salary and Pay Structure

In addition to the benefit of compensation for all or part of the costs of medical education, the military resident enjoys a compensation structure that is generally better than that in the civilian sector. Residents are entitled to salary commensurate with their rank. Rank generally starts at Captain for Air Force and Army residents and Lieutenant for Navy residents. Depending on the service member's state of residence, base pay may not be subject to state taxes. For the 1997-1998 academic year, the average military resident straight out of medical school earned about $33,000, exclusive of special pays and tax incentives, while the average civilian resident earned $30,000 (with tremendous variance by geographic area). In addition to base salary and tax incentives, military residents enjoy several special pays, including a nontaxable housing allowance. However, many prefer to live on the military base where rent and utilities are free in lieu of receiving the housing allowance. Residents also may receive variable housing pay designed to compensate individuals living in high cost-of-living locations.

After residency graduation, military physicians generally progress regularly in rank. Usually, the first promotion occurs 3 years after completing residency. Salary after graduation from residency is generally lower than that of civilian counterparts. However, it is still competitive when one considers tax benefits, scholarship benefits (for most, well over $150,000 in educational benefits), free comprehensive medical care for member and family (including medication, hospitalization, and both preventive and acute care), and student loan deferments. Dental care is also free for the active-duty member and offered at a substantial discount for family members. Loan deferments are allowed for 5 years of active duty time. Physicians also receive an extra $1,000 per year once board-certified and a specialty bonus that varies depending on service needs and is tied to civilian compensation (the most recent family medicine bonus was $6,000). In addition, once the service obligation has been fulfilled, a physician is eligible for an annual bonus of $15,000. The compensation package includes 30 days (includes weekends) of vacation and usually 1 week of paid continuing medical education. All aspects of compensation are subject to change. Life and disability insurance are available for minimal cost. The military offers generous retirement compensation for a minimum of 20 years of active duty service. However, if a member leaves at any time before that (unless having been offered an early retirement incentive) the member does not vest in the pension plan. An active duty member cannot enjoy the tax benefits of an Individual Retirement Account investment because of the existence of the pension.

Aside from the direct compensation benefits, military members also enjoy indirect benefits. At many of the military bases there are amenities available to service members and their families. These include grocery and department stores, recreational facilities, low-cost movie theatres, and gas stations. Most military retail facilities enjoy freedom from state tax requirements and often offer subsidized pricing. The military also provides opportunities for space-available travel throughout the world and low-cost hotel accommodations in many locations, including Tokyo, Germany, Honolulu, and Orlando.

Additional Duties During Training

All services provide military-specific training in addition to the usual family medicine residency curriculum. All students generally have completed a service-specific Officer Indoctrination program. This indoctrination comprises everything from learning the history of the service and its mission to how to salute and use a weapon. Service-specific rules and regulations, including dress, grooming, and fitness standards, are covered at this time. In some services, this indoctrination resembles basic training. All services include some type of survival training and combat medicine training which encompasses Advanced Trauma Life Support, chemical and biological warfare training, triage, and medical management of wartime emergencies. Service-specific training such as parachute training, water rescue, and ejection-seat training may be included. Team and leadership building exercises are common in military medicine. These include ''rope courses,'' which involve a series of obstacles and situations in which a team must determine a solution and then physically complete the task. These can be really fun and challenging experiences.

Each service also has specific fitness requirements that each officer must meet. The United States Army has a semiannual Army Physical Fitness Test. This consists of 3 events, including as many push-ups and sit-ups as you can perform in 2 minutes and a 2-mile run. The Navy requirement is similar. The Air Force currently requires a bicycle ergometer test. Failure to meet fitness requirements results in fitness training to bring a service member up to standards. There are specific weight standards, which, if not met, can result in denial of special and additional pay, inability to gain promotion, or eventually a less than honorable release from the service. All military members are subject to spot urine drug testing, annual HIV and tuberculosis testing, and required vaccinations and physical examinations as determined by each service or duty assignment. Military dress and grooming standards are specified. This provides the advantage of only needing a limited work wardrobe.

Rarely, military residency training may be interrupted for service requirements. During the Gulf War, the Army and Navy did remove some physicians from training for wartime deployments. The Air Force chose not to interrupt residency but programs were affected by deployment of many faculty during that engagement. Army and Air Force programs are continuous from internship through graduation. The Navy, however, may require physicians to complete a tour as a general medical officer (GMO) between internship and the completion of residency. This may be changing as family physicians are recognized as far more versatile and cost effective than those with more limited training.

FAMILY PRACTICE IN THE MILITARY

Practice Opportunities

Some individuals choose their service based on family influences, whereas others are interested in a particular practice location or opportunity. In general, Navy bases tend to be coastal for obvious reasons, and Navy physicians care for members of the Navy and Marines. Air Force and Army bases are scattered in a wide variety of geographic locations. All services provide care for retirees as well as active duty members and their families. Patient populations vary widely, depending on base location. Some military locations send retirees or even dependents to the civilian sector for care. All services have physician opportunities to serve as flight surgeons. This entails 6 weeks to 6 months of additional training covering the mechanics of flight with implications for the care of personnel assigned to airplanes. Flight surgeons care for flight crews and their families, stay with their unit when deployed, investigate flight crashes involving their unit, and have the opportunity to fly. Army and Navy family physicians can apply for a spot with one of the Special Forces teams for care of specialized troops. Any Uniformed Services physician may be nominated to serve as a White House physician and many are family physicians. They provide medical care for White House staff, which includes frequent travel.

There are service-specific differences in career opportunities that are now evident but subject to change. The Army tends to provide career tracks: clinical, academic, administrative/leadership, research, or operational. In general, Army physicians are more likely to stay in one location longer, provided the needs of the service and the individual's career goals are met. All services have family physicians as faculty at USUHS (the military medical school) and teaching in family medicine residency programs. All services approve additional fellowship training, provided it meets service needs. Camaraderie is perhaps the most advantageous aspect of a military practice, yet the least tangible.

Assignments Process

The graduate of a military family medicine program or a military physician entering a payback period submits a wish list of desired practice locations. An assignment officer then makes the assignment with needs of the service as the paramount priority. Many choose to do a remote assignment to a less than desirable location to get a guaranteed follow-on to the assignment of their choice. This option provides the most control over the assignment process. Some remote assignments are desirable in many respects. Sites in Turkey, Guam, and Asia provide an excellent opportunity for travel and outdoor activities. Almost all locations have a military base with security and amenities similar to the United States. The tour length for a remote assignment is generally shorter (12–18 months) if the service member is not accompanied by family. Some sites, such as Korea, allow only active duty personnel. Other clinical sites and hospitals are located throughout Europe and the United States. Navy assignments may well be aboard ship caring for Navy or Marine personnel. Military retirees are cared for at most United States and many overseas locations as well, providing for a reasonable geriatric experience.

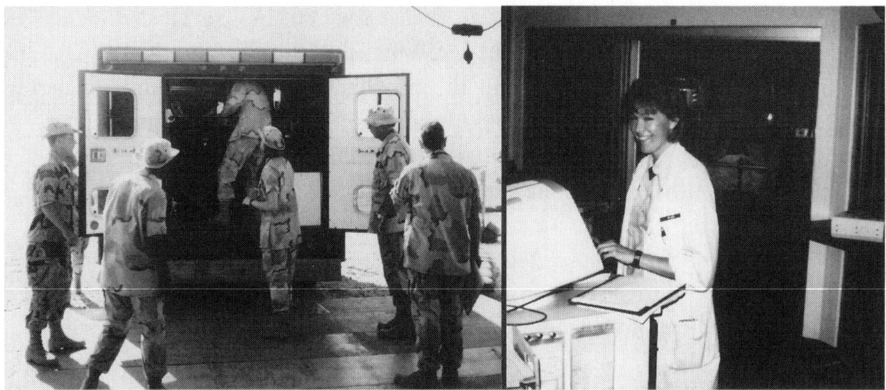

FIGURE 28-1
Family physicians in the military serve on the battlefield and in a more traditional role in clinics and hospital settings.

The realm of military family practice can range from functioning as an emergency physician, to purely outpatient family practice (general medical officer or flight surgeon), to full spectrum family practice, including obstetrics, pediatric and neonatal care, and inpatient and intensive care medicine (Fig. 28-1). Family physicians are coveted in many locations because of their versatility and ability to cover call for the Emergency Department and many other specialists (Box 28-1).

Procedural opportunities vary greatly from assignment to assignment. The highly motivated practitioner often can obtain the equipment needed to perform various procedures but must be prepared to justify the expense. It also is possible to come from a 3- to 4-year assignment in a purely outpatient practice without the ability to do certain procedures to a more comprehensive practice, which includes obstetrics and inpatient care. Access to quality continuing medical education can be challenging for those stationed overseas. The USUHS does provide overseas outreach courses and the Uniformed Services Academy of Family Physicians (USAFP) provides an exceptional annual Scientific Assembly for military family physicians. Many physicians use advanced information services such as on-line continuing medical education and CD-ROM options. Information technology is fairly advanced in the military, where the concept of telemedicine is being pioneered.

Information About Military Medical Opportunities

Students looking at HPSP options or civilian residents seeking sponsorship are encouraged to contact local military recruiting offices. Those interested

BOX 28-1 NAVY MEDICINE

John D. Pennington, M.D. *Senior Associate Consultant, Department of Family Medicine, Mayo Clinic Jacksonville, Jacksonville, Florida*

My first exposure to Navy medicine was in 1986 when I joined the Hospital Corps. Like all corpsmen, I was trained in patient care at the level of an LPN. I also held licenses in Emergency Vehicle Operations and as an Emergency Medical Technician. Additional training brought me to the level of a paramedic within 2 years of my enlistment. With promotion through the ranks came additional duties, such as training and education. I became a licensed instructor in Emergency Vehicle Operations, Emergency Medical Training, and Basic Cardiac Life Support. I had been in charge of immunizations, minor surgery, and finally of ambulance support services by the time I was discharged in 1990.

After graduate school and medical school, I began a residency in family practice. At that time, I sought to join the United States Naval Reserve Medical Corps as a licensed physician. I was commissioned as a Lieutenant (O-3, or Captain in other branches of the armed forces) and assigned to the PRIMUS unit at Naval Air Station Jacksonville. PRIMUS (Physician Reservists In Medical Universities and Schools) is a unique opportunity for medical support personnel. Members include physicians and nurses from several specialties, and the ultimate duty is to provide coverage in the naval facilities when active duty members are deployed to combat or special missions.

Instead of drilling one weekend per month, PRIMUS members have the option of substituting continuing medical education activity and teaching responsibilities for drill time. Therefore, 16 hours of lectures and teaching counts as a drill for the month. We still receive reservist pay, and time in service counts toward retirement. The unit meets twice per year for updating physical qualifications, including Physical Readiness Testing (sit-ups, push-ups, and a 1.5-mile run). Lectures during these drills include such topics as the Law of Armed Conflict and addresses from the Commanding Officer of the Reserve Center.

Since graduation from residency, I am in the process of being credentialed for privileges at Naval Hospital Jacksonville. I will be spending 16 hours a month in the labor and delivery section to remain current in obstetrics skills. Other duties have included sick call (walk-in clinic) for reservists and occasional invitations to perform annual physical examinations on reservists. These duties are performed in conjunction with corpsmen and nurses, and it is satisfying to think that I have participated on both sides of the medical team. My experiences are an excellent enhancement for my role as a staff physician in our residency program.

in the USUHS can contact the admissions office at (301) 295-3101 or via the Internet at http//www.usuhs.mil/.

The USAFP is the military chapter of the American Academy of Family Physicians (AAFP) and currently has more than 1,300 members. For information on military residency programs or the organization, call (804) 358-4002 or visit the home page at http//www.usafp.org/. They also can be accessed through a link from the AAFP home page.

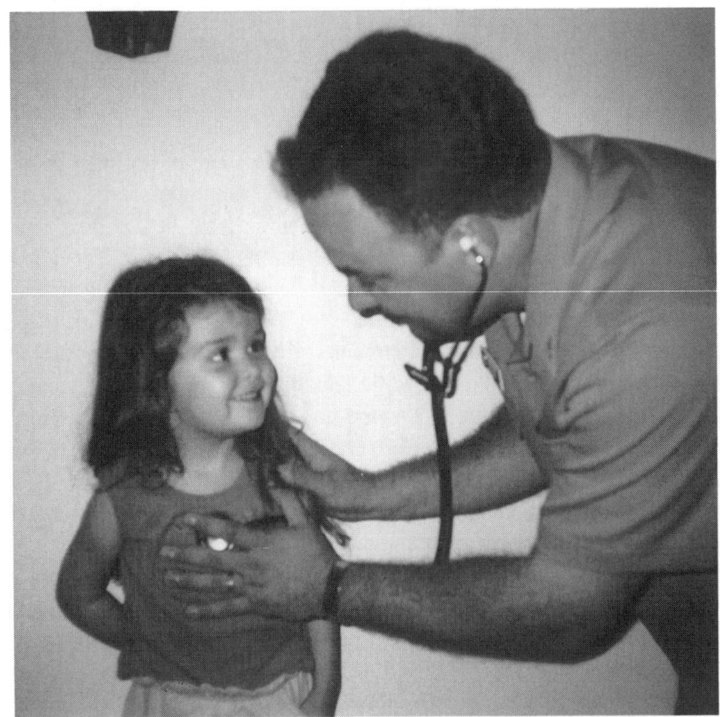

FIGURE 28-2
Serving as a family physician in the military has multiple benefits and can be very rewarding.

CONCLUSION

There are major changes occurring in the military as a tri-service unified health care system (managed care) is being implemented. This will change how the military serves patients and will impact residency education, but the specifics and extent of this are still uncertain. To date, military leadership maintains a strong commitment to graduate medical education and many predict the demand for family physicians will continue to grow in the future. It is definitely a great time to be a family physician in the armed services (Fig. 28-2).

29 PEARLS FOR FAMILY PHYSICIANS

The process of becoming a successful family physician does not come with an instruction manual. There are no set guidelines that ensure success and satisfaction with your practice of medicine. In most cases, the physician must test the waters before learning important information that may help to make life easier. Common sense and wisdom are not easily obtained and may take years to acquire. The following chapter is a collection of pearls offered by staff and resident physicians that may help to make your life easier as you develop into an experienced family physician (Fig. 29-1).

PEARLS FROM RESIDENTS

Ruel W. Scott, M.D.

1. The hospital admission process is one of the most stressful experiences that a patient ever faces. This process can be made less stressful if the intern or resident takes the time to discuss the patient's disease pathophysiology in terms of prognosis, complications, and treatment. The patient should be taught to identify important warning symptoms of the disease process. When we make the patient an active participant in medical care, it restores a measure of control to the patient and helps to alleviate anxiety. Allowing the patient to become a partner in care also makes the job of the intern or resident easier, because the patient discusses the disease from an educated perspective.
2. One of the most important responsibilities of the intern or resident is keeping track of a patient's medications. This responsibility can be facilitated if the names of the medications are written in the margin of each

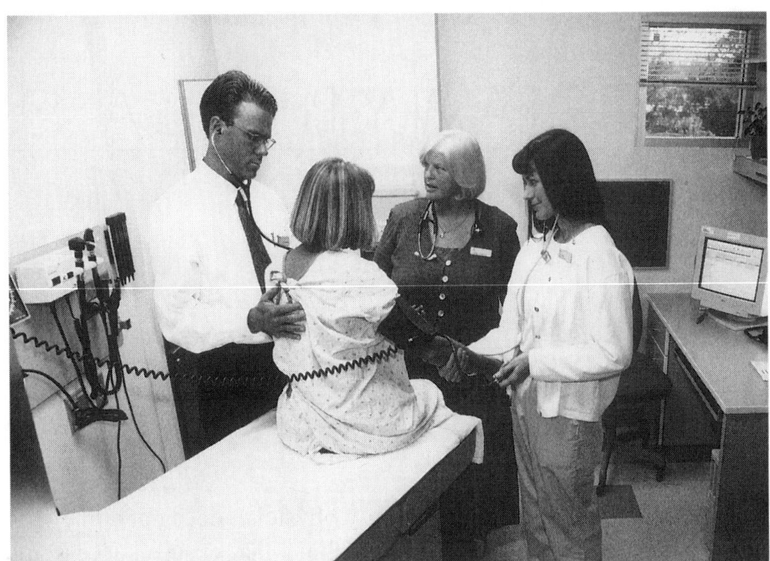

FIGURE 29-1 Family physicians in a group practice can learn from their colleagues and supervising staff physicians.

page of the medical record. During the admission process, take the time to write the patient's medication list in the margin of several blank pages in the medical record. This saves time in the mornings when the intern or resident is expected to write notes for morning rounds. If there are changes made to the medications, these changes also can be written in the margin on a daily basis.

''Instruction from teachers and books teaches a man what to think, but the great need is that he should learn how to think.''

—William J. Mayo

James R. Keene, Ph.D., D.O.

1. Take some time off for yourself on a regular basis. It is much too easy to get caught up in the rat race and ignore your personal needs. Do yourself a favor.
2. First, do no harm.
3. Fly the airplane (take control, do things yourself, be aggressive).
4. Ask a nurse ''What do you usually do in this situation?'' You will gain a friend and a nurse who appreciates your respect.
5. When a consultant or staff physician interrupts, it may be because you

aren't giving the proper information needed at the time. Listen when you are spoken to.

6. Direct questioning is a time-honored pastime of attending physicians and senior residents. It is also an excellent way to acquire an ulcer, presuming you are on the receiving end of continuous fulminating questions. Always remember that you get picked on simply because you are worth the questioner's time.
7. Eat as often as you can. Do not skip meals. When in doubt, eat (and eat healthy).
8. In general, you must obtain your attending physician's approval before ordering a consult.
9. Know when to refer. The more you are comfortably able to treat in your office, the more respect you will gain from your patients.
10. Read your own radiographs, computed tomographic scans, magnetic resonance images, and ultrasonograms.
11. Things will get better. Perhaps now you do not believe this, but experience shows it to be true. Keep a positive attitude, especially when things seem to be caving in on you and there is not enough time in the day to get everything done.
12. Always keep your attending physician informed. After all, the attending physician is the primary physician on the case.
13. Forget holidays. They are nothing more than calendar clutter. If you have call (which should be expected), they will likely be regular days at the hospital. Don't expect light days, unless you are such a fortunate soul as to be on an outpatient rotation or someone allows you a day off.
14. Residency can be summed up in 2 words: *pain* and *depression*. The antidote is a positive outlook on all things and an upbeat attitude. If this does not work, talk to your program director, behavioral scientist, or psychologist. He or she is a terrific resource and can be a close friend. Physicians are not immune to stress, anxiety, depression, and drug abuse.
15. The rumor that the second year is easier than the first year is a lie.

PEARLS FROM STAFF PHYSICIANS

Susan S. Wilder, M.D.

Rules to Live by in Family Practice

As family physicians, confidence in our identity is crucial to our survival as a specialty. I encourage everyone to own and read a textbook on family medicine. The rules that follow help clarify that identity and avert crises of insecurity.

1. You can't know everything, but you can know enough.
2. If you ever feel like you know everything, it's time to get out of the business.
3. Breadth of knowledge is every bit as valuable as depth. The neurosurgeons could no better do your job than you could do theirs.
4. Respect must be earned and to do so requires self-assurance, preparation, and diplomacy.
5. Know your limits. Never be afraid to say ''I don't know.''
6. If you learn anything, let it be where and how to look things up.

True Rewards

Enjoy the privileges of family practice: of becoming part of your patients' lives; of seeing them through births, marriages, childrearing, divorces, graduations, retirements, and deaths; and of finding, over time, that they care for you as much as you care for them. There are few careers so challenging and so rewarding.

Celebrate Life

In dealing with illness, death, and the excruciating burden of survival, you will be amazed at the incredible power of the human spirit. Learn from these traumas not to be paranoid, but simply to live. If you can bestow on others what an incredible gift each life represents, you will succeed as a true healer.

Keep Perspective

Every day, make note of something that

Inspired you,

Made you laugh,

Challenged you, and

Touched your heart

Try this for a while and share your thoughts with those close to you in place of daily negativism. It will change your life or at least your perception of it (from Dr. Joan Borysenko).

William J. O'Brien, M.D.

How to "Shine" as a Resident

1. Organize your patient data so your presentations and write-ups are concise!
2. Show your patient and your attending physician that you recognize how the illness impacts the patient and family.
3. Be willing, at least most of the time, to go a little beyond what you feel is expected of you by your patients, fellow residents, and attending physicians.
4. Remember that most nurses are more than willing to help keep you out of trouble, especially when you are receptive to their input regarding your mutual patients.
5. Be professional, but be yourself. An honest "I don't know, but I'll find out" is preferable to bluffing and, from an attending physician's viewpoint, much more trustworthy. The qualities I most value in the residents I rate highly are honesty, enthusiasm, empathy for patients, organization, and ability to apply academic knowledge to clinical situations.

"The aim of medicine is to prevent disease and prolong life; the ideal of medicine is to eliminate the need of a physician."

—William J. Mayo

Gregory A. Bartel, M.D.

1. When assisting in surgery, always ask the surgeon, "do you want the sutures cut long or short?"
2. Respect other people's time. If you are going to be late for clinic, call out of respect for your nurse and patients.
3. Learn to be cheerful even in the midst of being overworked and underpaid.
4. Spend your time on the patient's history; it's of utmost importance to the correct clinical assessment.
5. Listen to what the patient thinks is wrong.
6. Be humble enough to take medical advice from experienced nurses.
7. Practice defensive medicine by documenting what you say to the patient not just by ordering more tests.

8. As a resident, moonlighting is not only a good benefit financially but also a great learning experience, but moonlighting should never compromise your training program.
9. When considering your first job, don't let salary be the most important determinant.
10. If possible, spend an elective month as a resident with a group before you sign with them.
11. With so many job opportunities in family practice, narrow your choices by deciding what region you want to live in.
12. Death is inevitable for all; don't take it personally when a patient of yours dies.
13. Don't give up on the terminal patient; the time of death is often surprisingly delayed.
14. Heal a few, relieve much suffering, care for all.
15. Make contact with the family of the deceased for whom you have cared. They now are your patients and need your comfort.
16. Remember to nurture not only the mind but also the body and spirit.
17. No matter how dire the situation, keep your cool.
18. Take every opportunity to encourage your patients to change unhealthy habits, such as smoking.
19. As a resident, take a nap when you have a chance.
20. Be tactful. Learn to disagree without being disagreeable.
21. I have never heard a dying person exclaim, ''I sure wish I had spent more time at work,'' but plenty who wish they had spent more time with family and friends.
22. *Manual of Medical Therapeutics* (The Washington Manual)[1] and *The Harriet Lane Handbook*[2] are great reference books in the hospital for the busy family practice resident.
23. Early in medical school or residency start a small notebook as a reference for what to do in certain medical situations.
24. Read. Read. Read. *The American Family Physician* is a great monthly resource of medical information.
25. Wash. Wash. Wash. After each patient examination, wash to keep yourself and others from getting sick.
26. Remember no one makes it alone. As a family practitioner, don't be afraid to ask for help with a patient.
27. Have a pocket mask handy at all times. You never know when someone will need cardiopulmonary resuscitation.
28. Put first things first. Prioritize. Some things just have to wait for another day.
29. Show concern even to patient's trivial problems. It is not a small problem

to the patient, and say, "it is a good thing you came in to have that checked."

30. Don't make too many commitments, but keep the ones you do make.
31. There often is more than one way to treat the same problem. Don't be hesitant to ask questions of preceptors, even for seemingly simple problems. This is a great opportunity to pool knowledge that you can use for the future.
32. As a group of residents, care for one another; you are all going through the same battles. If you work as a team and help each other along the way, it makes the journey much more pleasant. This also builds good skills to help deal with partners when you go into practice.
33. Learn as much as you can about the business and management side of medicine while you are a student and resident. This is an area that is often notoriously weak in training the family physician.
34. Physicians are a target of self-serving financial planners and get-rich-quick schemes. Don't make hasty financial decisions. Allow yourself time to build a relationship of trust with someone who may be giving you financial advice.
35. As a family physician, there are certain medical decisions that have to be made quickly. This is especially true in cardiology and orthopedic trauma. Get as much experience in those areas as possible.
36. In family practice, take advantage of opportunities to get to know the patient's family and social history. This is part of what makes family practice unique and allows us to take better care of individuals.
37. There is something powerful about continuity of patient care. Your efficiency is improved by caring for your own patients. Patients are more satisfied if "their" physician takes care of them. This also leads to the physician being more satisfied.

Joseph W. Furst, M.D.

Remember that there are competing missions of any residency program. One mission is to provide health care to the patients, and the second mission is to educate the residents. Busy clinic days and large hospital services compete for time for education. Reviewing material before rounds in the hospital to ensure that all test results are available, vital signs checked, and nursing notes reviewed greatly enhances the value of your rounds when your preceptor arrives. The opportunity for education is significantly greater. Similarly, doing a thorough evaluation of the patient in the clinic before you review the case with your preceptor accomplishes the same goal. The time spent with your preceptor should be time spent learning and not simply gathering information together.

There will be rotations that seem irrelevant and preceptors with whom you don't click or who are less able teachers. I can't think of a rotation in medical school or residency training that did not have some value to me once I was in private practice. Further, I can't think of an individual preceptor from whom I didn't learn something. Much of medicine is not absolute, and you will benefit by becoming familiar with various approaches to problems. A good resident will be a good resident in any program—good or bad. A bad resident will be a bad resident in the same program as well. There is no substitute for personal initiative on the part of a resident.

Robert D. Sheeler, M.D.

Maximizing the Learner Role

1. Experience and examine team patients on hospital services.
   - By participating in the care of the whole team's patients, your database is greatly expanded.
   - Introduce yourself and ask to examine patients with positive findings (eg, thyroid nodules, heart murmurs, enlarged liver).
   - This will vastly increase your clinical acumen and database by the time you complete training.
2. Put yourself on the line.
   - State what you would consider doing in each clinical situation and find out the pros and cons of your approach.
   - It is easy to sit back and let others guide the decision process fully, but you do not learn command-level skills and ability to make the tough decisions by doing this.
   - You do not have to take risks with patients, just state what you would consider doing and ask what is good and bad about such an approach.
3. Think and plan discretely: diagnosis, therapy, and patient education.
   - Present each of these elements separately.
   - Diagnosis: What part of the plan will further diagnostics (eg, tests ordered)?
   - Therapy: What type of therapy—medication, physical modalities, counseling, or other—is planned?
   - Patient education and follow-up: What education, literature, and instructions has the patient been given? What are the follow-up instructions?
4. Seek and learn to accept constructive criticism.
   - This is hard to do. It requires learning to put your ego aside.
5. Learn to give concise presentations.
   - This greatly enhances your interactions and esteem in clinical medicine.

It is often key to leave out negative findings unless they are specifically pertinent.

6. Contribute to the team.
   Distribute articles and summaries from current literature to the team.
   Contribute a positive attitude, thanks, and chocolate.

Rhonda M. Medows, M.D.

Twenty-Five Things It's Taken Me 10 Years to Figure Out

1. Always introduce yourself
   Introduce yourself to a new patient or family member. Just because the individual has scheduled an appointment to see Dr. Jones, don't assume the person knows you. There are few things quite as frustrating as spending 30 minutes with a patient only to be asked, ''When will the doctor be coming in?''
2. Even if it's only for 5 minutes
   Try to sit down after entering the examination room to talk with a patient. Even though we know we are rushing to keep on schedule, we don't need to convey it. Standing at the door kind of gives it away.
3. When in doubt, ask
   Ask the patient to repeat history or concerns.
   Ask the nurse, physical therapist, or nutritionist for suggestions in finding creative solutions for an individual patient's special needs.
   Ask a colleague or consultant with more expertise or experience about particularly difficult diagnostic dilemmas.
4. Learn to trust your instincts
   Use everything in your arsenal—education, experience, and access to expert opinion, but always incorporate it with what you really know.
5. It's okay to say ''I don't know''
   It's even better to say ''I'll find out for you or help you find someone who does know.''
6. When interviewing or examining the agitated or reality impaired, never seat the patient between you and the door.
7. Learn to set limits
   Limits on what you will address
   Limits on how much of it you will address
   Limits on how you address it
8. Check your attitude at the door
   At the office examination room before entering

And at home (your 2-year-old can be blamed for a lot of things but probably not for Ms. Jones' recurrent 2:00 AM fever spikes)

9. Don't be afraid to ask the tough questions
   It may be uncomfortable for you personally to ask about spousal abuse or any kind of abuse, and you may perceive it to be potentially embarrassing to the patient. For those people who are victims, it may be the only chance to get help.
10. Five or more somatic complaints or office visits for the same complaint, in the healthy patient younger than 40 years, begs the question, Are you depressed? Are you being abused?
11. Beware of people bringing typed and laminated lists of concerns.
12. Document! Document! Document!
    Telephone calls, visits, changes in action plans
13. Gossip hurts!
    Avoid participating in patient-initiated conversations about mistakes or flaws of other physicians. Remember the term "passive-aggressive personality disorder." Remember you may be quoted later.
14. You cannot be all things to all people
    Sometimes a patient may "fire" you. That's reality.
    Satisfy yourself that this had nothing to do with a preventable and avoidable administrative-type problem (or if it was, initiate corrective changes).
    Realize that not every physician-patient relationship results in a perfect match.
15. Your title does not protect you from everything
    If you feel even a little bit uncomfortable about examining a patient alone (whether of the opposite sex or not), wait until you have a chaperone. Before the next visit is scheduled, decide if it's going to hinder further care. If so, find the patient another physician.
16. Avoid treating your family and close friends for serious illnesses
    Allow them the benefit of objective assessment and care by a medical professional.
    Allow yourself to assume the role of the patient's family member.
17. Say thank you
    Appreciate your office staff—secretary, receptionist, auxiliary staff, and nurse.
    Aside from making your daily work environment more pleasant (trust me—the day could be very long if they don't want to), this also encourages improvement in job performance. They need to know the things they did right as much as the things they did wrong.
18. Get a grip!

Know what is happening around you. Try to keep current with events and changes going on in general and especially in the health care industry. It's easy to get bogged down with the day-to-day responsibilities when your free time is limited. Consider a subscription to the *New York Times* Sunday edition, which contains a weekly summary of current events; listen to the news on the radio on your way home from work; or pick one of our news-reporting trade journals (*American Family Physician*) and make a point of reading it (eg, while waiting for an oil change for your car).

19. Just say no . . . and stick to it

    If you are approached by a patient with a request for a treatment course that does not seem reasonable to you (ie, diet pills for emergency weight loss), don't compromise. You are responsible for the possible consequences for therapy you prescribe.

20. The walls have ears

    The acoustics may not be what you think. Even muffled voices and laughter in the hall do nothing but fuel the imagination of the patient waiting anxiously for you.

21. Practice what you preach

    Most of us would be conscientious about making sure our loved ones receive the health care they need. Quality health care for our patients goes without saying. Don't forget we are also mere mortals. Keeping up and following through with our own age-appropriate physicals and health needs is just as important. Don't be a model for what not to do.

22. Major depression is a treatable medical illness

    It is not a fad to be treated by the media-hyped drug of the week. If you are not noting improvement with your patient's current therapy, consider consulting the appropriate mental health professional. You would do this with any other illness not responding to therapy.

23. Compile a list

    List services in the community that can assist and support your patients for problems you frequently see (ie, Eldercare programs, respite care, hospice, crisis hotlines, support groups, and local exercise programs like water aerobics for arthritis sufferers). Keep it posted where your staff and nurse can access it for your patients in your absence.

24. Get a life

    Presumably you went into medicine because you enjoyed learning and being able to apply this knowledge. Dealing with changes and increasing bureaucracy has dampened some of our enthusiasm. In

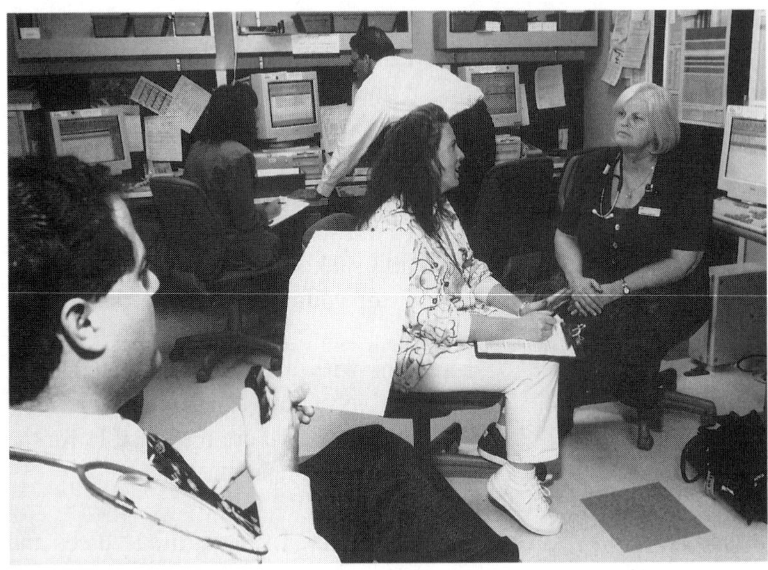

FIGURE 29-2
Clinical pearls can often be shared among fellow physicians and staff.

any case, our careers in medicine are just one part of our lives. Remember to live a little. Have a life. You'll be a happier person and a better physician.

25. Get some sleep
    There's always tomorrow!

CONCLUSIONS

These hard-earned pearls of wisdom are offered by the staff and residents of the Mayo Clinic. Although this list of reminders is comprehensive, it is by no means exhaustive. As you develop as a family physician, seek out mentors and more experienced family physicians for their advice (Fig. 29-2). A few minutes of attentive listening may prevent hassle and hardship. There is no substitute for experience. Take full advantage of the resources offered to you whether you're a resident in training or physician in practice—it's never too late to learn new approaches to old problems.

REFERENCES

1. Orland MJ, Saltman RJ, editors: Manual of Medical Therapeutics. Twenty-fifth edition. Boston, Little, Brown, 1986
2. Rowe PC, editor: The Harriet Lane Handbook: A Manual for Pediatric House Officers. Eleventh edition. Chicago, Year Book Medical Publishers, 1987

30

FUTURE OF FAMILY MEDICINE

Robert D. Sheeler, M.D.

The future of family medicine is resplendent. As a result of a strong heritage of accepting individuals and their needs as legitimate regardless of age, sex, or disease state, family medicine is in a unique position. The lineage of the family physician can be traced back to the times of broad generalists in many societies who served as personal physicians to individuals of all walks of life in their times of need. As technology continues to expand at an ever-increasing pace, the need for a sympathetic and caring interpreter of the human consequences of technologic choices becomes more important. Family physicians, with their long history of patient advocacy and longitudinal relationships with individuals and families, are ideally suited for this role.

Three separate aspects of technical evolution will dramatically influence the practice of medicine by the family physician (Fig. 30-1). Foremost is the computer and information revolution. Second is the development of more high-tech invasive and lifesaving procedures. Finally, the development of ultrahigh-tech procedures will bring the care of certain disease states back into primary care.

> *"The ills of today must not cloud the horizon of tomorrow."*
>
> —William J. Mayo

Social evolution favors more universal access to health care. This will be supported by family physicians, who know better than most the hard-hitting effects of solely profit-motivated health care systems on the weak and the sick, groups they are ethically committed to caring for as physicians.

Information technology continues to expand dramatically, and the effect on office practice will be no less than revolutionary. Continued pressure on

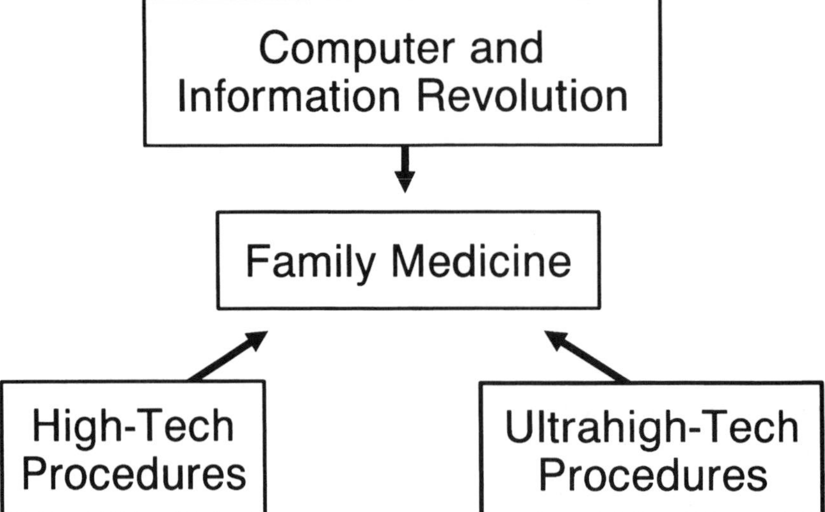

FIGURE 30-1 *Family medicine will be influenced by the computer and information revolution as well as by the development of high-tech and ultrahigh-tech procedures.*

cost efficiency will lead to changes in primary care–specialist relationships as well as continued growth of care teams within family practice offices. It is likely that access to medical records within offices and institutions as well as more formal channels of asynchronous communication such as e-mail will change the face of office practice.

The family physician will become involved in more intense case management, especially for outpatients. Teams of family physicians will likely work in concert with nurse practitioners and physician assistants, and expanded roles for other nurses will allow the family physician to have a larger patient panel. Resource utilization will demand the use of voice-interactive technologies as well as further delegation of other office interactions that include data gathering, patient tracking, and patient education.

This intensification of resource utilization will make the family physician's day more intense and demanding. However, the increased efficiency will help to maintain salary structure, albeit at the primary care end of the spectrum. It is likely that over time intellectual skills will become increasingly valued and thus physician incomes for primary care providers and specialists will become more homogeneous by regression toward the mean.

The marketplace will likely see to it that the higher-paid specialists do work that only they can accomplish. This will be a blessing for family physicians because it will be a force back in the direction of integrated patient care. Specialists will likely serve more often in a consulting role, outlining various viable treatment options, and family physicians will provide the ongoing follow-up. Consultations with specialists will evolve into a continuum rather than an all-or-none encounter. Various levels of communication with specialists and subspecialists will be possible, with more integrated medical information systems and systems that economically compensate the specialists for their intellectual expertise. Hence, a packaged electronic consultation might answer focused questions and review digital images, data, and treatment options. Smaller problems may be handled by electronic messaging to specialists and databases that are located remotely.

The availability of medical information to the layperson will continue to expand. This will serve more sophisticated consumers extremely well. However, a majority will be confused by information overload and need the help of an intermediary to sort out reliable and applicable data from the unedited random theories and sales pitches disguised as medical information that typify today's Internet. The family physician's role may continue to expand as a knowledgeable and trusted reference to help the consumer-patient sort through the information available.

> *''The romance of medicine lies in inductive philosophy, in which tomorrow is the great day.''*
>
> —William J. Mayo

The aggregation and affiliation of family medicine physicians into larger groups, many of which include specialists, will continue. Economically, it will make sense for narrowly focused specialists to provide specialized care in these settings rather than competing to do things their primary care colleagues can do especially well because of their ongoing relationships with their patients. Groups that use such efficiencies will surpass their counterparts. Similarly, disease management strategies will evolve to a state in which more uniform access to the most current and effective approaches will be available to virtually all physicians and their patients. Economics will again be the primary factor favoring their implementation, coupled with patient- or buyer-driven demand for quality.

The development of increasingly high-tech invasive procedures will ensure the role of the family physician. As some specialty fields become more technically oriented, the patient will feel increasing need for human contact and context within the medical environment. The family physicians' "high-touch" approach will complement the ongoing evolution of often perceived high tech. Additionally, the need for some specialists may decrease with this technologic evolution if such entities as robotic surgery and computer algorithmic interpretation of images and other tests increase the productivity of many different specialists.

Ultrahigh-tech developments will eventually bring care of some disease states back into routine office practice. Angioplasty and thrombolytics brought intervention in coronary artery disease out of the sole province of the operating room, transferring some care back from cardiac surgeons to cardiologists. Parallel evolution of treatment, prevention, and diagnostics toward integrated and nanotechnology will do the same for other disease states and will most certainly affect the delivery of primary care, allowing family physicians to provide more sophisticated and technology-based care. Genetic engineering will proceed at a frightening pace, expanding therapeutic and diagnostic options to unfathomable heights or depths, depending on your perspective. Again the family physician will have the opportunity to serve as guide and interpreter. Preventive medicine will make further strides on many fronts and will continue to be a cornerstone of primary care.

Many of the common diseases of today will succumb over time to integrated management. Infectious illnesses have diminished and have been replaced, in part, by diseases of affluence resulting from our gluttony, disjointed and stressful lives, and habits that soothe us in times of confusion and pain. However, as society continues to fragment and individuals become more isolated, care of the whole person will become paramount. This is a focus that is extremely well suited to family physicians.

Practices that have heretofore been relegated to the realms of alternative medicine, such as mind-body healing among others, will gain importance first within family medicine as a discipline. Much of the success of alternative medicine will be determined by the family physicians' success in integrating various treatment options. In this way and many others, family practice will become a more diverse specialty.

Family physicians will continue to be broadly trained, but their interests as well as dramatic increases in databases for each aspect of practice will encourage many to focus their attention on certain areas within the specialty. The percentage of family physicians doing obstetrics will decrease from the current 29 percent (U.S. figure) to the teens or below. Similarly, the percentage of family physicians practicing in the hospital environment will decrease. These trends will parallel overall decreased hospital utilization and declining birth rates. Such changes will be much less notable in rural areas, although they will be augmented by continued closure of rural hospitals unable to maintain the capital base to sustain technologic costs. Within both areas (obstetrics and hospital practice), interested individuals will maintain their privileges and ability to participate in such care by dedicating a significant portion of their practice to it.

Family medicine will struggle to some extent to maintain identity during the phases of diversification of the specialty. In many ways, the specialty will have come full circle. The unifying elements of family practice will become more philosophic based on an attitude of respect for patients and the opportunity to provide longitudinal and population-based care rather than on the close overlap of clinical practice parameters. Each physician will determine a focus of expertise but will remain true to the ideals of continuous and comprehensive care.

Although there may be divergent and sometimes difficult paths to navigate, this is an excellent time to be a family physician. You will be challenged to grow continuously and to commit to the ever-increasing needs of your patients as society at large changes. Change is sometimes difficult. However, with a positive attitude and the proper training and resources, family physicians can remain the leaders in the delivery of primary care.

''Individually, no man is respected more highly than the physician.''

—William J. Mayo

INDEX

NOTES

NOTES

NOTES

NOTES

NOTES

NOTES

NOTES

NOTES

NOTES

NOTES

NOTES

NOTES

NOTES

NOTES

NOTES

NOTES

NOTES

NOTES

NOTES